Sleep

of related interest

Sleep Difficulties and Autism Spectrum Disorders
A Guide for Parents and Professionals
Kenneth J. Aitken
ISBN 978 1 84905 259 7
eISBN 978 0 85700 550 2

Sleep

Multi-Professional Perspectives

*Edited by Andrew Green and
Alex Westcombe*

with Ved Varma

Foreword by Prof David Nutt

Jessica Kingsley *Publishers*
London and Philadelphia

Figure 2.5 on p.37 reprinted from Siegel 2005 with permission from Macmillan Publishers.
Figures 8.1–8.6 reprinted with permission from North Bristol NHS Trust.

First published in 2012
by Jessica Kingsley Publishers
116 Pentonville Road
London N1 9JB, UK
and
400 Market Street, Suite 400
Philadelphia, PA 19106, USA

www.jkp.com

Library of Congress Cataloging in Publication Data
Sleep : multi-professional perspectives / edited by Andrew Green and Alex Westcombe
with Ved Varma ;
foreword by David Nutt.
    p. ; cm.
Includes bibliographical references and index.
ISBN 978-1-84905-062-3 (alk. paper)
I. Green, Andrew, 1957 Feb. 4- II. Westcombe, Alex. III. Varma, Ved P.
[DNLM: 1. Sleep. 2. Sleep Disorders. WL 108]

    616.8'498--dc23

                        2012005235

British Library Cataloguing in Publication Data
A CIP catalogue record for this book is available from the British Library

ISBN 978 1 84905 062 3
eISBN 978 0 85700 257 0

Printed and bound in Great Britain

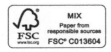

In memory of Ruth Green (1919–2012)

Contents

Foreword

In the UK, more than in other countries and for reasons that are unclear, sleep is the great forgotten aspect of human life. We all do it to a greater or lesser extent and for some up to a third of their lives are spent in this state, but thinking about sleep is not given the same relative importance as the things we get up to when awake. Often sleep is characterized as a nuisance, something that gets in the way of real life and which should be minimized and avoided – an attitude best exemplified by the expression 'sleep is for wimps'.

Yet sleep is a fascinating state which research has shown to impinge on all aspects of psychological life, from learning to self-awareness. Genes that regulate sleep and other clock processes show marked evolutionary conservation and, remarkably, appear to have a role in disorders such as depression and schizophrenia and in their response to treatment.

Moreover, sleep often goes wrong and this results in great distress to many people. Sometimes this is a primary problem and sometimes it is secondary to other disorders of the mind or brain. The magnitude of this issue is emphasized by the new ECNP/EBC (European College of Neuropsychopharmacology and the European Brain Council) survey of disorders of the brain which found that the prevalence of sleep disorders is very high, and exceptionally so in relation to the amount of money spent on research and treatment of these disorders. Insomnia (by far the major sleep disorder) came third to headaches and anxiety disorders in the table of prevalence. Across the 27 countries of Europe, 7 per cent of the population suffers insomnia each year, affecting a total of 44.7 million people. This is associated with considerable disability and costs, which a parallel report estimated as totalling €35 billion, of which €20 billion were in direct or non-medical health care costs and €15 billion in indirect costs such as loss of productivity.

These enormous figures belie the assumption that sleep is merely a transient, insignificant period between the days, and strongly suggest that more investment in diagnosis and treatment could pay dividends in terms of improved quality of life and enhanced work performance.

Certainly the almost complete absence of a proper insomnia assessment and treatment facility anywhere in the NHS is a great concern as we know that during their current medical training medical undergraduates receive about one hour of teaching on sleep and its disorders – so general practitioners (GPs) are largely under-skilled in this major element of their practice.

This book seeks to help remedy this situation by bringing together in a more easily digested form the experience of a number of experts in all aspects of sleep – from the philosophical to the clinical – under a lead editor who has pioneered group treatments of insomnia. It provides the necessary first step to understanding the nature and fascination of sleep for those outside the field. It is hoped that it will also inspire clinicians, and academics, to think more about engaging in this area and refresh the knowledge and enthusiasm of those already doing so. The editors and contributors are to be congratulated for this timely effort.

David Nutt FMedSci
Professor of Neuropsychopharmacology, Imperial College London
October 2011

Preface

The original suggestion for a book on sleep came from Dr Ved Varma, who has contributed to and edited a number of books in the last two decades. Although the completed book has migrated some distance from his original idea, it could not possibly have been produced at all without his cheerful optimism, persistence, encouragement and support. It was intended that Ved would co-edit this book but, sadly, he became unwell even before all the original contributors were recruited. As soon as chapters began to be submitted it became evident that a co-editor was essential and Alex Westcombe, who had already read some early drafts, agreed to take on the role.

We would like to say that the process of chapter selection for this book was in some way systematic; in reality, it was 'everything we could think of at the time'. For various reasons we were unable to secure, or keep, some topics that we wanted to include. However, the sole advantage of the project (inevitably) running late was that we were then able to include other perspectives on sleep, which we had not thought of or which became apparent as work progressed.

We acknowledge some duplication or overlap between the chapters, but we have endeavoured to reduce this where possible. Some cross-referencing is always necessary, but it would be tiresome to be continually referred to other chapters to find key information, and we also wanted each chapter to be able to stand independently. Furthermore, in some cases, to have complex material explained more than once in slightly different ways, or from different angles, can aid the process of understanding.

As for the selection of contributors, we hope the reader will agree that we have been able to assemble a diverse range of talent. The authors are people at various stages of their respective careers with a vast range of experience between them and a keen understanding of the way that sleep is studied in their particular discipline, and we are grateful that they have shared their knowledge in this way.

It is possible that as editors we have taken a more hands-on approach to our task than others might take, and it is likely that we tried the patience of some long-suffering contributors with our comments and questions on successive drafts. Complete agreement on how ideas are conveyed is unlikely, but we consider it has been a privilege to engage in such discussions. We have learned a lot in those exchanges and hope that the process has improved the book as a whole.

As well as acknowledging the contributors' efforts in producing their own chapters, we would like to thank them for offering their ideas and opinions in respect of other chapters, particularly when there was some conceptual overlap. Others who have helped in this way, and in many other ways, are too numerous to list – with the following exceptions. Claire Durant made a significant contribution in the final preparation of a number of chapters. Jessica Kingsley has been supportive from the outset and subsequently very patient. Finally, we would like to thank Sue Wilson, without whose help and support this would have been a lesser and later book.

Note: Terms in the glossary are marked in the text by an asterisk *.

1

Introduction

THE UNIVERSITY OF SLEEP

Andrew Green and Alex Westcombe

In recent years sleep has excited the interest of a range of disciplines. In fact, there seems to have been an explosion of interest, as can be judged by the variety of books that have been published in the last decade. There have, for example, been books on anthropology (Brunt and Steger 2008), sociology (Williams 2005) and 'popular science' (Horne 2006; Martin 2002). A chapter in a book on the history of the night-time has dealt with sleep in history (Ekirch 2006), there has been a history of insomnia (Summers-Bremner 2008) and a history of sleep research (Kroker 2007). There is also a book entitled *The Politics of Sleep* (Williams 2011). These have added to an existing and growing scientific and medical library with titles ranging from summaries of sleep disorders (Wilson and Nutt 2008) via an in-depth manual on the treatment of insomnia (Morin and Espie 2003) to detailed and specialized medical textbooks (Kryger, Roth and Dement 2011; Overeem and Reading 2010); it also includes such specialist titles as a book on the forensic aspects of sleep (Shapiro and McCall Smith 1997); and reproductions and reprints of classic works continue to be available (Kleitman 1987; Macnish n.d.). This prompts the question: why another book on sleep?

The reason for this book is precisely because of the increasing specialism in that increasing range of disciplines. Most readers could not hope to absorb such a wealth of information from so many different sources, and perhaps only a glutton would want to. However, it is the assertion of this book that the reader from one of the humanities may benefit by having the science carefully described and the terms explained – it would be an unwise sociologist, say, who addresses a scientific audience without understanding the rudiments of medication, for example. At the same time the scientist or doctor will be the richer for understanding more of the social, historical and cultural context of sleep, and, for example, be more alert to the risks of making assumptions about what is 'normal'. The principal aim of the book is therefore to enhance communication between science and the humanities – C.P. Snow's 'two cultures' (Snow 1959). For the more general reader the aim is simply to provide a wide-ranging and accessible introduction to the subject of sleep from a variety of angles.

It was originally intended that the book would deal systematically with all the disciplines in a fairly consistent manner. However, the range of material is so wide, and the voices so diverse, that such aspirations were soon discarded. Instead, we present the following collection of contributions and celebrate their variety; not only do they represent a range of perspectives on sleep, but their differing styles reflect the different academic traditions from which they come. This book might therefore be thought of as if it were an in-depth visit to a university specializing in sleep – where each department presents its work, or some aspect of it, to the visitor who would be struck not only by the different approaches, but also by the various personalities of the staff.

The visitor, or reader, is also likely to notice that whilst there are some scientific principles that regulate our sleep, there is also flexibility in the systems, and that boundaries are not always as clear as we may think. This flexibility is expressed in many ways – between societies and within societies – and for reasons of culture and for reasons that are regarded as disorder or the result of illness. Furthermore, sleep patterns have changed during the course of history and our knowledge of, or beliefs about, sleep have also changed.

In beginning a tour of such a range of departments it seems reasonable to start by looking at the scientific facts as they are currently understood. Chapter 2 serves as an introduction and begins by looking at the structure and regulation of sleep and considering its purpose. The flexibility of sleep systems is emphasized in an examination of the sleep of other animals that have evolved to sleep in a much wider range of circumstances. Chapter 3 also illustrates how some animals have adapted to extreme conditions, but the emphasis here is the timing of sleep. Chronobiology is perhaps a little known branch of science but it is nonetheless essential for understanding how humans maintain regular sleep despite environmental variation. The chapter explains in some detail how the mechanisms operate, and shows, for example, how there is natural variability between individuals in terms of preferred sleeping and waking times. Furthermore, it makes important connections between biological rhythms and mental well-being.

The next three chapters consider some of the variation that is possible despite the scientific norms. Chapter 4 takes an anthropological perspective and examines the way that sleep habits and practices vary around the world. A classification of sleep patterns is proposed, and there is a discussion of the rituals and routines people follow in preparation for sleep. A closely related subject is medical anthropology, and Chapter 5 looks at the way that expectations of sleep in modern society might be at odds with sleep as it has evolved over thousands of years – looking in particular at the sleep of children. It is argued that children have different needs for sleep and that parents may be unwise to attempt to manipulate their children's sleep patterns to match their own expectations and needs. The practices of parents can bring about sleep habits that are now defined as sleep disorders in a process known as medicalization. This is a concept from sociology, and from the perspective of sociology Chapter 6 shows how sleep is affected by the interaction between biological processes and the influence of *other* people. Sleep therefore varies within a culture, and the chapter highlights some of the ways that the sleep practices and attitudes might vary according to age and gender.

A discipline that might be thought to have little involvement with sleep is occupational therapy, but Chapter 7 argues that for three reasons it should. First, occupational therapy (or the related discipline of occupational science) is concerned with how people use time: sleep is part of this although its measurement in time-use studies is variable. Second, the quality of our sleep can affect our ability to perform activities (or to be 'occupied') during the day – for which there is clear evidence. Third, what people do *whilst awake* can affect the nature of their sleep although, in this case, the evidence is more tentative.

Much of the research that is described in the chapters thus far, and subsequently, depends on the recording of sleep in the laboratory. Chapter 8 is therefore indispensable to the understanding of the measurement of sleep. It provides an introduction to neurophysiology, including an explanation of how electroencephalography (EEG) developed, how it works, and what it can tell us about the science of sleep and the diagnosis of sleep disorders.

The next two chapters explore disrupted sleep from a medical perspective. Chapter 9 surveys a selection of sleep disorders. Insomnia is such a problem for so many people that the chapter deals with it in some detail. It also looks at excessive daytime sleepiness and some less common but equally disturbing sleep disorders, all of which demonstrate that the boundary between sleep and wakefulness is not as distinct as we may think. The delicate balance between wakefulness and sleep is explored more specifically from the standpoint of psychiatry in Chapter 10. Altered sleep is a feature of almost all mental disorders: in some cases, as in anxiety, it may be difficult to establish whether the disorder causes the sleep problem, or *vice versa*; in other cases, such as in dementia, the sleep mechanisms appear to be impaired. The two chapters show how easily the sleep/wake mechanism can be disrupted. The first line of treatment of sleep problems is often pharmacological, and Chapter 11 therefore outlines the way that some medications work, inevitably involving some of the scientific background. The main focus is on drugs that promote sleep, but the chapter also looks at medication designed to prevent sleep as well as at other substances – legally obtained and otherwise – that can influence sleep.

It could be argued that disordered sleep itself is not the greatest burden for individuals (or society) but that the consequences of that impaired sleep are. Chapter 12 looks at the specific relationships between sleep, sleepiness and fatigue in some detail, spending particular time on long-term fatigue. Some of the challenges of doing research into this area are acknowledged, as is the role of people's beliefs and expectations of what sleep should do for them.

Chapters 13 and 14 return to the humanities: providing historical, literary and religious perspectives. Whilst religious texts have not addressed sleep exhaustively, they contain numerous references to it; sleep is used in many instances to reflect or represent wider metaphysical and theological ideas. Chapter 13 addresses these ideas in a range of different religions and looks, for example, at the Protestant work ethic (that is, valuing productivity over sleep), the ideal timing of prayer for Sikhs, and the role of yoga and meditation in Buddhism. Looking at sleep in literature, Chapter 14 shows how writers have used sleep, or the lack of it, to explore our own relationship with natural rhythms, and it chronicles the shift from our alignment with nature to patterns driven by industrialization. It therefore also takes a historical perspective, and goes on to consider how sleep and sleeplessness are investigated and pathologized in contemporary society.

The final chapter attempts to take an overview of the material presented in other chapters and picks up on themes regarding different sleep practices and the clarity, or lack of it, of the boundaries between the three states of being (wakefulness, deep sleep and dream-sleep). It takes the opportunity to explore subject areas of other disciplines that are not represented here (such as perspectives from history and economics), and to stray back into the territory of some disciplines that are. It concludes by questioning what normality is when it comes to sleep – a question that is first addressed in Chapter 2 on the science of sleep.

References

Brunt, L. and Steger, B. (eds) (2008) *Worlds of Sleep*. Berlin: Frank & Timme.

Ekirch, A.R. (2006) *At Day's Close: a History of Nighttime*. London: Phoenix.

Horne, J. (2006) *Sleepfaring*. Oxford: Oxford University Press.

Kleitman, N. (1987) *Sleep and Wakefulness*. Chicago, IL: Midway Reprints, University of Chicago Press. (Original work published in 1963.)

Kroker, K. (2007) *The Sleep of Others and the Transformations of Sleep Research*. Toronto: Toronto University Press.

Kryger, M.H., Roth, T. and Dement, W.C. (eds) (2011) *Principles and Practice of Sleep Medicine*, 5th edn. St Louis, MO: Elsevier Saunders.

Macnish, R. (n.d.) *The Philosophy of Sleep*. BiblioLife. (Original work published in 1834.)

Martin, P. (2002) *Counting Sheep: The Science and Pleasures of Sleep and Dreams*. London: HarperCollins.

Morin, C.M. and Espie, C.A. (2003) *Insomnia: a Clinical Guide to Assessment and Treatment*. New York: Kluwer Academic.

Overeem, S. and Reading, P. (eds) (2010) *Sleep Disorders in Neurology: A Practical Approach*. Chichester: Wiley-Blackwell.

Shapiro, C. and McCall Smith, R.A. (eds) (1997) *Forensic Aspects of Sleep*. Chichester: John Wiley and Sons Ltd.

Snow, C.P. (1959) *The Two Cultures and the Scientific Revolution: The Rede Lecture*. Cambridge: Cambridge University Press.

Summers-Bremner, E. (2008) *Insomnia: a Cultural History*. London: Reaktion Books Ltd.

Williams, S.J. (2005) *Sleep and Society: Sociological Ventures into the (Un)Known*. London: Routledge.

Williams, S.J. (2011) *The Politics of Sleep: Governing (Un)consciousness in the Late Modern Age*. Basingstoke: Palgrave Macmillan.

Wilson, S. and Nutt, D. (2008) *Sleep Disorders*. Oxford: Oxford University Press.

2

The Science of Sleep

WHAT IS IT, WHAT MAKES IT HAPPEN AND WHY DO WE DO IT?

Louise M. Paterson

2.1. What is sleep?

Sleep occupies approximately a third of our lives and despite decades of study, we are only just beginning to understand its function. We now know that sleep is an active physiological process within the brain rather than a passive experience, and that it is highly regulated and controlled. It is also becoming apparent that good sleep is essential for normal brain function and for our overall health and well-being.

Sleep can be defined as a natural, periodic state of immobility where the individual is relatively unaware of the environment and unresponsive to external sensory stimuli. Nearly all voluntary muscles become inactive and metabolic rate is reduced. The brain, however, is far from inactive; brain waves display characteristic patterns that differ from those displayed during wakefulness or coma. It is important to make a clear distinction between sleep and other states of consciousness. For centuries it was wrongly assumed that consciousness ceased at sleep onset and resumed with waking. Sleep is better represented as a reorganization of brain activity where consciousness could be considered to be 'dulled'. Importantly, one is easily awoken from sleep, which also distinguishes it from coma, anaesthesia or from hibernation.[1] A particular sleeping position and sheltered site is usually adopted. Another important feature is that if sleep is lost or prevented, recovery sleep usually occurs in order to compensate for the loss.

The definition of sleep can be applied to humans as well as to most terrestrial mammals and birds, with only a few exceptions. There are notable differences for aquatic mammals, many of which can maintain mobility whilst asleep. A form of sleep that occurs in more primitive creatures requires more simplistic definitions.

Sleep appears important for humans for several reasons:

- we spend a large proportion of our time sleeping

- we cannot cope properly without sleep: sleep loss results in cognitive impairment, mood changes and hormonal abnormalities, and can exacerbate the symptoms of other mental and physical disorders

- we always try to make up for lost sleep: sleep loss is followed by a compensatory increase or rebound in sleep

- a rare disorder known as fatal familial insomnia (a prion disease) causes such severe sleep loss that it results in early death.

However, the desire to be well rested and to make up for lost sleep in order to maintain normal function does not account for the purpose of sleep. Scientists are still unsure about its precise functions. There may even be different functions for different species. The theories of the functions of sleep are discussed in more depth in Section 2.6.

2.2. How much sleep do we need?

The actual amount of sleep required is genetically determined and therefore varies between people. As individuals, we simply need enough sleep to feel refreshed and to be able to perform our daily tasks satisfactorily. Individual sleep need is dependent on biological processes that determine the timing, duration and depth of sleep. These are discussed in more detail in Section 2.4 and in Chapter 3.

It is generally considered that the 'optimal' amount of sleep for human adults is between 7 and 8 hours per night in a single consolidated period because this allows us to benefit most from alertness, improved mood, sound memory and good health (National Sleep Foundation 2002). Accordingly, the majority of people report that they would like to sleep for between 7 and 8 hours daily, but that the average amount of sleep they actually obtain is between 7 and 7.5 hours (see Figure 2.1).

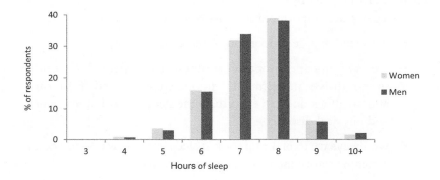

Figure 2.1. Average number of hours of sleep obtained per night
Data are taken from the responses of 1.1 million American women and men between the ages of 30 and 102 (Kripke *et al.* 2002).

Too little or too much sleep over prolonged periods can be detrimental, and both are associated with increased mortality (see Figure 2.2). Studies have consistently shown that those who typically sleep for about 7 hours experience the lowest risks for all-cause mortality, whereas those who sleep significantly longer or shorter have a higher risk of mortality, with the risk being slightly different between men and women (Grandner *et al.* 2010). Those who experience 6 hours or less per night are also more likely to be dissatisfied with their quality of life in general (Hublin *et al.* 2001; National Sleep Foundation 2002).

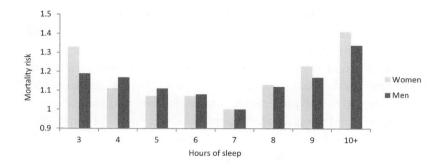

Figure 2.2. Relationship between sleep duration and mortality risk in women and men

Data are taken from the responses of 1.1 million Americans between the ages of 30 and 102 (Kripke *et al.* 2002). This study is one of many such examples reviewed by Grandner *et al.* (2010).

In practice, our sleep is often not optimal because of social constraints such as working hours, family commitments and societal structure that oblige us to sleep less or at times inappropriate to our biological clock (see also Chapter 3). This results in a sleep debt for which we are usually able to compensate by 'catching up' on lost sleep. For example, those who rely on an alarm clock to wake them for work will often 'sleep in' at the weekend, and those whose sleep is fragmented at night will often nap during the day, particularly in old age.

2.3. Sleep structure

In mammals and birds sleep is divided into two main types: rapid eye movement (REM) sleep and non-REM (NREM) sleep. In humans, non-REM sleep is further subdivided into four stages of increasing depth: stages 1 to 4, termed S1, S2, S3 and S4, according to sleep scoring criteria (Rechtschaffen and Kales 1968). The deepest stages of sleep (S3/S4) are also called delta sleep or *slow-wave sleep* (SWS). More recently, the American Academy of Sleep Medicine has produced an updated classification where stages N1, N2 and N3 broadly replace stages S1, S2 and S3/S4 respectively (Iber *et al.* 2007).[2] The vast majority of scientific sleep studies to date have used the original criteria, but this is expected to change in future as laboratories and clinics begin to adopt the new system.

The different sleep stages are determined in humans according to whether certain behavioural and/or physiological characteristics are present. Many characteristics can be observed without scientific instruments and include sleep posture, eye movements, mobility, responsivity and breathing rate. However, for measuring sleep stages accurately, the gold standard is polysomnography (PSG). This technique involves the recording of an individual's brain waves by electroencephalography (EEG), and is usually combined with measurements of eye movements by electrooculography (EOG) and of muscle activity by electromyography (EMG). A more detailed account of the sleep EEG and how it is measured is given in Chapter 8. Briefly, the EEG is described according to the size of the signal (voltage amplitude) and the number of oscillations per second (frequency). Frequencies are divided into bands which aid sleep scoring: delta, theta, alpha and beta. Alpha rhythm, for example, is particularly prominent in the waking EEG when eyes are closed, whereas delta rhythm predominates in SWS. The sleep EEG also features recognizable transient elements such as K-complexes (spikes resembling the letter K) and sleep spindles (oscillations of 12–14Hz) that help identify S2.

These patterns, along with EMG and EOG measurements, allow us to determine which stage of sleep is being experienced at any given time. Pictorial representations called hypnograms are used to illustrate the cycling of an individual through the different sleep stages throughout the sleep period. The course of a normal human sleep period is shown in Figure 2.3a and b. The characteristic 'skyline' that is produced is often referred to as sleep architecture or sleep structure.

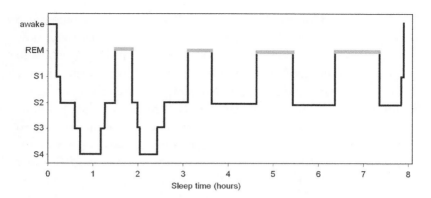

Figure 2.3a

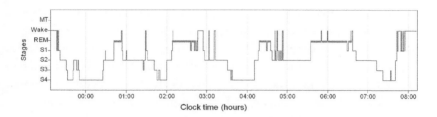

Figure 2.3b

Figure 2.3. Sleep structure in normal healthy adults

These graphs represent the cycling of sleep stages throughout the night: (a) an idealized hypnogram and (b) the actual hypnogram of a healthy 25-year-old male, showing the stages of sleep and their distribution over the course of a night. S1: stage 1, S2: stage 2, S3: stage 3, S4: stage 4, REM: rapid eye movement sleep, MT: movement.

During the night, sleep progresses between NREM and REM sleep stages in a series of sleep cycles. Progression through NREM stages followed by a REM episode is counted as one complete cycle. The cycle length in humans is normally between 90 and 110 minutes, with between three and six cycles per night.

The lightest stage of sleep is entered into first (S1), and this stage is associated with drowsiness and slow rolling eye movements. S1 is often disturbed by brief periods of wakefulness before S2 sleep commences. Sleep onset can be interrupted by those strange and sudden jerks, known as hypnic jerks, or involuntary muscle twitches that are often accompanied by the sensation of falling and can be a rude awakening for the sleeper and bed-partner. Sustained S2 sleep is identified when

K complexes and/or spindles occur (see Chapter 8), and signifies sleep onset proper. As sleep depth increases, breathing and heart rate slow down, muscle tone is reduced and the wave pattern slows (reduces in frequency) and increases in amplitude. These changes correlate with the decrease in arousal and increased synchrony between firing of nerves within the brain. The deeper stages of NREM sleep, or SWS, follow soon afterwards (S3 and S4). Heart rate and breathing are slowed and the EEG displays characteristic synchronous slow waves of large magnitude. The individual appears still and peaceful and it is more difficult to arouse someone from this stage of sleep. The amount and intensity of SWS is controlled by homeostatic mechanisms (see Section 2.4), and is very much dependent on the number of hours the person has been awake beforehand.

The first episode of REM sleep takes place 60 to 80 minutes after sleep onset, and the entry into REM happens quite abruptly with marked changes in the EEG. It is characterized by low-voltage EEG activity that resembles wakefulness: this is why REM sleep is often referred to as paradoxical sleep. However, REM sleep differs from wakefulness as it is accompanied by a complete loss of muscle tone or paralysis (atonia) and by the presence of the characteristic rapid eye movements. REM sleep is also most associated with the experience of dreaming. Indeed, muscle atonia during REM sleep is thought to prevent individuals from causing harm (or embarrassment) by acting out vivid dreams.

A greater proportion of NREM sleep is experienced in the early part of the night whereas REM sleep predominates in the latter part of the night (see Figure 2.3). A young healthy person would be expected to spend approximately 50 per cent of the night in S2, 20 per cent in SWS, 20–25 per cent in REM sleep, and the remainder in S1 or awake. It is quite usual to have several short periods of wakefulness throughout the night. Some waking episodes are remembered whereas others are not.

The amount, timing and structure of sleep changes throughout the lifespan, particularly during the first few years of life, but also during normal ageing. On the whole, these changes form an intrinsic part of brain development, but medical disorders can often cause unwanted changes to sleep architecture in old age.

The time and duration of babies' sleep tend to be chaotic during the first few weeks of life, but stabilize as the infants begin to develop a

24-hour circadian rhythm, strengthened by regular bedtimes and feeding times and a stable routine. Young children require more sleep in order to develop and function normally, with the required amount of sleep tending to decline as the child ages (see Table 2.1). Adolescents require more sleep than they might care to admit, and their sleep timing tends to be delayed compared with children and young adults. As the years progress through adulthood, sleep duration tends to shorten and sleep occurs earlier, particularly in old age. However, whilst consolidated night-time sleep appears much reduced in the elderly, it is often made up by daytime naps.

Table 2.1. Average sleep requirements throughout the lifespan

Age or condition	Average sleep required (hours)
Newborn	Up to 18 hours
1–12 months	14–18 hours
1–3 years	12–15 hours
3–5 years	10–13 hours
5–12 years	9–11 hours
Adolescents	9–11 hours
Adults	6–8 hours
Elderly	6–8 hours

The structure of sleep also changes during the lifespan. A newborn baby will spend up to 9 hours a day in *active* sleep resembling REM sleep, but by the age of five this has declined dramatically, with only slightly over 2 hours spent in REM. After that age, the proportion of REM sleep remains relatively stable (approximately 20%). The decline in NREM sleep is in line with the overall reduction in sleep duration with age, but the quality and depth of sleep is also reduced; elderly people tend to experience fragmented sleep and less deep sleep.

In general, women and men have similar sleep requirements, but women's sleep alters with the menstrual cycle, pregnancy and the menopause. This is because the secretion of certain hormones, such as oestrogens and androgens, affects sleep. These hormonal changes can, for example, cause premenstrual and post-menopausal insomnia, increased NREM sleep during early pregnancy and increased deep sleep during lactation (for a review see Paul, Turek and Kryger 2008).

2.4. Regulation of sleep timing

We tend to think of ourselves as able to decide when and where to sleep and for how long. Whilst this is true to a certain extent, there are two underlying biological processes controlled by the brain that play a large role in determining our sleep/wake cycle. These are the circadian process (C) (see below and Chapter 3) and the homeostatic recovery process (S). The circadian and homeostatic processes are separate but interacting and have become known as the two-process model of sleep (Borbély 1982). The combined processes ensure that the propensity for sleep is highest during hours of scheduled rest and lowest during waking hours when we are required to be alert. Figure 2.4 shows how in humans, the two processes work to promote the onset of sleep when both are high (at the usual bedtime), to maintain sleep when the C process is high and the S process is declining (in the small hours) and to promote wakefulness when the C process is low and sleep propensity is minimal.

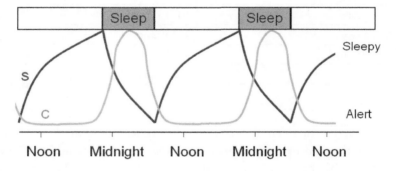

Figure 2.4. The two-process model of sleep

This graph demonstrates how the need to sleep changes throughout the 24-hour cycle in response to circadian and homeostatic processes. C is the circadian sleep drive which reaches a maximum around 4 a.m. and tails off in the morning, keeping us alert until early evening. S is the homeostatic sleep propensity which reaches a maximum after about 16 hours of wakefulness and rapidly declines during sleep.

The circadian and homeostatic mechanisms determine what time of day we are most likely to fall asleep, how deeply and for how long. In humans they make it easier to fall asleep at night during the hours of darkness, particularly if we have been sleep deprived, and make it difficult for us to sleep during daylight hours, or at night if we have had a long afternoon nap. For nocturnal and crepuscular animals (those awake at night and those awake at dawn and dusk respectively) these processes are similar, but work to promote sleep at different times, depending on the species.

The two processes are also able to compensate for one another: if, for example, you stay awake all night, the build-up of the S process will be overridden by the C process intervening in the early morning. This means that, even if you have gone without sleep for a night, you are still able to function the following day, albeit with reduced performance. Humans can manage to stay awake relatively well for periods of up to 72 hours. After this, our homeostatic drive to sleep is so strong that we can no longer force ourselves to stay awake.[3]

Maintaining a regular daily schedule strengthens the circadian drive and reinforces the homeostatic drive, making sleep easier to achieve at the chosen bedtime. Disruption of the circadian rhythm by keeping a chaotic sleep schedule, by doing night shift work or by regularly switching time zones can make sleeping difficult. This is clearly demonstrated by the effects of jet lag. Similarly, the process of being aroused, anxious or alert may overcome either of the sleep-promoting processes, and is one of the main mechanisms involved in the complaint of insomnia, particularly where the insomnia is long-standing and complicated by behaviours which weaken these processes such as irregular hours of sleep (see Chapter 9).

The circadian process

Circadian means approximately one day (*circa diem* in Latin), and describes the process that regulates the daily rhythms of the body and brain. The circadian rhythm is generated within the body by a pacemaker or master clock that is found in a group of cells in the suprachiasmatic nucleus (SCN) of the hypothalamus within the brain (see Chapter 3 and Figure 3.3). The SCN displays an oscillatory pattern of activity that has a period of about 24 hours. Remarkably, the oscillations are innate and self-sustaining – the cells continue to demonstrate cyclical activity even in isolation from the rest of the body. The circadian clock controls sleep/wake activity and all bodily rhythms such as hormone release and liver function. In fact, all other organs in the body co-ordinate their peripheral clocks with the SCN master clock in order to maintain normal function. The SCN is strongly influenced by light entering the eye and, to a lesser extent, by other time cues such as temperature. For humans, bright light in the early morning is necessary to set (entrain) the clock to a 24-hour rhythm; bright light in the evening will delay the clock. In the absence of external time cues, the SCN will 'free-run' to its own natural period; constant light or darkness reveals that the true biological cycle in humans is actually 24.3 hours in length. Many blind people can still entrain to the 24-hour day even though they do not have a conscious perception of light. This is because human eyes contain irradiance detectors that are able to sense light despite being incapable of producing a visible image. These receptors remain intact in many blind individuals, allowing entrainment to a 24-hour rhythm as usual. Blind people without eyes often have difficulty with entrainment and commonly suffer with circadian rhythm disorders of sleep (see also Chapter 3).

The homeostatic process

Homeostasis (from the Greek *homoios, stasis*) essentially means 'staying the same'. It is the property of a system that regulates its internal environment to maintain a stable, constant condition. Such a homeostatic mechanism is responsible for the brain's ability to recover lost sleep by increasing subsequent sleep. Unlike the circadian process, the homeostatic or recovery drive to sleep (the S process) is wake-dependent; it increases in proportion to the amount of time since the last sleep. When sleep has been shorter than usual, there is a 'sleep debt' which leads to an increase in the S process, which works to ensure that the debt is made up at the next sleep period by accelerating the time to sleep and by increasing sleep depth and duration. Conversely, if a lot of sleep has already been obtained (e.g. by napping) it may be difficult to get to sleep at night, and sleep depth will be reduced.

The allostatic process

More recently a third 'allostatic' process has been identified which is also involved in controlling the sleep/wake cycle – from the Greek (*allo, stasis*) meaning 'remaining stable by being variable'. Like homeostasis, allostasis achieves stability of a system but through multiple or variable physiological or behavioural changes. This is the mechanism by which sleep timing and duration can be controlled by external forces such as social and ecological cues. Clearly these allostatic mechanisms can override the circadian and homeostatic propensity for sleep if it is necessary to stay awake. Sleep researchers have started to investigate these allostatic mechanisms but so far they are poorly understood (Saper, Scammell and Lu 2005b).

Genetic control of circadian drive

Recent research has revealed that the genes responsible for maintaining the circadian rhythm within cells are common to many species including fruit flies, rodents and primates (including humans). These 'clock' genes have been shown to produce cyclical patterns of activity, because the biochemical pathway for gene activation eventually leads to inactivation of the same gene (see Chapter 3). Clock gene mutations (polymorphisms) can lead to alterations in circadian function and are particularly easy to identify in fruit flies. Similar gene variants have subsequently been found in people with circadian rhythm disorders such as delayed sleep phase syndrome (see Chapter 9). Genetic make-up can also have an influence on our chronotype (our preferred time for activity), sometimes referred to as diurnal preference. Normal chronotypes lie on a continuum, with evening types ('owls') and morning types ('larks') having a distinct preference for activity when they are naturally more alert according to their genes (see Chapter 3).

2.5. What are the brain mechanisms of sleep?

Certain features of sleep are shared between species which suggests that brain mechanisms are also shared, having been preserved and developed through evolution. This is supported by the conservation of the clock genes controlling timing of rest and activity that exist throughout the animal (and plant) kingdoms.

In birds and mammals, including humans, sleep and wakefulness are controlled by a network of brain regions, collectively referred to as the wake and sleep centres (Dijk and von Schantz 2005; Saper *et al.* 2005a, 2005b). These networks are driven by the actions of chemical messengers – neurotransmitters – which communicate messages between brain regions via nerves in order to co-ordinate an appropriate response. In the case of sleep, the signals resulting from circadian rhythms, homeostatic processes and external stimuli are directed to the wake and sleep centres of the brain. Here, the signals are integrated and the relative strength of activity in the 'wake' versus the 'sleep' centres will determine whether an individual is awake or asleep. This is known as the 'sleep switch'. The whole process is stabilized by another brain system which prevents an individual from switching between wake and sleep states inappropriately. A more complex description of the main brain regions related to sleep and wake, and the major neurotransmitters involved in sleep regulation, is shown in Figure 3.3.

The circadian system feeds into the wake and sleep centres in the brain. However, the SCN is always active during daylight hours and the sleep centre is always active during sleep, so the intervening brain circuitry alters in order that the circadian peak will produce sleep at the appropriate times. This will differ, depending on whether an animal is diurnal, nocturnal or crepuscular.

It is possible to see how disruption of one or many of these brain pathways might lead to sleep/wake disturbance. The neurotransmitter systems are also influenced by drugs – illicit and medicinal – and are the subject of intense study in order to develop novel pharmaceuticals for sleep/wake disorders such as insomnia, parasomnias and excessive daytime sleepiness.

2.6. Theories on the purpose of sleep

Historically it has been assumed that sleep must serve some universal, essential purpose. However, emerging evidence suggests that this is not necessarily the case. Instead, sleep has evolved multiple functions to cope with the increasing sophistication of the nervous system and the ever-increasing volume of sensory information that must be processed in complex species.

Numerous theories regarding specific sleep functions have been proposed, but none is well established (Siegel 2005). Energy conservation appears to be an important sleep function for many animals as this serves to optimize the timing and duration of behaviour and therefore prevents unnecessary activity at inopportune times. Nervous system recuperation and restoration is another important consideration – that sleep somehow reverses wake-related changes in brain function that may otherwise cause damage, such as depletion of energy stores and neuronal death. The role for sleep in neurogenesis, thermoregulation and the regulation of emotion is also being investigated.

In humans, the 'information-processing' theories have been most studied so far. Sleep has a role in the reinforcement of learning and consolidation of memory, with distinct roles for NREM and REM sleep. Some research supports the formation of new brain connections during sleep whilst other research suggests that they are removed during sleep, thereby retaining important information and discarding non-essential information (Crick and Mitchison 1983; Meerlo *et al.* 2009). Studies have suggested that memories are replayed, modified, stabilized and enhanced during sleep, although there is disagreement about whether NREM, REM or both are required and to what extent they are involved (Stickgold 2005, 2006). Such research gives us reason to believe that there may be some truth in the concept of 'sleeping on a problem' and the saying, 'sleep on it'. The importance of sleep for cognitive function is discussed in Chapter 7.

Whereas slow-wave sleep is most closely associated with sleep's restorative effects, REM sleep is thought to play an important role in development because it is maximal in the young. Other data suggest that REM sleep may have a role in facilitating entry into the wake state following NREM sleep. One of the more fascinating aspects of REM sleep is its relationship to dreaming. Whilst dreaming can occur in the other stages of sleep, it most often happens during REM, and these REM dreams have the imaginative story-like quality that often prompts us to recount the experience to our sleeping partner upon waking. Dreams are most often remembered when interrupted by a period of wakefulness during or at the end of the REM episode, and may not be remembered otherwise.

The content of dreams, their purpose and underlying brain mechanisms have been the subject of much discussion for many decades. Freud maintained that dreams were an attempt at wish fulfilment. Others believe that dreams may facilitate the incorporation of new ideas or experiences into existing brain networks, thereby assisting problem-solving. It is certainly true that the memories of daily life are sometimes reflected in our dreams. However, they are often fragmented in time and place, and cannot easily be predicted or studied scientifically. Current research is exploring the link between dreaming and memory and how our experiences during sleep relate to brain activity (Nir and Tononi 2010). For example, brain imaging studies have demonstrated that the visual cortex and memory-related brain regions are activated during REM sleep, consistent with vivid visual imagery during dreaming, and the possible incorporation of prior memories into dreams.

2.7. When sleep goes wrong

We have seen that there are many factors affecting sleep including age, hormonal cycle and the strength of circadian, homeostatic and allostatic drives. However, sleep can also be altered by other external factors. Illness can change sleep, particularly serious chronic psychiatric and neurological disorders. The drugs that are often used to treat these disorders and other medical conditions might also affect sleep, as might some recreational drugs and over-the-counter medicines. This is because all these factors affect the brain pathways controlling the sleep/wake cycle in some way. Some may affect the circadian or homeostatic processes and others may affect specific neurotransmitter systems. If the brain circuits are disturbed, progression into or out of sleep, the transition between sleep stages or the presence or absence of muscle tone may be disrupted leading to a lack of sleep, too much sleep, sleep at inappropriate times or strange sleep phenomena.

The brain circuitry controlling the sleep/wake cycle is very tightly controlled (Figure 3.3), so if one or more of the pathways is damaged or disturbed, a multitude of sleep disorders can result. Further descriptions of sleep phenomena and sleep disorders are given in Chapter 9. Similarly, illness or disease can affect sleep by altering one or multiple components of the sleep pathways in the brain, particularly psychiatric and neurological disorders such as depression, schizophrenia, Parkinson's or Alzheimer's disease which can have very marked effects on sleep (see Chapter 10).

Many drugs affect sleep, whether they are prescription medications targeting sleep or otherwise. Drugs that treat sleep disorders are designed to target a particular neurochemical sleep pathway (see Chapter 11), whereas illicit and other drugs are not, but their effects may overlap with certain sleep pathways anyway, often causing sleep disturbance. For example, two of the most heavily consumed drugs on the planet, alcohol and caffeine, can have profound effects on sleep.

Caffeine consumed close to bedtime can increase the time it takes to fall asleep and reduce the deeper stages of sleep thereby reducing total sleep time and efficiency. It is thought to increase arousal by inhibiting adenosine, a neurotransmitter that is involved in the development of sleep propensity as part of the homeostatic mechanism, but may also involve other arousal mechanisms. Small amounts of alcohol tend to make one feel sleepier and can aid the onset of sleep in light drinkers. However, at higher doses it often causes sleep fragmentation as its effects wear off in the latter part of the night. Alcohol can also disrupt sleep through its diuretic effects.

2.8. Sleep in other animals

Sleep in one form or another is common to all vertebrates: mammals, birds, reptiles, amphibians and fish. The definition of sleep cannot be extended to include lower order animals such as invertebrates, unicellular organisms or plants, but changes in activity are measurable even in invertebrate insects such as ants and fruit flies. Such species may display rest/activity cycles or periods of dormancy, but do not 'sleep' as such. The complexity of sleep largely depends on the complexity of the organism, with humans displaying complex changes in brain activity patterns and fruit flies displaying a simple rest/activity pattern. For an illustrated introduction to animal sleep, see Lacrampe (2003).

Humans are usually able to alter sleep to fit personal circumstances. Whilst biological factors (circadian and homeostatic drive) play a role in controlling sleep, its timing and duration are often dictated by social factors such as work, family and societal structure. In animals that are reliant on foraging, hunting or maintaining vigilance for survival, the opportunity for sleep is much reduced. Ecological factors such as habitat, light, food, warmth, shelter and the presence of young become more important drivers that determine the timing and duration of sleep, or indeed whether sleep can be obtained at all, if at the expense of more pressing needs. These are all known as allostatic factors (see Section 2.4). Because of these external pressures the nature of sleep has evolved to be flexible: sleep adaptations have allowed species to adopt different habitats and to maintain a balance with their other vital needs such as feeding and reproduction (Siegel 2009). Sleep structure therefore varies greatly between animals; for example there are notable differences between the sleep of land dwelling and aquatic mammals, between carnivorous and herbivorous mammals and with even more striking differences between warm- and cold-blooded animals.

It is also becoming clear that some sleep functions are present in some species and absent in others, possibly because they are not required or because the same function can be achieved in wakefulness instead. The differences can be quite marked. In rats, for example, sleep loss can prove fatal over a shorter time than even food deprivation would, suggesting that at least one of the possible functions of sleep is absolutely essential to them. Conversely, several species of fish such as schooling tuna are active continuously, and do not appear to sleep at all (Kavanau 1998). Similarly, whales and other aquatic mammals seem capable of managing without sleep for weeks when looking after their newborn.

Mammals and birds

In general, the kind of sleep that we observe in humans is associated with warm-bloodedness. In mammals and birds, sleep can be determined easily using behavioural observations such as movement, sleeping posture and non-responsiveness to external stimuli, but the EEG can be used to determine sleep stages more accurately. Sleep EEG shows that there are structural similarities between the sleep of most mammals and birds. Indeed, much of what we have learned about human sleep is derived from performing laboratory experiments in other terrestrial mammals (particularly rats, whose brain mechanisms for sleep appear to be very similar to our own) or from performing field studies of animal sleep in the natural environment.

Almost all mammals and birds that have been studied show regular cycles of NREM and REM sleep throughout the sleep period. The pattern is similar to those measured in humans, although birds' cycles are much shorter, and birds do not lose muscle tone to the same extent as most mammals. Mammals that do not show clear NREM/REM cycles include the monotremes (egg-laying mammals) such as the platypus, where REM sleep is thought to be localized to the brain stem, and not to project to the brain cortices, representing a more primitive form of sleep than is observed in other mammals.

Some mammals and birds sleep more than humans and others sleep less (for a review, see Siegel 2005). Sleep time for any given species cannot be easily predicted. It is related to multiple factors including age, body size, environment, diet, behaviour of predators or prey, safety and availability of the sleeping site (Allison and Cicchetti 1976). For example, bats sleep for 18–20 hours per day, hanging upside down and entirely safe within caves, whereas horses appear to need only 2–3 hours sleep, and can do so standing up. Terrestrial carnivores at the top of the food chain are able to obtain long periods of deep sleep as they eat infrequently and spend relatively little time hunting, feeding, mating or defending themselves. Smaller herbivores tend to spend more time foraging, eat more frequently and must remain alert to potential predators so spend much less time sleeping. Newborn terrestrial mammals tend to sleep for longer than adults, whereas neonatal aquatic mammals show very little sign of sleep at all. This is thought to reflect the urgent need for the aquatic youngsters to learn to swim and grow rapidly. The mother also refrains from sleep during the early days postpartum to allow her to continue nursing and hunting.

The sleep cycle length also differs between species. Smaller mammals tend to have shorter sleep cycles than the larger species; for example, cycle length is approximately 8 minutes in the shrew, 1.5 hours in an adult human and 1.8 hours in the elephant, and sleep may be obtained in several bursts rather than in one session. Humans have the opportunity to sleep in one consolidated period, whereas most other mammals and birds do not have this luxury; fragmented sleep and sleep obtained in multiple sessions are common, and allow the animal to balance its need for sleep with those of feeding, mating and vigilance. For example, the shrew can only sleep for very short periods of time as it must feed almost continuously to maintain its energy levels; failure to feed could result in starvation within a matter of hours. It remains unclear whether sleep in those species with short sleep performs the same functions as those in longer sleepers, and perhaps sleep does perform different functions for different species.

Reptiles, amphibians, fish and lower species
In other species with nervous systems, such as reptiles, amphibians and fish, neurological sleep states are very difficult to define. Sleep studies indicate that NREM and REM sleep are not a feature of sleep in these animals. Although changes in brain activity can be recorded, they cannot be reliably attributed to a particular sleep state. A more primitive form of sleep/wake cycle, or rest/activity cycle, is usually

observed using behavioural measures instead, such as mobility, posture and responsiveness.

The great differences in complexity of sleep between lower and higher order species support the notion that sleep does not perform the same function(s) for all species, as noted earlier. Whereas the EEG patterns of mammals and birds point to complex mechanisms for brain restoration and the facilitation of learning and memory, rest/activity cycles may simply serve as a mechanism to preserve energy. However, this is not to say that the study of sleep in simple species is not worthwhile: much of the information we now have about the genetic control of the circadian sleep/wake cycles comes from experiments with fruit flies (Cirelli 2009).

Special sleep adaptations

Adaptation of sleep has enabled species to sleep in obscure ways in order to fill a particular ecological niche, or to help ensure their survival. Sometimes specific mechanisms have evolved that allow sleep in difficult environmental conditions. For example, although horses and giraffes can sleep whilst standing, they must lie down for short periods of REM sleep when muscle tone is lost. Many birds also sleep standing up and can remain standing to obtain REM sleep because they do not lose muscle tone to the same extent as mammals. King penguins sleep on their feet whilst incubating their single precious egg; they remain standing for several months, and sleep hunched over for only a few minutes each day. In whales and dolphins REM sleep has not yet been reliably observed, which raises questions about its function (or lack of it) in these animals.

By far the most impressive sleep adaptation is the ability of some aquatic mammals and birds to sleep with only one half of the brain at a time. This is known as unihemispheric slow-wave sleep. Slow-wave EEG activity can be recorded in one brain hemisphere whilst simultaneously recording waking EEG in the other hemisphere (see Figure 2.5a and b). Essentially this means that one half of the brain and the contralateral side of the body can remain awake, allowing essential tasks to be performed, whilst sleep can perform its restorative functions in the other.

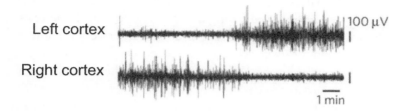

Figure 2.5a

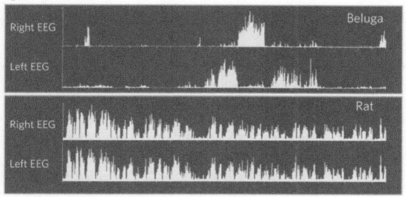

Figure 2.5b

Figure 2.5. Unihemispheric sleep in cetaceans

(a) Example of an EEG recording an immature beluga whale during
unihemispheric sleep of the left, followed by right brain hemisphere.
(b) Spectral plots of brain activity in the beluga whale in comparison with
the rat. The graphs show the amount of activity in the 1–3 Hz frequency
band (slow-wave activity) in both cortical hemispheres over a 12-hour period.
The pattern of unihemispheric sleep in the beluga contrasts with the bilateral
pattern of slow waves seen in the rat, a terrestrial mammal. Reprinted by
permission from Macmillan Publishers Ltd: Siegel, J.M. 'Clues to the functions
of mammalian sleep.' *Nature 437*, 7063, 1264–1271. Copyright © 2005.

Unihemispheric sleep allows aquatic mammals such as whales and
dolphins (cetaceans) to be almost continuously mobile, to maintain
vigilance and to continue surfacing for air whilst half asleep (Lyamin *et
al.* 2008). It has been recorded in all cetaceans that have been tested so

far. Because one half of the brain and body remains asleep, asymmetric activity can often be observed during unihemispheric sleep. In fur seals, asymmetric motor tasks such as flipper and whisker action allow it to constantly monitor its position, to continue swimming and remain afloat whilst in unihemispheric sleep. Interestingly, the fur seal reverts to a bilateral pattern as soon as it sleeps on land. Its regulation of REM sleep is also remarkable. It spends very little time in REM whilst in water, but roughly equal time in both NREM and REM sleep when on land.

Some birds are also capable of both forms of sleep. Mallard ducks can sleep with both hemispheres when they feel safe, and will do so in a tucked up position with both eyes closed, but if they feel threatened they can adopt unihemispheric sleep, with one eye open and thus can alternate sleep between hemispheres. Similarly birds on the edge of a group of sleeping companions can adopt unihemispheric sleep in order that the outward-facing eye can remain vigilant for the protection of the flock. It has even been suggested that unihemispheric sleep may allow certain birds to obtain sleep on the wing. This might be particularly relevant for migrating species, or those spending most of their lives at sea such as the albatross, although this has not yet been confirmed (Rattenborg 2006).

2.9. The future of sleep science

Our understanding of the function and regulation of sleep has been accelerated by the development of new technology. Techniques such as PSG which measure sleep structure in humans can now be combined with sensitive functional brain imaging techniques such as magnetic resonance imaging (MRI) and positron emission tomography (PET) which measure regional brain activity. These techniques allow researchers to pose many questions, for example: Which brain structures are involved in the control of NREM and REM sleep? How do they interact? What are the effects of loss of sleep or too much sleep? What are the functions of sleep phenomena such as spindles and slow waves? The potential for imaging techniques to increase our understanding of the brain is summarized in research reviews (Dang-Vu *et al.* 2007).

Technology known as radiotelemetry is now available and allows the continuous recording of an animal's EEG, and other measures, in its own environment. Electrodes can record EEG, EMG, body temperature and movement and transmit the radio signals to a receiver which can store all the information in real-time. Animals in captivity have been shown to display different sleep patterns from those in the wild (see Chapter 7), so recording sleep and behaviour undisturbed in the natural habitat is very important if we are fully to understand the multiple functions of sleep in different species.

There have also been major advances in understanding the brain neurochemistry mechanisms that cause and influence sleep. This research is facilitated by the ability of sleep researchers to measure and manipulate the sleep/wake cycle in animals (particularly rodents) and to extrapolate the results to humans and other species. Understanding the neurochemistry of sleep is particularly important for informing drug development. The discoveries that come about through these techniques help us to piece together the puzzle surrounding the science of sleep, its functions and mechanisms. Ultimately the research helps us to understand why sleep is important, how much we should be getting and when, and how to improve it if necessary.

This chapter was completed in October 2010.

Notes

1. Coma, anaesthesia and hibernation are very different from normal sleep. Coma is a state of prolonged unconsciousness, usually caused by injury or illness, from which the subject cannot be aroused. Anaesthesia is a pharmacologically induced, reversible state characterized by analgesia and a varying degree of consciousness, depending on the type of anaesthetic. Hibernation is a kind of very deep sleep, from which an animal cannot be easily woken, and is characterized by a profound reduction in metabolic processes.
2. Distinction between the two stages S3 and S4 was considered to be arbitrary and sleep researchers could not agree on how they should be distinguished, so they were merged to form a single sleep stage, N3.
3. The record for wakefulness is held by Randy Gardner who, in 1964, managed to stay awake for a continuous 264 hours (11 days). This was not without consequences for his behaviour and cognitive abilities: during the challenge he suffered from mood swings, memory loss, paranoia and hallucinations. However, he recovered fully after obtaining subsequent sleep.

References

Allison, T. and Cicchetti, D.V. (1976) 'Sleep in mammals: ecological and constitutional correlates.' *Science 194*, 4266, 732–734.

Borbély, A.A. (1982) 'A two process model of sleep regulation.' *Human Neurobiology 1*, 3, 195–204.

Cirelli, C. (2009) 'The genetic and molecular regulation of sleep: from fruit flies to humans.' *Nature Reviews Neuroscience 10*, 8, 549–560.

Crick, F. and Mitchison, G. (1983) 'The function of dream sleep.' *Nature 304*, 5922, 111–114.

Dang-Vu, T.T., Desseilles, M., Petit, D., Mazza, S., Montplaisir, J. and Maquet, P. (2007) 'Neuroimaging in sleep medicine.' *Sleep Medicine 8*, 4, 349–372.

Dijk, D.-J. and von Schantz, M. (2005) 'Timing and consolidation of human sleep, wakefulness, and performance by a symphony of oscillators.' *Journal of Biological Rhythms 20*, 4, 279–290.

Grandner, M.A., Hale, L., Moore, M. and Patel, N.P. (2010) 'Mortality associated with short sleep duration: the evidence, the possible mechanisms, and the future.' *Sleep Medicine Reviews 14*, 3, 191–203.

Hublin, C., Kaprio, J., Partinen, M. and Koskenvuo, M. (2001) 'Insufficient sleep – a population-based study in adults.' *Sleep 24*, 4, 392–400.

Iber, C., Ancoli-Israel, S., Chesson, A. and Quan, S.F. (2007) *The AASM Manual for the Scoring of Sleep and Associated Events: Rules, Terminology and Technical Specification.* Westchester, IL: American Academy of Sleep Medicine.

Kavanau, J.L. (1998) 'Vertebrates that never sleep: implications for sleep's basic function.' *Brain Research Bulletin 46*, 4, 269–279.

Kripke, D.F., Garfinkel, L., Wingard, D.L., Klauber, M.R. and Marler, M.R. (2002) 'Mortality associated with sleep duration and insomnia.' *Archives of General Psychiatry 59*, 2, 131–136.

Lacrampe, C. (2003) *Sleep and Rest in Animals.* Richmond Hill, ON: Firefly Books.

Lyamin, O.I., Manger, P.R., Ridgway, S.H., Mukhametov, L.M. and Siegel, J.M. (2008) 'Cetacean sleep: an unusual form of mammalian sleep.' *Neuroscience and Biobehavioural Reviews 32*, 8, 1451–1484.

Meerlo, P., Mistlberger, R.E., Jacobs, B.L., Heller, H.C. and McGinty, D. (2009) 'New neurons in the adult brain: the role of sleep and consequences of sleep loss.' *Sleep Medicine Reviews 13*, 3, 187–194.

National Sleep Foundation (2002) *National Sleep Foundation Sleep in America Poll 2002.* Available at www.sleepfoundation.org/sites/default/files/2002SleepInAmericaPoll.pdf, accessed on 21 August 2010.

Nir, Y. and Tononi, G. (2010) 'Dreaming and the brain: from phenomenology to neurophysiology.' *Trends in Cognitive Science 14*, 2, 88–100.

Paul, K.N., Turek, F.W. and Kryger, M.H. (2008) 'Influence of sex on sleep regulatory mechanisms.' *Journal of Women's Health 17*, 7, 1201–1208.

Rattenborg, N.C. (2006) 'Do birds sleep in flight?' *Naturwissenschaften 93*, 9, 413–425.

Rechtschaffen, A. and Kales, A. (1968) *A Manual of Standardised Terminology, Techniques and Scoring System for Sleep Stages in Normal Subjects.* Washington, DC: United States Department of Health and Welfare.

Saper, C.B., Lu, J., Chou, T.C. and Gooley, J. (2005a) 'The hypothalamic integrator for circadian rhythms.' *Trends in Neurosciences 28*, 3, 152–157.

Saper, C.B., Scammell, T.E. and Lu, J. (2005b) 'Hypothalamic regulation of sleep and circadian rhythms.' *Nature 437*, 7063, 1257–1263.

Siegel, J.M. (2005) 'Clues to the functions of mammalian sleep.' *Nature 437*, 7063, 1264–1271.

Siegel, J.M. (2009) 'Sleep viewed as a state of adaptive inactivity.' *Nature Reviews Neuroscience 10*, 10, 747–753.

Stickgold, R. (2005) 'Sleep-dependent memory consolidation.' *Nature 437*, 7063, 1272–1278.

Stickgold, R. (2006) 'Neuroscience: a memory boost while you sleep.' *Nature 444*, 7119, 559–560.

3

Chronobiology

BIOLOGICAL RHYTHMS THAT INFLUENCE SLEEP

Katharina Wulff

3.1. Introduction

Chronobiology is the scientific study of biological rhythms in living organisms. Whereas humans have divided time into units of seconds, minutes, hours, weeks, months and years, nature follows 'biological time'. This is determined by alternations in light/dark phases and high/low temperatures driven by the rotation of the earth around its axis. Because of the tilt of the axis as the earth orbits the sun, environmental conditions cycle in a seasonal fashion from the poles to the tropical zone at the equator.

All living plants and animals have developed biological clocks that permit them to survive under these rhythmic conditions. The mechanisms that control rhythmic processes are manifested at every level of biological organization – from genes to neuronal networks and other secondary messengers, such as hormones. Evolved over millions of years, the genetic code holds a blueprint for a biological clock, which tracks the passage of approximately 24 hours. Biological or 'circadian clocks' (from *circa* = about, and *diem* = a day) drive physiological and behavioural processes such as blood pressure, body temperature and hormone production, as well as sleep, alertness and mood. In temperate and tropical zones, we experience a 24-hour pattern in light/dark exposure, which our circadian clock uses to adjust its internal clock work, thereby aligning internal biological time to the environmental day/night cycle. The clock's output signals are used to anticipate predictable environmental changes and to adapt physiology for forthcoming behavioural changes.

This chapter describes how organisms use internal circadian timekeeping to adapt to a periodic environment by using physiological processes that track time and help anticipate predictable local changes, such as the quality of light. First, it describes the principles of measuring biological time and how biological clocks work. Then it illustrates how these clocks regulate human sleep/wake timing and how our sleep/wake cycle responds to disruptions of internal clocks. In the last part of the chapter, attempts are made to explore medical implications of unrecognized circadian problems and their effects on sleep, mental health and well-being.

3.2. Biological oscillatory control systems
Biological systems are dynamic
The theory of oscillations is a branch of physics in which all temporal-periodic procedures are described; these range from mechanical to electromagnetic oscillatory systems, such as a pendulum or alternating current. Man-made oscillating systems are a familiar part of our technical world (such as a driving crank in any motor vehicle), and these engineered systems share the same principles with biological oscillatory systems. They alternate between state A and state B as a periodic function of time with a certain amplitude and frequency. Similarly, our vigilance 'swings' between low during sleep and high during wakefulness, whilst our metabolic states alternate between 'hunger' and 'satiation'. Many physiological processes such as the release of pineal melatonin and the drop of core body temperature before sleep onset occur repetitively with a particular internal reference time to each other.

Importantly, if two circuits (e.g. morning cortisol increase and melatonin decrease) are combined into a system in which they interact, the assembled entity shows properties that arise entirely from the *coupling* of actual states. Coupling enhances stability and adjusts the period length of the oscillating system. All oscillating systems have three basic requirements: a positive input signal to drive a change, an output signal and a feedback. A feedback occurs whenever an output signal of the system 'feeds back' to the input signal. The capacity to oscillate is a property of all biological systems with *feedback loops*. There are two types of feedback loops – positive and negative – which can occur separately or in combination. Positive feedback means to 'accelerate' and negative to 'slow down' a process. If combined, they create multiple loops, which provide more robust oscillations, so the system is more fault-tolerant.

Fundamental properties of biological clocks

Intracellular circadian clock mechanisms in mammals involve an interaction of multiple positive and negative loops, and these loops provide a self-sustaining cycle of the molecular clock using transcription-translational feedback, which takes 24 hours to complete a full oscillation. The aim is to keep the system oscillating in a bordered bandwidth that has to be meaningful for a species – that is, about a day. Another key property of all biological clocks is that they are temperature-compensated; that is, their period is constant irrespective of environmental temperature. If this were not the case, our clocks would run slower on a cold day and faster on a hot day, and clocks of reptiles or amphibians would be useless. The dynamics of circadian rhythms are identical to a periodic change explained by formal natural laws, as illustrated in the elongation-time diagram (see Figure 3.1). These laws penetrate into all layers of biological rhythms, from molecular to behavioural levels, and their basic principles are fundamental to the understanding of biological clocks.

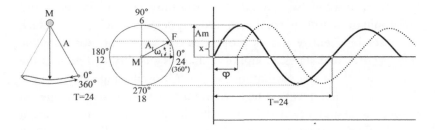

Figure 3.1. Properties of oscillating systems

The regular swing of a pendulum (left) illustrates a periodic movement that can be translated into a circle (middle) and then into a harmonic oscillation curve (right). Φ is a measure for shifts in time of a second oscillator (liver tissue) relative to the first oscillator (SCN) (dotted curve). A clock works in the same way as a harmonic oscillation that consists of a vector A (e.g. pendulum) that swings with the same angular speed ω around a central point M (anchor of the pendulum). After lapse of time t the vector has moved with its angle speed ωt from M0° into a different position MF. The biggest peak-to-trough difference M6 = M18 = Am is called amplitude. Each complete cycle (360°) of the vector A, or the time it takes the vector to return to its original position after release, is named period T of the oscillation (e.g. from sunrise to next sunrise = 24 hours). The reciprocal value of the period T is the frequency f = 1/T of the oscillation. Its unit is Hertz (Hz). The swing 0° to F equals x, and the equation for this swing is x = A sin ωt, where A is the length of the vector. If the vector A is not in the horizontal position at the beginning (that is at time point t = 0°) but in a tilted position of a certain angle φ in relation to the horizontal position (e.g. time point t = 23°), this shift is defined as the phase angle φ.

The principles of biological rhythms

The basic principle of rhythms is the law of conservation of mass, by which biological rhythm generators can be distinguished into *passive* or *active* oscillators. In *passive* oscillators the rhythms dampen out after a number of cycles, like an abandoned swing. If an oscillator has a constant source of energy and a regulator within the organism that generates and keeps the beat of the rhythm, this is an *active, endogenous* system that is capable of *self-sustained* regular oscillations and not reliant on environmental input. This is the hallmark of a clock, whether biological or man-made. For a biological clock to work, it needs a setting mechanism that connects its internal oscillation to external cycles of the geophysical environment, for example, light/dark or tidal changes, and a means that makes the output of the clock biologically useful (Foster 2004).

Taken together, *endogenous* timekeeping describes the internal representation of time that originates from within an organism. Internal clocks enable organisms to exploit ecological circuits by anticipating environmental changes (e.g. dusk/dawn), driven by an evolutionary advantage for individual organisms. Animals, plants, bacteria, algae, fungi – all have developed biological clocks that first emerged more than three billion years ago. The next part of this chapter describes the mechanism by which biological clocks work.

3.3. Cellular mechanisms of circadian rhythm generation

Anatomical sites and properties of biological clocks in mammals

Biological rhythms are categorized with respect to their frequency. For example, in *ultradian* rhythms (of less than 24 hours), the event occurs more frequently than daily, whereas in *infradian* rhythms, the event occurs less than daily; *circannual* rhythms have a describing cycle with a period of about a year.

Daily rhythms with a 24-hour period are universal and, with only a few exceptions, they exist in all organisms with a true cell nucleus (Eukaryota) – from fungi, and single-cell animals (protozoa) such as malaria parasites, to complex aquatic and terrestrial animals. They govern many of the organism's basic functions such as cell division, capacity for photosynthesis and phototaxis (movement in response to a light stimulus), but also very specific functions such as the glow in the bioluminescent dinoflagellate algae *Gonyaulax polyedra* or the readiness for mating in the protozoa *Paramecium*.

Daily rhythms are the most intensively studied and also the most significant rhythms for human well-being. In the traditional model of the mammalian circadian system, endogenous circadian rhythms result from a single master pacemaker that ensures that physiological processes of the body run on time and in the correct order. This master clock was discovered to be a small cluster of about 20,000 cells situated above the optic chiasm (where the optic nerves cross) in the anterior part of the hypothalamus of the brain (Stephan and Zucker 1972); it is therefore called the *suprachiasmatic nuclei* (SCN).

Early experiments showed that eliminating the SCN caused regular circadian rhythms to disappear in all behavioural and endocrine functions. For example, consolidated sleep and wake periods broke up into smaller bouts of sleep across the 24-hour period. Until recently, it was the widespread belief that only the SCN contains the circadian molecular machinery.[1] It came much to everyone's surprise that 24-hour oscillation of gene expression was also found in cultured connective tissue after treating the cultured cells with serum (Balsalobre, Damiola and Schibler 1998). This circadian rhythm in gene expression continued for a few cycles before dampening out, comparable to a *passive* oscillator. Further experiments in peripheral tissues such as the heart and liver provided unequivocal evidence that individual cells in the body contain the mechanism to drive circadian rhythms in gene expression, used for protein synthesis (Hastings, O'Neill and Maywood 2007). Recently, a number of neural circadian oscillators have been identified in a wide variety of mammalian brain regions including olfactory bulb, amygdala, hippocampus, thalamus, cerebellum and nuclei in the hypothalamus (Guilding and Piggins 2007). All these structures show circadian rhythms in core clock gene expression, hormone output and electrical activity, but are they master circadian clocks?

A master clock is considered a 'true' clock if the tissue is capable of producing *self-sustained* circadian output rhythms (i.e. in isolation from all other tissue and when excluded from external cues), and to be able to synchronize its self-sustained rhythm to an external rhythm, for example, that of light and dark. The SCN fulfils both these criteria: under light/dark conditions, the electrical activity of SCN neurons alternates in accordance with the light/dark exposure, and this activity can be shifted by the same cue, for example, a shift in light exposure. This rhythmic activity continues under constant darkness and even when the SCN is isolated from the surrounding tissue: the SCN is therefore deemed a master clock.

Outside the SCN, the first robust rhythms were found in the olfactory bulb and the retina. All principal brain regions and peripheral organ systems (including liver, heart, kidney, skeletal muscles) are now known to contain intrinsic circadian clocks, which can express circadian cycles of clock gene expression. Importantly, these cycles are not driven passively by efferent signals from the SCN. Instead, each individual cell in this tissue generates oscillations of 24 hours at high amplitude *in vitro* but they are not timed to be in tune with each other (see Figure 3.1). Desynchrony (individual cells being out of beat with each other) causes the culture to appear arrhythmic (Liu *et al.* 2007). Therefore the tissue cells depend on SCN input to get in step with each other and with the light/dark cycle. This dependency on the SCN input makes them semi-autonomous and not master clocks and differentiates them from the SCN. The SCN is the only structure known so far that has the property to entrain its period to solar time (e.g. after a transatlantic flight). But what type of signal does the SCN provide to the rest of the body and how is it conveyed?

SCN output and signalling of internal circadian time

Neural projections from the SCN drive endocrine and other circadian cycles via polysynaptic connections (Buijs and Kalsbeek 2001). Major relay areas lie adjacent to the SCN (e.g. the sub-paraventricular zone) extending into the dorsomedial hypothalamus (Saper, Scammell and Lu 2005). These relay areas are connected to sleep and arousal-regulatory regions and to the parasympathetic and sympathetic nervous systems, through which peripheral clocks, including heart, liver and adrenal gland, receive SCN-dependent circadian time cues (Kalsbeek *et al.* 2006) (see Figure 3.2). One SCN molecule, prokineticin 2, is particularly important in consolidating sleep, which shows the wider role of circadian signalling in sleep regulation[2] beyond the timing of sleep (Prosser *et al.* 2007). This demonstrates the SCN's ability to secrete a sequence of 'time-stamped' factors, which are taken up by local intrinsic clocks in other brain regions and peripheral organs to reconstruct phases of the circadian cycle. Consequently, if local clock mechanisms are being disrupted, behaviours depending on these regions will be impaired. Support for this assumption comes from studies of polymorphisms in clock genes. These studies show that people with a specific gene variant have cognitive deficits after 24 hours without sleep, whilst people without this variant appear to have compensatory mechanisms that keeps cognitive performance within the normal range (Viola *et al.* 2007).

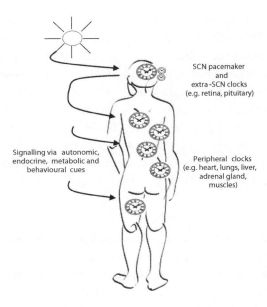

SCN pacemaker
and
extra-SCN clocks
(e.g. retina, pituitary)

Signalling via autonomic,
endocrine, metabolic and
behavioural cues

Peripheral clocks
(e.g. heart, lungs, liver,
adrenal gland,
muscles)

Figure 3.2. Schematic illustrating circadian hierarchical coordination across the body

The master pacemaker (SCN) entrains to the natural light/dark cycle by light information received through retinal projections from the eyes. The SCN synchronizes clocks in other brain regions and peripheral clocks in major body organs via autonomic, endocrine, metabolic and behavioural (e.g. exercise, food intake) cues.

One of the best characterized SCN output pathways is the circadian regulation of pineal enzymatic activity. This produces a pronounced daily variation in melatonin secretion, with serum concentrations of melatonin at night exceeding the daytime values by as much as 50-fold in mammalians, including humans (Dunlap, Loros and DeCoursey 2004). Melatonin synthesis is driven by a multisynaptic pathway extending from the medial hypothalamus to the sympathetic afferents of the pineal gland. The synthesis is light-dependent and the nocturnal rise is substantially delayed by artificial light exposure, which can also delay the SCN rhythms relative to the rigid conventional 24-hour/7-day clock (Santhi *et al.* 2011). In all mammals studied, whether a nocturnal or diurnal species, the duration of elevated melatonin secretion is directly proportional to the length of the dark phase of the natural day/night schedule. This *photoperiodic* regulation of the melatonin rhythm creates a pattern in hormone concentrations that serves as an endocrine seasonal calendar. The target organs are informed of the season of the year by the changing length of the melatonin synthesis. This neurohormone is involved in mediating a time signal such as changes in day length, seasonal or annual cycles, which are important cues for physiological processes underlying thermoregulation, reproduction, appetite, sleep or hibernation.

In humans, the SCN is a brain region with one of the highest density of melatonin receptors. Upon melatonin release from the pineal gland, these receptors become occupied and suppress SCN neuronal activity during the dark phase when sleep occurs. This is another example of a negative feedback loop, whereby melatonin release has a dampening effect on SCN activity. It is increasingly apparent that this complex interplay between the SCN and other clocks in the brain and body has consequences for brain-specific disease processes. For example, any type of depression – whether unipolar, bipolar or seasonal type – is often associated with disturbances of the sleep/wake cycle, including sleep fragmentation, excessive sleepiness or delayed sleep phases (see Chapter 10). Newer antidepressant medications, such as agomelatine, now target the circadian system using melatonergic agonists to consolidate the oscillatory clock work of the brain with promising results (de Bodinat *et al.* 2010; Kasper *et al.* 2010).

Circadian dysfunction has also been shown to relate to sleep/wake disruptions in various neurodevelopmental diseases, such as schizophrenia, and neurodegenerative diseases, for example, dementia of Alzheimer's type or Huntington's disease (Wulff *et al.* 2010). Schizophrenia patients with long-term, self-reported sleep disturbances show highly abnormal and diverse sleep/wake cycles and less exposure to daytime light when compared with a group of healthy but unemployed individuals without external routines being imposed upon them (Wulff *et al.* 2012). These sleep and circadian rhythm disturbances persisted independently of mental state and antipsychotic medication, and could not be explained by the patients' level of everyday function, indicating that symptoms of psychosis and sleep/circadian rhythm disturbances may share a common origin. In support of this hypothesis, schizophrenia patients with fragmented sleep and activity patterns performed worse in cognitive tasks than those with a high amplitude in sleep/activity (Bromundt *et al.* 2011). If one could correct the circadian dysfunction by pharmacological imposition of selective endocrine mechanisms, this could in turn slow down cognitive decline. This has not yet been explored in psychosis but has been successfully tested in a mouse model for Huntington's disease (Pallier *et al.* 2007).

In conclusion, most major organs contain a molecular clock mechanism comparable to that of the SCN. The key difference between a local oscillator and the SCN is that only the SCN is able to entrain to the solar day, whilst tissue-based oscillators are synchronized by endocrine, autonomic and behavioural cues that are dependent on the SCN. The SCN regulates a temporal agenda that enables specific phase relationships between multiple peripheral/brain oscillators and the SCN. Conversely, temporal disorganization in the circadian system can underlie mental disorders and consequently, the circadian system could be utilized for targeted therapies. The next section describes the most important signals that set biological clocks.

3.4. Regulation of biological rhythms by light
Setting circadian clocks to the local environment
The endogenous 24-hour period starts *free-running*, which means it deviates from exactly 24 hours, when cut off from any time-of-day information, namely constant light levels, no social cues and constant temperature. Although organisms continue their circadian oscillations in physiology and behaviour, the range their biological clocks are able to adjust to is limited to 3 hours either shorter or longer than 24 hours, which is called the *range of entrainment*. If an artificial light/ dark cycle outside this range were created, for example, a 28-hour light/dark cycle, the biological clock could not follow such a long period and would disconnect from the artificial light/dark cycle and free-run with its endogenous period. In humans, the clock's endogenous period ranges from 23.8 to 24.5 hours (Czeisler *et al.* 1999).

The cues that have the ability to synchronize endogenous (internal) clocks of plants and animals are called *zeitgebers* (German = *time giver*). Light is the most powerful *zeitgeber*, but there are also non-photic *zeitgebers* including temperature, exercise and food, to which the circadian clock can be entrained. The human circadian system is no exception and it is sensitive to light as in other mammalian species. Notwithstanding the importance of social cues and food availability, even low levels of light have an effect on the human clock. The neuronal activity of the circadian pacemaker alternates between high activity during hours of light (day) and low activity during the dark (night), to maintain clock–environment synchrony.

When human volunteers participated in an experiment (Czeisler and Gooley 2007), where they stayed in constant dim light across many days and nights, they were given bright light ranging from 200 to 2000 lux for six hours at different phases of their internal circadian clock cycle. If light was delivered during their internal phase of decreasing neuronal pacemaker activity, their phase became *delayed* at the next cycle. If light was delivered during their internal phase of rising neuronal pacemaker activity, their phase became *advanced* at the next cycle. This is known as a light-dependent circadian phase-response curve. The same happens under ordinary environmental conditions: if we expose ourselves to early morning bright light, we will generally experience an earlier sleep onset and start activity earlier the following morning. If we extend our light exposure into the first part of the night, we will experience a later sleep onset and activity start the following day. Taken together, the point in time that the light hits the person's endogenous circadian cycle determines the direction and size of the phase shift. The duration and intensity of the light exposure also determines the size of the phase shift.[3]

The importance of the mammalian eye
for visual and non-visual tasks

Since the period length of the SCN is not exactly 24 hours, the clock must adjust every day. The *zeitgeber* rhythm and the SCN's rhythm are coupled in a way that one rhythm is independent (light/dark cycle) and the other dependent (biological clock). If light information is essential for circadian entrainment, there has to be a connection from light-receptive organs to the SCN. In mammals, light is detected through the eyes, and if both eyes are lost, all visual sense and alignment of circadian rhythmicity to local time is lost too. The animal's sleep/wake pattern dissociates from the environmental light/dark cycle and starts to free-run. About one-third of SCN neurons are light-responsive and receive light information via direct projections from the retina.

When light levels change, these SCN neurons gradually change their electrical activity: the majority increase discharge rate in response to light and a minority decrease discharge rate. The response of SCN neurons is sustained for the full duration of retinal light exposure and this response is essential to the SCN's function to code for the varying length of light across seasons.

The retina is the layer of light-sensing and light-processing cells at the back of the eye. Typical photoreceptors in mammals are rods and cones, but evidence for another light-sensing system in the eye came from studies in blind mole rats and mouse mutants, where all rods and cones were ablated.[4] Whilst the lack of the known rods and cones had little effect on the animals' ability to entrain to light, the loss of the eyes abolished this ability (Hankins, Peirson and Foster 2008). A small subset (around 1%) of retinal ganglion cells has been found to detect light, and in subsequent experiments, the molecule responsible for brightness detection was discovered, and named melanopsin. Only these melanopsin-containing retinal ganglion cells project directly to the SCN (Hattar et al. 2003; Provencio, Rollag and Castrucci 2002). These newly found light-sensitive ganglion cells (pRGCs) not only project to the SCN but also to other areas of the brain, thereby having implications for widespread functions beyond the SCN, for example, pupil constriction, heart rate variability and sleep (Lupi et al. 2008).

In conclusion, the eye provides two parallel outputs, one for forming images of the world and one for detecting brightness. The knowledge of the dual function of the eye has clinical implications for people with ocular diseases. Although blind people may lack visual acuity, their pRGCs may remain intact and most can still adjust their circadian clock to the environmental light/dark cycle and therefore keep body functions and behaviour occurring at specific times of the day (Lockley et al. 1997). In contrast, completely blind people often complain of sleep disturbances, take sleeping pills and suffer from daytime sleepiness. This most likely occurs as a consequence of desynchronization between body clocks and the environmental light/dark cycle, leading to free-running sleep/wake cycles, which are getting in and out of phase with the environmental day/night cycle. Clinically, this implies that every attempt should be made to preserve the eyes in people suffering from certain types of eye diseases to maintain circadian entrainment and thereby mental and physical well-being.

Jet lag – a phenomenon in response to an artificial phase jump of zeitgebers

If one shifts the light pulse by a few hours (as in flights across several time zones), it takes the master and peripheral clocks some time to synchronize to the new local schedule. The direction of the flight prolongs or shortens the exposure to daylight, and the distance travelled determines the speed with which the clock synchronizes and establishes a stable phase relationship to the new local light/dark cycle. For westward travellers across ten time zones, adjustment takes about 11 days, and about 14 days after eastward flights (Klein and Weller 1972). This temporary loss of synchrony within and between body clocks and local time leads to a mismatch of temporal processes and causes general discomfort, a phenomenon that is well known as jet lag. It does not occur after long-haul north–south flights where no time zone changes occur.

Symptoms of jet lag are transient and include tiredness with the inability to initiate sleep at the desired time, disturbed digestion with appetite at inappropriate times, difficulties concentrating, headaches or general malaise. The symptoms fade as the internal clock adjusts to the new time zone through entrainment. Some travellers suffer from jet lag more than others for reasons that are still unclear. It seems that morning-type individuals, typically energized and fully functioning at the start of the day, have less trouble with eastward flights than evening-type individuals, because an advance of their internal clock is required. The opposite should occur for evening types and westward flights, but there is no strong empirical evidence. However, some evidence indicates that the shorter the time interval between last sleep period before departure and next sleep period upon arrival in the new time zone determines the extent and duration of jet lag – the shorter the interval the fewer the jet lag symptoms (Dunlap et al. 2004). This requires careful planning of travel arrangements.

Remedial measures to alleviate symptoms include exposure to bright light to advance or delay the phase of the endogenous clock, but this must be carefully scheduled, depending on the direction of the flight and the times of departure and arrival. Portable light sources (light visors) and strong sunglasses are available, although evidence of the effectiveness of such applications is limited. The administration of melatonin can alleviate symptoms of jet lag by improving sleep quality and promoting rapid entrainment of the master clock to local time. However, the optimal dose and time of administration have yet to be determined, and it is unclear whether the benefit is derived from melatonin's sleep-inducing effect or from phase-shifting the master circadian clock.

In summary, light facilitates the adaptation of circadian behaviour to the local environment. Most living organisms also organize their lives on a seasonal schedule. Even humans are receptive to photoperiodic changes, albeit without conscious awareness (Zaidi *et al.* 2007). The next subsection describes seasonal and circannual rhythms and how circadian timing is also part of mammalian *photoperiodism* – the timekeeping regulation of seasonal rhythms using changes in light.

Photoperiodism and the seasonal schedule

Because of the earth's changing position relative to the sun during the year, it is exposed to marked seasonal changes in light and temperature. The temperature difference between January and June in northern polar regions is 40°C, whilst in temperate regions (latitude 50°N) it is 25°C and at the equator, less than 1°C. Along with the temperature variation, there are other changes in climatic conditions, such as solar energy (UV-rate), air pressure, atmospheric humidity and amount of precipitation. The lives of most living organisms are organized on a seasonal schedule whereby they generally concentrate reproductive effort during seasons of abundant food supply that favour the survival of their offspring.[5]

The most reliable indicator of the season favoured by natural selection is the change in *phase* and *duration* of light because these change predictably over the year. With increasing distance from the equator, the duration of daylight increases or decreases gradually towards the extremes of half-yearly constant light or darkness at the poles. Photoperiod has a direct effect on physiological processes that influence reproductive status in many species and is called a *proximate* factor for seasonal reproduction. However, it is important to distinguish proximate factors from *ultimate* factors which are the other cyclic environmental factors directly affecting reproductive fitness, such as energy expenditure. This is why high rainfall and food availability in a tropical climate became more important for timed reproduction than photoperiod – photoperiod is relatively stable in tropical forests.

For seasonal rhythms, the same retinal light-sensing system and the same master clock (SCN) are used as in coding daily rhythms. The intimate link between the circadian system and the photoperiodic timing has been demonstrated in mammals whose SCN has been destroyed and that can no longer regulate reproduction according to changes in the duration of daylight. Under normal conditions, the SCN's electrical activity adjusts to daily photoperiod: high during the hours of daylight and low during darkness. If the SCN signals a photoperiod of a short day and long night, as in winter, the pineal releases melatonin for a *longer* period, whilst on a long summer day, and short night, melatonin is released for a *shorter* period. Melatonin receptors, consisting of two forms (MT1 and MT2), are not only found in the SCN, but also in many other tissues including the reticular thalamic nucleus (MT2 only) – known to be involved in promoting non-rapid eye movement (NREM) sleep – or the pars tuberalis of the pituitary gland, involved in triggering a cascade of reproductive activity. Since the occupancy of melatonin receptors is equivalent to seasonal light, melatonin influences the regulation of all kinds of activities.

In conclusion, photoperiodic signals in mammals are relayed by ocular photoreceptors to the circadian clock and from there to the pineal, where the timed release of melatonin acts as photoperiodic messenger for other neuronal and neuroendocrine regulation centres (e.g. for sleep and for reproduction). Light also determines the duration of melatonin release through acute inhibitory effects on melatonin synthesis. Disruption of seasonal patterns by artificial means may trigger conflicting signals that are deleterious for the body, for example, poor sleep quality. However, if so, this could easily be ameliorated by developing light sources excluding wavelengths that are absorbed by melanopsin-sensitive ganglion cells.

Extreme seasonal environments that may impose difficulties in circadian entrainment

In northern polar regions, organisms live in constant darkness between November and February and constant light from April to September. This presents a special difficulty to the circadian system, which has evolved to use daily changes in light as its primary *zeitgeber*. Before the arrival of Europeans, groups of native people lived peacefully in very small shelters and in geographical isolation for many months. The records of expeditions suggest that these people were happy and had a balanced mood and sleep/wake pattern with no sign of depression during the long winter darkness (now known as seasonal affective disorder). However, about 25 per cent of non-native groups living in northern Alaska experience mild symptoms of seasonal affective disorder, including sleepiness, irritability and loss of interest in social interaction (Dunlap *et al.* 2004). When non-native people are working on polar research bases over several months, they are unable to entrain under these conditions and show free-running rhythms in their sleep/wake behaviour. Workers regularly use bright light boxes to prevent symptoms of depression and for keeping entrained (Francis *et al.* 2008).[6]

3.5. Co-ordination of circadian timing in peripheral tissues

Physiological and metabolic processes are dynamic and therefore need to be organized in a temporal order to prevent chaos. Rest/activity, sensory perception, memory function or electroencephalographic (EEG) brain activity, to name a few, oscillate in a daily manner as much as cardiovascular functions, blood composition, hormone production, excretion or cell metabolism. Internal synchrony between different physiological and metabolic systems is established via signalling circadian time through a hierarchy of autonomous cellular oscillators distributed across different tissues of the body, which are synchronized by SCN-dependent circadian time cues (see Figure 3.2).

On the cellular tissue level, the clock gene *Per2* appears to be a potential sensor of rhythmic cues and a possible mediator of internal synchronization, but multiple mechanisms are likely to subserve internal synchrony, including body temperature, autonomic pathways and hormones (Hastings *et al.* 2007). Amongst them, corticosteroids seem to play a major role because their activation can phase shift circadian timekeeping in cells and tissues (Balsalobre *et al.* 2000) – although not in the SCN because it lacks the necessary glucocorticoid receptors. Internal synchrony may be viewed as a hierarchical axis from the SCN to the adrenal gland-producing glucocorticoids. This mediates circadian gene expression in clocks of peripheral tissue. These in turn direct the expression of their own target genes (e.g. enzymes), whose rhythmic expression is critical for vital body functions, such as detoxification, and needs to match in time with the rest/activity rhythm.

Circadian factors affecting temporal regulation of sleep

Humans are more aware of their daily sleep/wake rhythm than of any other circadian rhythm. Sleep is timed to occur at a specific phase of the endogenous circadian cycle, and aligned to the external light/dark cycle. Under entrained light/dark conditions a young adult's sleep starts about 1 to 2 hours after the rise of melatonin. Core body temperature (CBT) decreases during sleep and reaches its minimum about 6 hours after the rise in melatonin. However, under free-running conditions sleep starts later, close to CBT minimum, with *rising* CBT. This change in internal phase relationship provides an insight into the circadian regulation of sleep architecture. Whilst the time course of slow-wave sleep (SWS) remains unaltered, REM sleep shifts towards the beginning of the sleep period under free-running conditions. Furthermore, spontaneous *internal desynchronization*, as described earlier, can be observed. CBT continues to cycle with a near-24-hour period, whilst the sleep/wake cycle lengthens its period to up to 32 hours. Wake periods become much longer, up to 24 hours followed by 8 hours of sleep. This indicates that the two cycles, which are usually coupled under 24-hour light/dark cycles, become uncoupled in the absence of an entrainment cue, or when light cannot be received because of severe eye diseases. From experiments in which the sleep/wake cycle has been forced to decouple from the SCN's 24-hour period, important mechanistic explanations can be drawn for the circadian regulation of sleep (Dijk and Czeisler 1995). For example, the phase of the circadian CBT cycle at which sleep is initiated during desynchronization determines the duration of sleep. The longest consolidated sleep episode is initiated around CBT minimum. But sleep is not always initiated with the same intensity. It varies along the body clock's phases. A 2-hour period where sleep is almost impossible to initiate is about 6–8 hours before CBT minimum, the so-called 'wake maintenance zone' (Cajochen *et al.* 2002).[7] Under entrained conditions, this would relate to evening hours.

Once sleep is initiated, SWS and REM sleep are also differently affected by the circadian phase at which sleep occurs. SWS always declines over the sleep period regardless of circadian phase. In contrast, REM sleep propensity is modulated by the circadian phase at which sleep occurs, with a peak in REM propensity at or shortly after the minimum of CBT. Falling asleep in ordinary conditions is also determined by circadian clock phase: it is easier to get to sleep during the second part of the night when body temperature is low, and it gets harder the higher the CBT. Taken together, sleep needs to occur at a specific phase of the circadian clock, otherwise sleep quality is poor. Poor sleep is a frequent complaint and problem for sleep-deprived night-shift workers, who attempt to catch up sleep during the day, but cannot because it is at the wrong circadian time and coincides with the drive for wakefulness of the circadian cycle.

Sleep processes are also influenced by the duration of wakefulness. If an individual gets sleep-deprived for half or the total of the subjective night, SWS rebound will occur in the undisturbed part of the night or at the subsequent sleep period, respectively. The principle is that the longer the waking period, the more intense the SWS rebound, which makes the need for an *extended* sleep period unnecessary. Conversely, if a person takes a nap in the afternoon, this will decrease the intensity of SWS in the following night-sleep period. However, lost REM sleep will only be compensated by longer REM sleep at the next opportunity. Continuous REM sleep deprivation, without the opportunity to catch up, puts individuals at risk of developing depressed mood. During sleep deprivation, sleep pressure accumulates progressively the longer the waking period, whilst the drive for wakefulness also increases progressively to counteract sleepiness. During sleep, the accumulated sleep pressure dissipates and only starts accumulating again at waking. The interaction of the two processes determines the timing, duration and quality of both sleep and wakefulness (Dijk and Franken 2005). It demonstrates that there is an intimate link between the circadian system and sleep physiology. So how are circadian and sleep physiology functionally linked?

3.6. Brain circuits connecting circadian and sleep processes

Circadian regulation acts on many layers and sleep is also a highly complex state. Both arise from interactions amongst multiple brain regions, neurotransmitter systems and modulatory actions of hormones, but none of the systems involved is exclusive to the generation of sleep (Wulff *et al.* 2010). The major brain structures and neurotransmitters involved are shown in Figure 3.3. This complexity makes sleep very vulnerable to disruption. Disrupted sleep can lead to a number of health problems, including stress, and emotional, attentional and cognitive problems. Many of the health problems that arise from sleep disturbances also occur in mental disorders, but sleep disturbances are rarely suspected as a cause of these problems. Parallel brain pathways might be affected both in sleep/circadian disruption and in mental disorders.

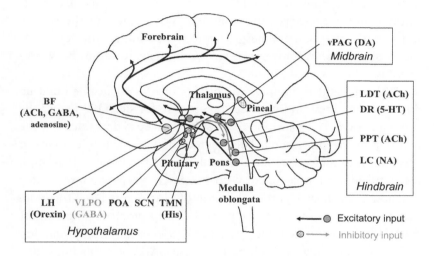

Figure 3.3. Schematic sagittal view of the human brain highlighting the circuits involved in the regulation of sleep/wake timing and arousal[8]

Abbreviations: 5-HT = 5-hydroxytryptamine (serotonin); ACh = acetylcholine; BF = basal forebrain; DA = dopamine; DR = dorsal raphe nucleus; GABA = gamma-amino-butyric acid; His = histamine; LH = lateral hypothalamus; LDT = laterodorsal tegmental nuclei; LC = locus coeruleus; NA = noradrenaline (norepinephrine); POA = preoptic area; PPT = pedunculopontine tegmental nuclei; SCN = suprachismatic nuclei; TMN = tuberomammilary nucleus; VLPO = ventrolateral preoptic area; vPAG = ventral periaqueductal grey matter.

Sleep and wakefulness are two mutually exclusive states that alternate with each other on the basis of alternating excitatory and inhibitory systems (see Figure 3.3). During sleep, the ventrolateral preoptic nucleus (VLPO) is activated and releases the neurotransmitter gamma-aminobutyic acid (GABA) and galanin to inhibit wake-promoting orexin neurons in the lateral hypothalamus and excitatory aminergic as well as cholinergic neurons in the brain stem. The NREM-REM flip/flop every 80–100 minutes is driven by neurons in the midbrain and the brain stem. During REM sleep, aminergic neurons remain inhibited, but cholinergic neurons are activated. REM-on neurons project to the spinal cord and drive muscle paralysis (atonia). During wakefulness, the excitatory neurotransmitters noradrenaline, serotonin, histamine, acetylcholine and orexin are released from their respective neurons in the brain stem, midbrain and basal forebrain structures. These neurotransmitters drive conscious wakefulness in the cortex. Importantly, the monoaminergic neurons also inhibit the release of the inhibitory neurotransmitters GABA and galanin from the VLPO neurons.

Wake-dependent homeostatic drivers such as adenosine build up during wakefulness and increase the pressure for sleep the longer the waking period. The transition from wake to sleep is dependent on the build-up of 'sleep pressure'. The accumulation of adenosine occurs in specific brain regions, especially in the basal forebrain, where high levels of adenosine correlate with increased sleep pressure. A key function of adenosine is the inhibition of GABAergic basal forebrain neurons, because they act to suppress the sleep-promoting neurons of the VLPO (during wakefulness). Disinihibition of the sleep-promoting VLPO neurons allows the VLPO to release GABA and galanin, which is needed to inhibit the arousal-promoting systems in the brain stem, midbrain and basal forebrain, thereby initiating sleep (Pace-Schott and Hobson 2002).

The SCN receives feedback from several brain structures involved in regulating sleep and arousal, such as the VLPO in the anterior hypothalamus, and the brain stem (e.g. dorsal raphe nuclei). Their function is likely to provide the SCN with current status of the body and for tuning its neuronal activity, for example, a change in amplitude, phase or period. Recognition of the temporal dynamics of sleep physiology, its underlying control by the circadian clock and the role of neurotransmitters and hormonal programmes provides a new perspective on the relationship between circadian clocks and sleep and the impact on well-being and economy.

3.7. Impact of biological timing on subjective and economic well-being

Although all human beings are diurnal, the genetic make-up of circadian clock genes determines whether one is more a 'morning' or an 'evening' person. Morning people prefer to get up early and to do things first thing in the morning and have an early bedtime, whilst evening people prefer to rise late, do things later during the day and go to bed late.

Questionnaires have been developed to assess one's so-called 'chronotype' based on their individual preferences, if they were entirely free to choose (Dunlap *et al.* 2004; Horne and Ostberg 1976), or by asking questions regarding their real bedtimes and rising times on work days and free days (Roenneberg, Wirz-Justice and Merrow 2003). Surveys using these questionnaires have shown that most people are near the mean, the so-called intermediate types, whilst at the two ends of the bell-shaped curve of normal distribution are the morning types ('larks') and the evening types ('owls'). Physiological phase markers of the clock, for example, the peak in melatonin production or the minimum in CBT, corresponded to the questionnaire results – the peak in melatonin occurs earlier in morning types and later in evening types. Therefore, the circadian system plays a critical role in human daily performance. Being an extreme morning or evening type does not normally cause any problems as long as one can plan the day accordingly. However, problems do occur if people are forced to perform at inappropriate phases, for example, an evening person having to work early morning shifts. Living against one's biological clock by activating or suppressing processes at the wrong time of the day may undermine our mental and physical well-being and increases the risk of certain disease conditions such as hypertension, diabetes or depression (Wulff *et al.* 2010). As an example, sleep problems and an increased risk for hypertension and cancer are amongst those clock-related functions that have been studied in shift workers, because shift work causes desynchronized conditions similar to jet lag. Furthermore, our body shows time-of-day dependent responses towards drugs, toxic substances, hormones and radiotherapy. Circadian processes at a cellular level, such as cell proliferation or metabolic and enzymatic activity, are thought to be responsible for this susceptibility because drugs, hormones or radiation act on all or a few specific cells.

Many diseases are also cyclic in their activity. As a consequence, physicians need to be able to predict the correct time of a medical event for a particular illness. For example, a rapid rise in blood pressure, angina attacks and strokes occur most frequently in mid-morning.[9] Timed drug intake becomes very important for a drug to be most effective. Today, most drugs are not administered on the basis of body clock time but for convenience. Drugs are also often developed to survive for a long period in the body ('retard'), and only vaguely coincide with the peak of the disease, but they often increase undesired potential side effects. To reduce the risk of these side effects and to maximize the desired disease-modifying actions, the *right drug* with the *right dosage* needs to be given at the *right time* to each individual. Successful *chronotherapy* – that is, when treatment is customized on the basis of the individual's chronotype, or body clock time, and disease cycle – has been found to improve clinical outcome in childhood leukaemia (Rivard *et al.* 1993), adrenal insufficiency (Johannsson *et al.* 2009) and ischemic heart disease (Portaluppi and Lemmer 2007).

Increased knowledge of the molecular and cellular bases of biological clocks has brought circadian time to the forefront of biomedicine, and has shown how temporal disorganization can underlie compromised sleep and overall health. Chronomedicine is likely to offer opportunities for the development of targeted therapies, including melatonin agonists to improve sleep, which utilize the circadian timing system.

3.8. Concluding remarks

The understanding of the complexity, diversity and adaptability of biological clocks has gradually grown over the past decades. Awareness of the importance of biological timing for human health has been achieved by discoveries and cross-species breakthroughs – for example, that the mouse and the fly still share the same clock gene components, whilst all organisms, even separated by billions of years of evolution, employ similar feedback loops for generating 24-hour rhythms. Collaboration between chronobiological research and sleep research is increasing, based on growing knowledge of circadian rhythms and sleep being closely linked to metabolic and mental activities by their co-evolution over millions of years.

Sleep is universal and it is the most obvious aspect of circadian timing for people, but there are still many gaps in our understanding of its function and mechanism. Basic and clinical research highlight major health issues related to chronic partial sleep loss in modern societies (Foster and Wulff 2005). Sleep deficit affects millions of people and it is directly related to suboptimal performance at school, work and at home. With the growing awareness of the adaptability of biological timing – and the increasing pressures on individuals in westernized societies where productivity is valued over creativity and play – the integration of sleep into human society using the understanding of the circadian basis of sleep will be an important area for future study.

Notes

1. At the molecular level, genetic information stored in the DNA inside the cell nucleus activates the expression of amino acid sequences of messenger RNA and subsequent accumulation of proteins of clock genes. Specific protein products translocate from the cell body into the nucleus and bind to a specific set of genes and accelerate their transcription (Clock/Bmal1, positive feedback), whilst other specific protein-binding products translocate into the nucleus, bind to specific genes and inactivate transcription, thereby suppressing the synthesis of their own enzymes (Cry/Per negative feedback). Once the protein products are cleared a new cycle starts.

2. Rhythmic glucocorticoid signalling also plays a prominent role in mediating SCN output and internal synchronization. Additional diffusible paracrine factors, such as transforming growth factor alpha (TGFα) and cardiotrophin-like cytokine, are likely translators of SCN output.

3. This was first shown in a dinoflagellate algae *Gonyaulax polyedra* (Hastings and Sweeney 1958).

4. Whilst cones are associated with colour vision in bright light, rods are associated with night vision in dim light, motion detection and peripheral vision. It was long thought that rods and cones were the only photoreceptors in the eye that convey light information to the brain. Whilst this is true for image-forming vision, it is not so for measuring brightness (Foster, Hankins and Peirson 2007).

5. An example of this is the breeding times in birds, which vary with latitude. In equatorial regions birds breed year-round, but progressively later with increasing distance from the equator – in spring in temperate and early summer in outer regions (Dunlap *et al.* 2004). Other activities, such as growth, moulting, migration and hibernation are also timed relative to a seasonal environment. Temporal co-ordination between season, behaviour and physiology is essential for survival and must not get out of balance; for example, migration and moulting must not occur simultaneously.

6. Animals native to the polar regions, such as reindeer, are unconstrained by circadian entrainment and show ultradian phases of activity. It has been suggested

that this lack of overt circadian rhythmicity might be an adaptive strategy to allow foraging whenever food is available in this unpredictable and extreme environment (van Oort *et al.* 2005). Migrating birds that are only in the polar region in summer for breeding do not show these ultradian patterns; they show entrained circadian activity. The circadian-based photoperiodic mechanism of regulating circannual behaviours such as reproduction, hibernation or migration is only *one* way of co-ordinating circannual timing. For example, SCN lesions in hibernating animals eliminate all circadian rhythms of behaviour but do not abolish circannual hibernation. The mechanism by which these rhythms are co-ordinated is not known, but it points to another endogenous timing system in the absence of anatomical identification of a discrete circannual pacemaker.

7. This is the time when the circadian drive for wakefulness is highest. Melatonin is not high enough to occupy the SCN receptors, and adenosine does not quite inhibit GABA-containing basal forebrain neurons, which in turn triggers sleep-promoting disinhibition of neurons in the ventrolateral preoptic area.

8. The circuits involved in the regulation of sleep/wake timing and arousal span across several functional complexes of the brain, e.g. brainstem (pons and medulla), thalamus, hypothalamus and forebrain. Sleep-promoting neurons in the ventrolateral preoptic area (VLPO) and wake-promoting neurons in the lateral hypothalamus (LH) interact with components of the ascending arousal system (LTD, PPT, DR, LC, TMN) to keep the sleep/wake phases in balance. During waking, the orexinergic neurons of the LH activate the arousal system to maintain wakefulness. During sleep the GABA-ergic neurons of the VLPO inhibit orexinergic neurons and the arousal system to maintain sleep. The suprachiasmatic nuclei (SCN) are important for the initiation of sleep onset and wake onset. The SCN contains many neurotransmitters, peptides and diffusible biochemicals, which originate either from incoming (glutamate, PACAP), outgoing (AVP, PK2, TGFα, VIP) or intrinsic (ANG II, AVP, CalB, CALR, Gal, GRP, melatonin, NPY, PHI, SS, VIP) neurons with many neurons not having only one neurotransmitter but co-localizing with peptides and neurotransmitters (Reghunandanan and Reghunandanan 2006). Accumulation of adenosine in the basal forebrain is essential for inhibiting GABA-containing basal forebrain neurons, which suppress the VLPO. Disinhibition of the VLPO neurons enables them to release GABA and galanin to suppress arousal systems and thereby initiate sleep (Strecker *et al.* 2000).

    Abbreviations: AH = anterior hypothalamus; ANG II = angiotensin II, possible neuromodulatory role in the SCN; AVP = vasopressin, excitatory role in increasing firing rates in the SCN; CalB = calbindin (calcium-bining protein), function as gates to relay photic signals; CALR = calretinin (calcium-binding protein); Gal = galanin; GRP = gastrin releasing peptide, putative role in photic entrainment; NPY = neuropeptide Y, involved in synaptic transmission; PACAP = pituitary adenylate cyclease-activating polypeptide; PHI = peptide histidine isoleucine; PK2 = prokineticin 2, role in photic entrainment; SS = somatostatin, regulatory role in modulating SCN phase by interconnections with VIP and AVP neurons; TGFα = transforming growth factor alpha, humoral diffusible output substance; VIP = vasoactive intestinal polypeptide, involved in SCN function and light-induced resetting

9. The maximum susceptibility for allergic reactions towards house dust and penicillin is in the evening. It has been suggested that these allergic reactions relate to the corticoid level in the blood, which shows a circadian-driven minimum in the evening (Reinberg 1989).

References

Balsalobre, A., Damiola, F. and Schibler, U. (1998) 'A serum shock induces circadian gene expression in mammalian tissue culture cells.' *Cell 93*, 12, 929–937.

Balsalobre, A., Brown, S.A., Marcacci, L., Tronche, F. *et al.* (2000) 'Resetting of circadian time in peripheral tissues by glucocorticoid signaling.' *Science 289*, 5488, 2344–2347.

Bromundt, V., Köster, M., Georgiev-Kill, A., Opwis, K. *et al.* (2011) 'Sleep-wake cycles and cognitive functioning in schizophrenia.' *British Journal of Psychiatry 198*, 4, 269–276.

Buijs, R.M. and Kalsbeek, A. (2001) 'Hypothalamic integration of central and peripheral clocks.' *Nature Reviews Neuroscience 2*, 7, 521–526.

Cajochen, C., Wyatt, J.K., Czeisler, C.A. and Dijk, D.-J. (2002) 'Separation of circadian and wake duration-dependent modulation of EEG activation during wakefulness.' *Neuroscience 114*, 4, 1047–1060.

Czeisler, C.A. and Gooley, J.J. (2007) 'Sleep and circadian rhythms in humans.' *Cold Spring Harbour Symposia on Quantitative Biology 72*, 579–597.

Czeisler, C.A., Duffy, J.F., Shanahan, T.L., Brown, E.M. *et al.* (1999) 'Stability, precision, and near-24-hour period of the human circadian pacemaker.' *Science 284*, 5423, 2177–2181.

de Bodinat, C., Guardiola-Lemaitre, B., Mocaër, E., Renard, P., Muñoz, C. and Millan, M.J. (2010) 'Agomelatine, the first melatonergic antidepressant: discovery, characterization and development.' *Nature Reviews Drug Discovery 9*, 8, 628–642.

Dijk, D.-J. and Czeisler, C.A. (1995) 'Contribution of the circadian pacemaker and the sleep homeostat to sleep propensity, sleep structure, electroencephalographic slow waves, and sleep spindle activity in humans.' *Journal of Neuroscience 15*, 5, 3526–3538.

Dijk, D.-J. and Franken, P. (2005) 'Interaction of Sleep Homeostasis and Circadian Rhythmicity: Dependent or Independent System?' In M.H. Kryger, T. Roth and W.C. Dement (eds) *Principles and Practice of Sleep Medicine*, 4th edn. Philadelphia, PA: Elsevier Saunders.

Dunlap, J.C., Loros, J.J. and DeCoursey, P.J. (eds) (2004) *Chronobiology: Biological Timekeeping*. Sunderland, MA: Sinauer Associates.

Foster, R.G. (2004) 'Oscillators, Clocks and Hourglasses.' In R.G. Foster and L. Kreitzman (eds) *Rhythms of Life: The Biological Clocks that Control the Daily Lives of Every Living Thing*. London: Yale University Press Profile Books.

Foster, R.G. and Wulff, K.L. (2005) 'The rhythm of rest and excess.' *Nature Reviews Neurosciences 6*, 5, 407–414.

Foster, R.G., Hankins, M.W. and Peirson, S.N. (2007) 'Light, photoreceptors, and circadian clocks.' *Methods in Molecular Biology 362*, 1, 3–28.

Francis, G., Bishop, L., Luke, C., Middleton, B., Williams, P. and Arendt, J. (2008) 'Sleep during the Antarctic winter: preliminary observations on changing the spectral composition of artificial light.' *Journal of Sleep Research 17*, 3, 354–360.

Guilding, C. and Piggins, H.D. (2007) 'Challenging the omnipotence of the suprachiasmatic timekeeper: are circadian oscillators present throughout the mammalian brain?' *European Journal of Neuroscience 25*, 11, 3195–3216.

Hankins, M.W., Peirson, S.N. and Foster, R.G. (2008) 'Melanopsin: an exciting photopigment.' *Trends in Neurosciences 31*, 1, 27–36.

Hastings, J.W. and Sweeney, B.M. (1958) 'A persistent diurnal rhythm on luminescence in Gonyaulax Polyedra.' *The Biological Bulletin 115*, 3, 440–458.

Hastings, M., O'Neill, J.S. and Maywood, E.S. (2007) 'Circadian clocks: regulators of endocrine and metabolic rhythms.' *Journal of Endocrinology 195*, 2, 187–198.

Hattar, S., Lucas, R.J., Mrosovsky, N., Thomson, S. *et al.* (2003) 'Melanopsin and rod-cone photoreceptive systems account for all major accessory visual functions in mice.' *Nature 424*, 6944, 76–81.

Horne, J.A. and Ostberg, O. (1976) 'A self-assessment questionnaire to determine morningness-eveningness in human circadian rhythms.' *International Journal of Chronobiology 4*, 2, 97–110.

Johannsson, G., Bergthorsdottir, R., Nilsson, A.G., Lennernas, H., Hedner, T. and Skrtic, S. (2009) 'Improving glucocorticoid replacement therapy using a novel modified-release hydrocortisone tablet: a pharmacokinetic study.' *European Journal of Endocrinology 161*, 1, 119–130.

Kalsbeek, A., Palm, I.F., La Fleur, S.E., Scheer, F.A.J.L. *et al.* (2006) 'SCN outputs and the hypothalamic balance of life.' *Journal of Biological Rhythms 21*, 6, 458–469.

Kasper, S., Hajak, G., Wulff, K.L., Hoogendijk, W.J.G. *et al.* (2010) 'Efficacy of the novel antidepressant agomelatine on the circadian rest-activity cycle and depressive and anxiety symptoms in patients with major depressive disorder: a randomized, double-blind comparison with sertraline.' *Journal of Clinical Psychiatry 71*, 2, 109–120.

Klein, D.C. and Weller, J.L. (1972) 'Rapid light-induced decrease in pineal serotonin N-acetyltransferase activity.' *Science 177*, 4048, 532–533.

Liu, A.C., Welsh, D.K., Ko, C.H., Tran, H.G. *et al.* (2007) 'Intercellular coupling confers robustness against mutations in the SCN circadian clock network.' *Cell 129*, 3, 605–616.

Lockley, S.W., Skene, D.J., Arendt, J., Tabandeh, H., Bird, A.C. and Defrance, R. (1997) 'Relationship between melatonin rhythms and visual loss in the blind.' *Journal of Clinical Endocrinology and Metabolism 82*, 11, 3763–3770.

Lupi, D., Oster, H., Thompson, S. and Foster, R.G. (2008) 'The acute light-induction of sleep is mediated by OPN4-based photoreception.' *Nature Neuroscience 11*, 9, 1068–1073.

Pace-Schott, E.F. and Hobson, J.A. (2002) 'The neurobiology of sleep: genetics, cellular physiology and subcortical networks.' *Nature Reviews Neuroscience 3*, 8, 591–605.

Pallier, P.N., Maywood, E.S., Zheng, Z., Chesham, J.E. *et al.* (2007) 'Pharmacological imposition of sleep slows cognitive decline and reverses dysregulation of circadian gene expression in a transgenic mouse model of Huntington's disease.' *Journal of Neuroscience 27*, 29, 7869–7878.

Portaluppi, F. and Lemmer, B. (2007) 'Chronobiology and chronotherapy of ischemic heart disease.' *Advanced Drug Delivery Reviews 59*, 9–10, 952–965.

Prosser, H.M., Bradley, A., Chesham, J.E., Ebling, F.J.P., Hastings, M.H. and Maywood, E.S. (2007) 'Prokineticin receptor 2 (Prokr2) is essential for the regulation of circadian behavior by the suprachiasmatic nuclei.' *Proceedings of the National Academy of Sciences of the USA 104*, 2, 648–653.

Provencio, I., Rollag, M.D. and Castrucci, A.M. (2002) 'Photoreceptive net in the mammalian retina. This mesh of cells may explain how some blind mice can still tell day from night.' *Nature 415*, 6871, 493.

Reghunandanan, V. and Reghunandanan, R. (2006) 'Neurotransmitters of the suprachiasmatic nuclei.' *Journal of Circadian Rhythms 4*, 2.

Reinberg, A. (1989) 'Chronopharmacology of H-antihistamines.' In B. Lemmer (ed.) *Chronopharmacology: Cellular and Biochemical Interaction.* New York, NY: Marcel Dekker.

Rivard, G.E., Infante-Rivard, C., Dresse, M.-F., Leclerc, J.-M. and Champagne, J. (1993) 'Circadian time-dependent response of childhood lymphoblastic leukemia to chemotherapy: a long-term follow-up study of survival.' *Chronobiology International 10*, 3, 201–204.

Roenneberg, T., Wirz-Justice, A. and Merrow, M. (2003) 'Life between clocks: daily temporal patterns of human chronotypes.' *Journal of Biological Rhythms 18*, 1, 80–90.

Santhi, N., Thorne, H.C., van der Veen, D.R., Johnsen, S. *et al.* (2011) 'The spectral composition of evening light and individual differences in the suppression of melatonin and delay of sleep in humans.' *Journal of Pineal Research* doi: 10.1111/j.1600-079X.2011.00970.x.

Saper, C.B., Scammell, T.E. and Lu, J. (2005) 'Hypothalamic regulation of sleep and circadian rhythms.' *Nature 437*, 7063, 1257–1263.

Stephan, F. and Zucker, I. (1972) 'Circadian rhythms in drinking behavior and locomotor activity of rats are eliminated by hypothalamic lesions.' *Proceedings of the National Academy of Sciences of the USA 69*, 6, 1583–1586.

Strecker, R.E., Morairty, S., Thakkar, M.M., Porkka-Heiskanen, T. *et al.* (2000) 'Adenosinergic modulation of basal forebrain and preoptic/anterior hypothalamic neuronal activity in the control of behavioral state.' *Behavioural Brain Research 115*, 2, 183–204.

van Oort, B.E.H., Tyler, N.J.C., Gerkema, M.P., Folkow, L., Blix, A.S. and Stokkan, K.-A. (2005) 'Circadian organization in reindeer.' *Nature 438*, 7071, 1095–1096.

Viola, A.U., Archer, S.N., James, L.M., Groeger, J.A. *et al.* (2007) 'PER3 polymorphism predicts sleep structure and waking performance.' *Current Biology 17*, 7, 613–618.

Wulff, K.L., Gatti, S., Wettstein, J.G. and Foster, R.G. (2010) 'Sleep and circadian rhythm disruption in psychiatric and neurodegenerative disease.' *Nature Reviews Neuroscience 11*, 8, 589–599.

Wulff, K.L., Dijk, D.-J., Middleton, B., Foster, R.G. and Joyce, E.M. (2012) 'Sleep and circadian rhythm disruption in schizophrenia.' *British Journal of Psychiatry 200*. (Published online 22 December 2011.)

Zaidi, F.H., Hull, J.T., Peirson, S.N., Wulff, K.L. *et al.* (2007) 'Short-wavelength light sensitivity of circadian, pupillary, and visual awareness in humans lacking an outer retina.' *Current Biology 17*, 24, 2122–2128.

Further reading

Dunlap, J.C., Loros, J.J. and DeCoursey, P.J. (eds) (2004) *Chronobiology: Biological Timekeeping.* Sunderland, MA: Sinauer Associates.

Foster, R. and Kreitzman, L. (eds) (2004) *Rhythms of Life: the Biological Clocks that Control the Daily Lives of Every Living Thing.* London: Yale University Press Profile Books.

4

Cultures of Sleep

Brigitte Steger

4.1. Introduction

Many factors influence a good night's sleep. As elaborated elsewhere in this volume, these may include physical factors, such as biological rhythms or physical or mental health, or environmental factors, such as light and sound. Some of the broader sociocultural issues, however, are also worthy of attention, as they have an impact both on what people consider desirable sleep to be and on how it can be achieved.

During sleep, we are only marginally aware of what is going on around us and subject ourselves to potential dangers such as physical attacks or nightmares. We are vulnerable and may feel out of control. *How* we deal with the insecurity of sleep and *when* we sleep are decisions that may strike us as neutral. Yet these questions are markers of culture, closely tied to the values a community shares about appropriate work and social behaviour. This chapter first explores how people in different cultures ensure a good night's sleep. It then goes on to discuss sleep patterns in different societies and asks what socioeconomic and cultural circumstances such as work organization and religious beliefs influence people's sleep arrangements.

4.2. Ensuring a good night's sleep

Those who do not live in secure housing, such as, for example, the homeless of Amsterdam who sleep outside, are particularly vulnerable; they are exposed not only to wind and weather, but also to attacks and attention from the police. And because many of them carry all their documents on their person, a robbery can mean the loss of identity. Even though many people believe that the homeless lead a lazy life, stress-related sleep problems are more common for homeless people than for people in senior management positions (Rensen 2003). Similarly, victims of disasters and refugees are often traumatized by their experience of violence and dislocation which disrupts their sleep. And there can be additional problems: for example, the Karenni in refugee camps at the Thai–Burma border suffer from the permeability of their bamboo huts – welfare organizations allow only certain building materials to be used and most people are poor. The threat of storms, fire and landslides affects sleepers, as does the threat of attacks by people and by animals – from mosquitoes and bedbugs to snakes and wild boars (Vogler 2008).

Fleas and bedbugs were also common bed companions in European history. Glasgow experienced a doubling of the population during the Industrial Revolution, between 1801 and 1821. This led to a severe housing shortage, miserable living conditions for the newly arrived low-wage labourers, poor hygiene conditions and the spread of diseases (Maver 2003). Scenes of large numbers of people in unwashed bedding and without ventilation were considered 'an antithesis of order, rationality and sensory lucidity' (Crook 2008, p.21). Yet the hygiene movements of the eighteenth and nineteenth centuries added more insecurity to sleep even as they tried to clean up. Sanitary inspectors entered overcrowded tenements at night to make sure that there were not more than 15 people sleeping in one room, but of course, the neighbourhoods were well organized and people warned each other when the inspector was arriving (Douglas 2001).

In Germany and the Netherlands the situation was less dramatic, and the authorities found different approaches to improve hygiene. They gave financial incentives to encourage people to throw out their box-beds and, in their place, build bedrooms with windows. Housewives were educated to air the rooms, change their sheets more frequently and to boil them (Schimek 1997); in the 1940s the more radical hygienists used DDT to get rid of the bugs.[1] Flea bites on children's soft skin became a sign of bad housekeeping, social backwardness and low social class. A 'master bedroom' with ironed sheets became a symbol and central feature of a bourgeois household. In the nineteenth-century Netherlands, even the working class wanted to have one room for representation and one for sleep. However, social reformers and hygienists – themselves coming from the higher classes – considered this kind of luxury inappropriate for the lower classes; it was felt to be an attempt to overthrow social order. They worked against it by putting toilets into the rooms, which, it was supposed, made the rooms unsuitable for hosting guests but still suitable for sleep (Montijn 2008).

In other parts of the world, we also see a relationship between sleeping place and social status. People who sleep on the street or in their rickshaw in India do so because they do not have a house. Remarkably, however, they appear hardly to be afraid of attacks or robbery (by sleeping on their belongings, though, they add another level of security). Neither the presence of strangers nor the noise in the street cause sleepless nights. On the contrary, sleeping alone, in silence, and sheltered from the outside world would keep many Indian people awake with fear, whereas the presence of people seems to protect the sleepers from hazards and fear of attacks by supernatural beings (Brunt 2008).

In European medieval and early modern literature, one of the greatest fears of sleeping was to die during sleep without having prepared for it; the unguarded soul would have been in danger of suffering eternally in hell (Klug 2008). People had to anticipate this eventuality every evening by confessing their wrongdoings, asking for forgiveness and praying. As sociologists Aubert and White (1959, p.51) put it, 'we may view the bed as a training ground for dying'. People without religion also sometimes experience difficulty getting to sleep whilst lying in bed, calm, no longer distracted by everyday life: repressed problems and conflicts may rear their ugly heads. All kinds of troubles and emotions arise: worry, loneliness, *angst*, sorrow or pain. Job-related and personal stress, including a fear of failure, job loss or a feeling of desolation, can underlie problems in falling or staying asleep, which increases stress in its own right.

As these examples show, sleepers are vulnerable in physical, social, mental and spiritual ways, and in different historical periods and societies sleepers have found different means of protection from such threats. In this chapter I argue that how people protect themselves during sleep reveals some of the key values and assumptions within a given society. Theoretically, I suggest, there are four major sources of the emotional security that is required for a relaxing and peaceful sleep: first, the stability of the physical sleep environment, the sleeping place; second, the presence of trusted people (whether known in person or not); third, recurring rituals or routines; and fourth, social acceptance of certain sleep behaviour. Whilst all these factors appear to shape sleep around the world, their particular manifestation and importance may vary in different cultural contexts (cf. Steger 2004).

When North Americans and Europeans suffer from insomnia and consult their doctor, they are often advised to use their bedroom exclusively for sleeping, to keep away noise and distraction, and there is a long tradition of having some items around the bed that help them to sleep, such as teddy bears, alarm clocks, pictures of loved ones or symbols of spiritual protection. This means that the sleeping room not only provides protection against actual attacks, but the familiarity of the sleeping environment also conveys reassurance and a feeling of belonging. This 'sleep hygiene' is learned from earliest childhood. It seems to be common sense to provide a sleeping room for every child almost from birth – children are supposed to sleep alone in order to become independent. However, the reality is more complex. A study in England has shown that breastfeeding mothers are more likely to co-sleep[2] with their child in the same room than mothers who bottle feed. But mothers usually do not admit this to the midwife, because they are afraid of social disapproval (Hooker, Ball and Kelly 2001). When young Americans come to university, it is likewise taken for granted that they share a room, often with a complete stranger. My students at the University of Pennsylvania discovered in interviews with their peers that room sharing was a major reason for sleep disruption. This was, however, only true for those who had grown up from early childhood with a bedroom of their own. Students of South Asian or African descent told the interviewers that they had no problem sleeping in a shared room: on the contrary, they felt very comfortable.

In most countries, however, it would be simply unthinkable to leave a baby or toddler to sleep alone in a room. In Japan mothers and paediatricians have read Dr Spock's advice to firmly put the baby to bed and to let the child cry in order to learn to sleep alone (Spock and Rothenberg 1992), but are convinced that it is important to convey a sense of security and belonging to the children by sharing the sleeping place with them. It is also easier for the mother to make sure that the children are properly covered and have no other problems when they sleep in the same room (Tsuneyoshi and Boocock 1997; on India see Shweder 2003). The connection between co-sleeping, emotional security and feelings of belonging is not limited to Japan, of course. In the USA, psychologist John Selby points out that insomnia is:

> almost always associated with a disruption of one's sense of communal security and belonging…as soon as something happens in our life, either emotionally or economically, which threatens our sense of ongoing communal security, we begin to experience an inability to relax into sleep. (Selby 1999, p.7)

It is thus not only the room or physical environment that is supposed to convey the emotional security to sleep well, but also the presence of trusted people. By extension, this may include people who are not physically present. Whilst medical sleep researchers tend to see the mobile phone as a disruption to sleep (as Venn and Arber 2008 observe), many Japanese teenagers use their mobile phone as a kind of 'teddy bear', constantly reassuring them that they can connect to their friends if needed (Kaji and Shigeta 2007).

Routines and rituals also reassure people that they will – like every night before – reawaken from their sleep. Such a routine can consist of one last telephone call, a glass of wine, putting on night clothes, washing, praying, watching television, reading or many other things. The habit of reading to children at bedtime has spread from Europe and the USA to middle and upper-middle classes around the world (Ben-Ari 2008). Children often want to hear the same story over and over to feel reassurance. However, it is not the case that children get special attention in every society, and people have also developed rituals less familiar to Europeans.[3] In Japan, for instance, some people sleep best after cleaning their ears, which reminds them of their childhood when their mother did it after the daily bath (Kaji and Shigeta 2007). Routines or rituals are thus related to the physical environment or to people. Such routines help to switch from active life to sleep mode. We not only go to sleep because we are tired, but also become sleepy because we prepare for bedtime (cf. Schwartz 1973).

The reassurance that certain sleep behaviour is allowed or healthy can also improve sleep. Someone who has 'earned' rest after a productive work day is satisfied and likely to sleep well. When people frequently wake up during the night, a referral to the sleep laboratory can help, partly because they get advice on sleep routines, but often because they are simply reassured by the result of the electroencephalogram (EEG) that their sleep is – after all – not as bad as they had thought and that interrupted sleep is 'normal' (Jürgen Zulley, personal communication). The fear of not getting enough (or occasionally, of too much) sleep is a worry for many Americans. It is the doctors who now tell us how to sleep; they become 'moral entrepreneurs'. Their advice is based on scientific research, but their cultural environment also influences their views and their research questions. From a sociocultural perspective, there are differences in how to deal with sleep problems, and to consider certain sleep patterns as problematic or not is to a large extent a matter of cultural interpretation. For example, Japanese popular advice books on sleep, written by sleep researchers and physicians, emphasize environmental aspects, they take both co-sleeping and daytime sleep for granted, and see them in a much more positive light.

This leads to another issue. Social approval of certain sleep behaviour is not only necessary for nocturnal sleep, but more generally for sleep patterns, especially for daytime naps. Naps are subject to social rules, however tacit and sometimes difficult to obey those rules may be.

4.3. Timing sleep

If sound sleep is maintained by factors that vary across time and space, how is sleep actually organized in various societies? What influences different sleep patterns and how are they evaluated? I argue that socioeconomic, cultural, climatic and other environmental conditions have an influence, both on the amount of time and the way in which we sleep. Furthermore, sleep arrangements point to people's priorities and key values, not least about time use, work ethics and social behaviour. In principle, three different patterns can be found, which I categorize as the following 'sleep cultures'.

The first category is the *monophasic sleep culture* with a single sleep phase during the night, usually of about eight hours. Social constraints allow only marginal social groups (e.g. children or sick people) and those working in occupations requiring night shifts to sleep during the day. The second category is the *siesta culture*. Belonging to this group are societies in which biphasic sleep (two-phase sleep) comprises the principal sleep pattern, with a socially determined time period for both night and midday rest. Social life quiets down not only during the night, but also in the early afternoon. The third category is the *napping culture*, which is characterized by polyphasic sleep with individually selected, often irregular, sleep times during the day in addition to the regulated night-time sleep. Polyphasic naps can be subdivided into two varieties. First there are mono*chronic* naps that are clearly distinct from social life. These naps are a 'spate during which one is unavailable' to social life (Pugh 2000, p.261) and retreats to privacy. Second there are poly*chronic* naps, when people doze in the presence of other people who are awake and remain – at least in part – socially aware of what is going on and always prepared to engage with the social situation at hand if necessary.[4] Such naps are called *inemuri* in Japanese, literally 'the sleep taken whilst present in a situation that is not oriented around sleep', such as naps during a train ride or in business meetings.

It goes without saying that these are idealized types. In reality, there are people with different sleep patterns in every society simultaneously, and the Indian subcontinent is a prime example (cf. Brunt 2008). Moreover, individuals themselves may also change their sleep patterns depending on circumstances, maintaining monophasic sleep during the week and taking a nap at weekends. Although daytime sleep helps to combat afternoon fatigue, in biphasic and polyphasic sleep cultures it is not primarily compensation for lack of night rest, as is implicitly or explicitly assumed in most studies of sleep behaviour. These three types are, instead, merely different arrangements for consuming sleep. None is more 'normal' than the other. They have developed in and of their own right and all stand on equal footing with one another.

Monophasic sleep culture

Monophasic sleep seems so self-evident and natural to most westerners that it is often elevated to the *physiological* norm. Alexander Borbély, a Swiss pharmacologist and sleep scientist, explains how human development runs from polyphasic sleep in infancy through biphasic amongst children to monophasic sleep amongst adults (Borbély 1986). With reference to the siesta in the Mediterranean and in China, he qualifies his schema by adding that certain 'climatic conditions can… cause adults to maintain the biphasic sleep characteristic of preschool children' (Borbély 1986, p.35). By this, he seems to imply that Mediterranean countries and China are 'stuck' at an earlier stage of development, likening physiological development of humans with a country's socioeconomic development.

In European history, one can indeed detect a development from polyphasic to monophasic sleep patterns. Pictures and anecdotes indicate that in the Europe of centuries prior to the Industrial Revolution, public daytime sleep was common (cf. Gleichman 1980). However, daytime sleep was not completely unregulated and did not go unnoticed. In early German literature (written by and addressed to the nobility), for an exhausted knight to fall asleep outside in the fields would place him in danger, and such naps usually represented a highly dramatic point in medieval stories, when the fate of the hero was determined. At King Arthur's court it was considered extremely rude to sleep in the company of knights and ladies. When the legends describe someone dozing during a court dinner, it severely damaged his honour (Klug 2008). Similar rules were increasingly applied in Italy as well. As shown by Elias (1997), Giovanni della Casa's *Galateo* (1558), a treatise of manners and behaviour, listed various bad habits meant to be avoided: 'One should not fall asleep in the society of others'; 'One should not pull out letters and read them; one should not cut and clean the fingernails in public' (cited in Elias 1997, p.278). These guidelines allow us to conclude that disapproval of public sleep was by no means self-evident, but it was increasingly considered undesirable, at least amongst higher social classes.

In religious writings, sleep was considered 'a potentially sinful kind of sluggishness' (Klug 2008, p.37) and daytime sleep in particular was thought likely to deprive people of their chance for salvation. In later centuries and other places in the world, Christian preachers likewise warned their parish not to nod off during mass. They made their point with the story of the Agony of Christ in the garden of Gethsemane in the night before his crucifixion. Jesus severely scolded his disciples for twice falling asleep rather than praying so that they would not fall into temptation (Matthew 26:41). This was especially poignant because Peter did in fact fall into temptation, even denying his acquaintance with Jesus. Perhaps particularly concerned was the typical minister of colonial New England who feared sluggishness and the neglect of prayers on which the salvation of his parish and their soul depended (Cox 2008).[5]

At the same time, the literature offers numerous accounts of daytime naps that do not condemn the midday sleeper. Withdrawing to take an afternoon nap for people of higher rank appears to have been daily routine. The schedule for taking a nap at noon was prompted by personal duties. Members of the upper class had to attend to their business interests in the morning and to the many social events in the evening. A prominent napper in English literature was Hamlet's father who, in his Ghost speech, referred to his habit thus: 'Sleeping within my orchard, my custom always of the afternoon' (Hamlet, I. v. 59–60). Daytime sleep was not very regulated for the lower classes who were hardly at leisure to attend dinner parties and other social events, but as can be judged from visual sources as well as stories, in early modern Europe they would rarely hesitate to take an opportunity for a break and sleep, including in public (Gleichmann 1980).

This situation gradually changed with industrialization. Monophasic sleep patterns are best suited to match industrial work structures as machines must be used continuously in order to utilize them efficiently, and work is strictly measured and remunerated by the hour. Work that is in unison with machines must be oriented to fixed schedules. The lazy, inactive body was defined as a threat to this early capitalist culture, and 'sleeping on the job' was strictly prohibited (cf. Thompson 1967). Taylorism[6] added further pressure to adjust sleep. Over the course of the proletarianization of the rural population and the accompanying pressure to conform to industrial work processes, they had less opportunity for individual napping. Office work gradually followed such industrial work patterns. Moreover, with increasing urbanization, commuting times to the workplace increased. Most workers (whatever colour their collar) no longer had the possibility of going home for lunch to rest, fearing that to lose any time at midday would extend the work day into the evening. During the twentieth century, the midday break has been nominally reduced to 30 minutes in many offices all over Europe and the USA, even in administrative bodies. This allows for free time after work but not for a nap during the working day. Moreover, public sleep declined ever more amongst the petit bourgeoisie as they aspired to the habits of the upper classes and refrained from sleeping in public.

Nevertheless, as I discuss in more detail below, even in societies where it is widely accepted that the normal sleep rhythm for adults is monophasic, people still withdraw to rest, particularly after lunch and at weekends. Even though many medical doctors declare it the norm, not everyone sticks to the monophasic sleep pattern all the time.

Siesta culture

Siesta cultures are marked by biphasic sleep. In addition to night rest, there is also a socially institutionalized midday rest period. The word *siesta* comes from Latin *sexta hora*, the sixth hour, which identifies the middle of the day (Paquot 2000). Siesta cultures can be found all over the world. Webb and Dinges draw the general conclusion that more agriculturally organized, settled ethnic groups tend to regulate the times for daytime sleep (i.e. siesta), whereas nomads nap at irregular times (Webb and Dinges 1989), often adjusting to the needs of their animals during travels. Sometimes they walk for days with hardly any sleep. Yet when they reach an oasis, they sleep for very long stretches of time. Despite an inner clock that regulates sleep rhythms and regardless of climatic influences, people are flexible and adjust their sleep to the demands of work organization or social obligations.

On the other hand, there is no mandatory link between specific work structures and certain sleep patterns. A comparison also shows that people react differently to the same kinds of socioeconomic pressures and developments, like industrialization and globalization. Recent data from the Harmonised European Time Use Survey (HETUS) indicate a relationship between the midday nap and the midday meal. In Spain, Italy, France and Bulgaria, people take time to sit down for lunch, and consequently, with the exception of France, an afternoon nap is more prevalent, although by no means ubiquitous. Compared to this, for countries like Finland, Germany and Latvia, the data hardly show any significant concentration of workers taking extended lunch breaks, and there is no concentration of nap taking either. Yet at any one time during the day, at least 5 per cent of the adult population (aged between 20 and 78) are asleep. This is not the case in the south, where fewer people than that are asleep before lunch or in the later afternoon.[7] It is unclear how many of those sleepers are shift workers and how many are nappers. Further investigation is necessary to analyse the meaning of these statistical relationships, but my hypothesis is that the siesta is not mainly a result of the heat or sleep-inducing heavy meals nor of work content. Instead, both ideas – having a proper meal and a rest period in the middle of the day – are connected to a similar understanding of how one should live a proper life.

In regions further from the equator, midday naps are more widespread in summer than in the colder seasons, not only because of the warmer temperatures, but also because of the relatively shorter nights, as is also the case in Mongolia. However, in Inner Mongolia there are people who keep a midday nap, whereas others reject this as a Chinese tradition (Konagaya 2001), indicating that political motives are also involved in the decision of whether or not to sleep during the day. And indeed, the question of taking a midday nap has long been a political one in China itself. In the 1950 constitution, Mao Zedong established 'the right of the workers to rest' (*xiuxi*), and thereby institutionalized the centuries-old custom of the midday nap (*wushui*) that the literati of the Song period (960–1279) had already celebrated in their verses (Li 2003).

With increasing globalization and the expansion of urban centres, the siesta is being increasingly questioned, even in Spain. In part, this is due to socioeconomic changes: increasing commuting times, couples who both work, air conditioners (keeping the air temperature cooler), the necessity to communicate with other European Union (EU) countries, and people wanting more quality time at home in the evening. However, ideology also plays a role. The siesta has an image of being a relic of a somewhat backward society of idle sleepy villages (cf. Steger and Brunt 2003).

There are similar developments and attitudes in China. After the death of Mao, and with an increasing orientation towards American ideas of modernization and business, the long midday break has come under question. A translated article by American journalist Linda Mathews in 1980 hit a raw nerve and was widely discussed, stirring great controversy. The article claimed that the communist system, symbolized by the midday sleep, was the reason for China's economic backwardness. America, on the contrary, used its technology 24 hours a day, and was therefore efficient, economically successful, and well-off. Consequently more and more Chinese – mainly those who had international business relations – became accustomed to conducting business without taking a proper break. In 1984, the government announced an official change of work hours – the midday break was reduced to an hour. However, after the massacres at Tiananmen Square in 1989, and the critical international reaction, anti-American sentiments rose and the contempt towards the afternoon nap was increasingly questioned although the long break was never reinstated. In later years ideological considerations have been put aside, and the issue of the midday break has increasingly become a personal and medical affair – people now nap at any time when they find an opportunity, but at least in the cities they no longer have a common break. It seems that most people are willing to sacrifice sleep if they are able to earn some extra cash (Li 2003).

In Taiwan there is no official siesta but, from primary school onwards, teachers ask the entire class to nap at their desks for about 15 minutes after lunch. In practically all offices the lights are switched off for a time after the midday meal. Employees lay their heads down on their desks and take a short nap. The doors remain open, but potential visitors know that they should not disturb anyone at this time. Such napping might be an economized and reduced form of the institutionalized siesta, but it is still a collective period of sleep and must be distinguished from individual forms of napping.

Napping culture

The third form of sleep organization, to take a nap during the day whenever one wants and has a chance to, is found throughout the world, just like siesta cultures. As indicated before, napping cultures are often associated with pre-industrial societies and countries of the south. However, in Japan napping can also be observed, especially in family restaurants, coffee shops and internet-manga cafés (where customers can surf the web or read *manga* – comic books or print cartoons). Another popular option is on trains, where many consider it an efficient way to use their commuting time. Besides, closing one's eyes in public transport also protects against the prying eyes of fellow train passengers and thus creates some private space in the midst of a crowd. In schools and offices, lectures and meetings provide a regular opportunity for naps or *inemuri*.[8] Although physiologically sleep, sociologically speaking, *inemuri* is not sleep. It should be compared to daydreaming and follows similar rules of engagement (cf. Steger 2003, 2006). *Inemuri* is a polychronic form of napping. Shoes and clothes are not generally taken off, the places chosen for napping are not marked as sleeping places and the body posture of the sleeper hardly differs from those around who are not asleep. The frequent occurrence of napping is explained by the busy lifestyle in contemporary Japan, but *inemuri* has been common throughout history, regardless of lifestyle and social class.

Irregular napping is also a much more common phenomenon in the so-called western world than is publicly acknowledged. Around 2000 a boom in 'power napping', a term coined by David Dinges,[9] was emerging in the USA. This was closely linked to the development of sleep science. Consulting firms translated knowledge on sleep and chronobiology into 'opportunities to enhance safety and performance in our 24/7 global society',[10] and more companies are now willing to allow their employees a power nap. Workplace naps in North America, however, are controlled and partially regulated. They are a monochronic event and normally take place either in a room set aside for this particular function or perhaps in an unused meeting room. The goal of this strategic nap is to avoid a drop in work quality and to prevent an increase in accidents caused by fatigue and as such, might be seen as a further development of the Taylor model to organize work time in a more efficient way, even if Taylor's early followers would have been horrified to hear about napping on the job. This strategic nap as a management method has arisen parallel to a change in work organization conditioned by globalization, 24-hour businesses, technological changes and the dominance of information technologies (IT) and other service sectors that support industrial production. These changes demand increasing worker flexibility. For example, management expects that, if necessary, employees work late into the night and at weekends. Meanwhile, freelancers, who must organize their own work hours, simply have to ensure that contracts are completed on time regardless of how long it takes; they are therefore free to take a break and a short nap to overcome their fatigue if their deadline allows.

The American public has been enthusiastic in their reception of arguments in favour of napping. And the message of the benefits of napping has rapidly crossed the Atlantic and the Pacific, with more and more workplaces equipped with sofas, allowing a short rest to cope with the hectic pace of work. Research has been booming ever since, and in popular publications all over the world people are increasingly advised to take a short nap during the day (cf. Brunt and Steger 2008). Japan has caught up with this trend. Many self-help books with titles such as *The Short-sleep Method that Makes You Smart* (Matsubara 1993) suggest shortening nocturnal sleep and introducing short sleep periods during the day whenever possible or necessary. In reality, many have always followed this pattern by doing *inemuri*, even if they had not recognized it as a sleep method.

Although there is a high degree of tolerance towards napping in many societies, it is always subject to social rules. These rules, however, are not uniform, and are sometimes difficult to obey, even for those raised in that culture. There are situations, like train journeys, where napping is perfectly acceptable in most countries. However, taking a nap in school classes would provoke different reactions depending on the country and age grade. An Indian or British pupil is likely to be scolded or even punished, whereas the likely reaction of a Japanese school teacher would be to pity the exhausted student who would be assumed to have worked hard the previous night. *Inemuri* during work meetings would hardly be acceptable in most countries, but in Japan, it depends very much on the social rank of the sleeper. Established employees often take naps; their presence at the meeting is important, but young people who want to climb the career ladder must show more active engagement in the discussion (cf. Brunt and Steger 2008, pp.18–21).

4.4. Conclusion
Sleepers are vulnerable to physical, emotional and social predicaments. The kind of fears people connect with sleep reveal some of their most central concerns and key values, be it the fear of perdition of their soul

or the loss of property, be it concerns with their work or with family and love relationships. The worry of getting enough healthy sleep has spread more recently, starting in North America, spreading to Europe and East Asia, because medical sleep researchers have now emphasized the importance of sleep and started to prescribe or suggest specific sleep hygiene measures.

Around the globe, people have found different ways to ensure a good night's sleep. They have built secure housing and surrounded themselves with familiar items; they take care of each other by co-sleeping or keeping in contact by telephone and the internet. Bedtime routines give insights into the cultural and social significance of sleep arrangements. Whilst Europeans used to bring their day to a close by praying to God to grant good sleep, they now listen to medical advice when they have difficulties falling or remaining asleep – doctors have become the new moral authorities. People are, however, more receptive to some advice than other, depending on their own needs and values. The positive effects of midday napping have been particularly easy to popularize, and in some work environments, 'power napping' has become acceptable.

The trend in power napping suggests that polyphasic sleep (a napping culture) is not necessarily an early state of social development, as has often been suggested. Sociologists Baxter and Kroll-Smith (2005) argue in their study of daytime sleep in North and South America that, along with the transfer of industrial production to southern countries, the custom of the siesta has increasingly declined in these countries, whereas in North America, daytime sleep is moving toward ever more acceptance. Similarly, based on a study of mainland China, Hong Kong and Taiwan, historian Li (2006) suggests that modernization has a tendency of impacting and eroding the traditional practice of co-ordinated afternoon naps, or siesta. But as modernization continues, new socioeconomic factors are causing a reintroduction of daytime napping, albeit on an individual basis. There is a clear connection between a polyphasic sleep arrangement and post-industrial economic structures. There is, however, no imperative link between polyphasic sleep and post-industrial societies; it can often be found in pre-industrial societies as well, as can be seen in the Japanese case. But a monochronic understanding of time and manual labour, as can typically be found in modern industrial societies, favours a monochronic sleep pattern, whether there is one single sleep phase during the night (monophasic sleep) or two socially sanctioned sleep phases (biphasic sleep in siesta cultures). The variables of climate, work organization, the commute to work, and primarily cultural and ideological influences are important here. The new *strategic* naps in major American companies are built on a Taylorist work ethic, and are employed in a controlled manner to increase efficiency and effectiveness. Not all forms of polyphasic sleep are goal-oriented: often those who are tired simply use any available opportunity to sleep (cf. Richter 2003).

Sleep patterns are certainly influenced by practical questions of adaptation to socioeconomic conditions. Yet work organization is not only a question of industrial needs. Ideology is also important and includes the question of how 'work ethics' are defined, whether, for instance, efficiency is a virtue and how it is to be achieved; how commitment to work is evaluated; what is considered to be proper behaviour in public; how important care for body and health is; and even what is considered good health. The overview of worldwide sleep patterns also shows that human bodies are capable of adjusting to a variety of sleep patterns.

This chapter was completed in August 2010.

Notes

1. From a poster displayed at the exhibition 'Schlaf und Traum' ('Sleeping and Dreaming') at the Deutsche Hygienemuseum, Dresden, Germany, 2007.
2. The term 'co-sleeping' is used in different ways, but generally refers to a parent (usually the mother) and child sharing a sleeping room, usually in close proximity, and sometimes also the sharing of a bed.
3. For more information on children's sleep habits around the world see, for example, Owens (2004) and Gianotti and Cortesi (2009).
4. Historian A. Roger Ekirch (2001) has described another form of polyphasic sleep. What he aptly calls 'segmented sleep' is not, however, the equivalent of my term 'polyphasic sleep', but is rather a 'segmented nocturnal sleep'.
5. A connection to Protestant work ethics is recognizable. However, demands to control one's sleep were and are known in most religions, including Islam, Buddhism and Hinduism.
6. In *The Principles of Scientific Management* (1911) Frederick Taylor devised a means of detailing a division of labour in time-and-motion studies and a wage system based on performance. His teachings became the basis for scientific management known as Taylorism. The central aim was to make use of employees' work time as efficiently as possible.

7.   Data from studies in 2007 and 2007–2008 of the Harmonised European time use surveys (HETUS) available at: www.h2.scb.se/tus/tus/AreaGraphCID.html, accessed on 31 May 2012.

8.   The Japanese noun *inemuri* literally means: sleeping while being present; it refers to napping in public transportation, at meetings, during classes and lectures.

9.   See: www.med.upenn.edu/uep/faculty_dinges.html, accessed on 1 February 2011.

10. See: www.alertsol.com/qry/page.taf?id=15, accessed on 30 March 2012.

References

Aubert, V. and White, H. (1959) 'Sleep: a sociological interpretation I.' *Acta Sociologica 4*, 2, 46–54.

Baxter, V. and Kroll-Smith, S. (2005) 'Normalizing the workplace nap: blurring the boundaries between public and private space and time.' *Current Sociology 53*, 1, 33–55.

Ben-Ari, E. (2008) '"It's Bedtime" in the World's Urban Middle Classes: Children, Families and Sleep.' In L. Brunt and B. Steger (eds) *Worlds of Sleep*. Berlin: Frank & Timme.

Borbély, A. (1986) *Secrets of Sleep*. New York, NY: Basic Publications.

Brunt, L. (2008) '*Sote hue log*: In and Out of Sleep in India.' In L. Brunt and B. Steger (eds) *Worlds of Sleep*. Berlin: Frank & Timme.

Brunt, L. and Steger, B. (2008) 'Introduction.' In L. Brunt and B. Steger (eds) *Worlds of Sleep*. Berlin: Frank & Timme.

Cox, R. (2008) 'The Suburbs of Eternity: On Visionaries and Miraculous Sleepers.' In L. Brunt and B. Steger (eds) *Worlds of Sleep*. Berlin: Frank & Timme.

Crook, T. (2008) 'Norms, forms and beds: spatializing sleep in Victorian Britain.' *Body & Society 14*, 4, 15–35.

Douglas, P. (2001) 'The evolution of the Glasgow tenement.' *Dennistoun Online*. Available at www.dennistoun.co.uk/Page.asp?Title=Digest&Section=22&Page=4, accessed on 29 July 2010.

Ekirch, A.R. (2001) 'Sleep we have lost: pre-industrial slumber in the British Isles.' *American Historical Review 106*, 2, 343–385.

Elias, N. (1997) *Über den Prozeß der Zivilisation. Soziogenetische und psychogenetische Untersuchungen. Vol. 1: Wandlungen des Verhaltens in den weltlichen Oberschichten des Abendlandes*. Frankfurt am Main: Suhrkamp. (Original work published in 1936.)

Gianotti, F. and Cortesi, F. (2009) 'Family and cultural influences on sleep development.' *Child and Adolescent Psychiatric Clinics of North America 18*, 4, 849–861.

Gleichmann, P. (1980) 'Einige soziale Wandlungen des Schlafens.' *Zeitschrift für Soziologie 9*, 3, 236–250.

Hooker, E., Ball, H. and Kelly, P. (2001) 'Sleeping like a baby: attitudes and experiences in northeast England.' *Medical Anthropology 19*, 3, 203–222.

Kaji, M. and Shigeta, M. (2007) 'Knick-knacks for sleeping (*nemuri-komono*) in contemporary Japan.' Unpublished manuscript for the workshop 'New Directions in the Social and Cultural Study of Sleep', University of Vienna, 7–9 June.

Klug, G. (2008) 'Dangerous Doze: Sleep and Vulnerability in Medieval German Literature.' In L. Brunt and B. Steger (eds) *Worlds of Sleep*. Berlin: Frank & Timme.

Konagaya, Y. (2001) 'Mongoru yūboku sekai ni okeru suimin jikū' ['Time and Space to Sleep in the World of the Mongol Nomads']. In S. Yoshida (ed.) *Suimin bunka-ron [Treatise on Sleep Culture]*. Tōkyō: Heibonsha.

Li, Y. (2003) 'Discourse of Mid-day Napping. A Political Windsock in Contemporary China.' In B. Steger and L. Brunt (eds) *Night-Time and Sleep in Asia and the West: Exploring the Dark Side of Life*. London: RoutledgeCurzon.

Li, Y. (2006) 'To nap or not to nap: traditional *wushui* practice in the modernizing and modernized Chinese worlds: reflections of its public discourses.' Unpublished manuscript. Conference of the European Sleep Research Society, Innsbruck, 6 September.

Matsubara, E. (1993) *Atama o yoku suru tanmin-hō* [*The Short-sleep Method that Makes You Smart*]. Tōkyō: Mikage Shobō.

Maver, I. (2003) "'The Mirk Shades o' Nicht." Nocturnal Representations of Urban Scotland in the Nineteenth Century.' In B. Steger and L. Brunt (eds) *Night-Time and Sleep in Asia and the West: Exploring the Dark Side of Life*. London: RoutledgeCurzon.

Montijn, I. (2008) 'Beds Visible and Invisible: Hygiene, Morals and Status in Dutch Bedrooms.' In L. Brunt and B. Steger (eds) *Worlds of Sleep*. Berlin: Frank & Timme.

Owens, J. (2004) 'Sleep in children: cross-cultural perspectives.' *Sleep and Biological Rhythms 2*, 3, 165–173.

Paquot, T. (2000) *Siesta: Die Kunst des Mittagsschlafes*. Köln: vgs.

Pugh, A. (2000) 'Sleep in a Sleepless Age. A Sociology of Sleep, Work, and Family.' In E. Balka and R.K. Smith (eds) *Women, Work, and Computerization: Charting a Course to the Future*. Boston, MA: Kluwer Academic Publishers.

Rensen, P. (2003) 'Sleep Without a Home. The Embedment of Sleep in the Lives of the Roughsleeping Homeless in Amsterdam.' In B. Steger and L. Brunt (eds) *Night-Time and Sleep in Asia and the West: Exploring the Dark Side of Life*. London: RoutledgeCurzon.

Richter, A. (2003) 'Sleeping Time in Early Chinese Literature'. In B. Steger and L. Brunt (eds) *Night-Time and Sleep in Asia and the West: Exploring the Dark Side of Life*. London: RoutledgeCurzon.

Schimek, M. (1997) 'Im Interesse der Förderung der Volksgesundheit…: Staatliche Maßnahmen zur Abschaffung von Alkoven in Nordwestdeutschland, dargestellt anhand des Freistaates Oldenburg.' In N. Hennig and H. Mehl (eds) *Bettgeschichte(n). Zur Kulturgeschichte des Bettes und des Schlafens*. Schleswig: Volkskundliche Sammlungen des Schleswig-Holsteinischen Landesmuseums, 215–234.

Schwartz, B. (1973) 'Notes on the Sociology of Sleep.' In A. Birenbaum and E. Sangrin (eds) *People in Places. The Sociology of the Familiar*. London: Nelson.

Selby, J. (1999) *Secrets of a Good Night's Sleep. Natural, Pleasurable Techniques Designed to Help Cure Insomnia*. New York, NY: Excel.

Shweder, R. (with Balle-Jensen, L. and Goldstein, W.) (2003) 'Who Sleeps by Whom Revisited.' In R. Shweder, *Why Do Men Barbecue? Recipes for Cultural Psychology*. Cambridge, MA and London: Harvard University Press.

Spock, B. and Rothenberg, M. (1992) *Supokku hakase no akachan to kodomo no ikuji (Dr. Spock's Baby and Child Care)*. Tōkyō: Kurashi no techō-sha. (Originally published in 1945.)

Steger, B. (2003) 'Getting away with sleep – social and cultural aspects of dozing in parliament.' *Social Science Japan Journal 6*, 2, 181–197.

Steger, B. (2004) *(Keine) Zeit zum Schlafen? Sozialhistorische und kulturanthropologische Erkundungen japanischer Schlafgewohnheiten*. Münster: LIT Verlag.

Steger, B. (2006) 'Sleeping through class to success: Japanese notions of time and diligence.' *Time & Society 15*, 2–3, 197–214.

Steger, B. and Brunt, L. (2003) 'Introduction: Into the Night and the World of Sleep.' In B. Steger and L. Brunt (eds) *Night-Time and Sleep in Asia and the West: Exploring the Dark Side of Life*. London: RoutledgeCurzon.

Taylor, F.W. (1911) *The Principles of Scientific Management*. New York, NY: Harper & Brothers.

Thompson, E.P. (1967) 'Time, work-discipline and industrial capitalism.' *Past and Present 38*, 1, 56–97.

Tsuneyoshi, R. and Boocock, S.S. (1997) *Ikuji no kokusai hikaku. Kodomo shakai to oyatachi* [*International Comparison of Child Rearing. The World of Children and their Parents*]. Tōkyō: NHK Books.

Venn, S. and Arber, S. (2008) 'Conflicting Sleep Demands: Parents and Young People in UK Households.' In L. Brunt and B. Steger (eds) *Worlds of Sleep*. Berlin: Frank & Timme.

Vogler, P. (2008) 'Sleeping as a Refuge? Embodied Vulnerability and Corporeal Security during Refugees' Sleep at the Thai-Burma Border.' In L. Brunt and B. Steger (eds) *Worlds of Sleep*. Berlin: Frank & Timme.

Webb, W. and Dinges, D. (1989) 'Cultural Perspectives on Napping and the Siesta.' In D. Dinges and R. Broughton (eds) *Sleep and Alertness. Chronobiological, Behavioral and Medical Aspects of Napping*. New York, NY: Raven Press.

5

Medical Anthropology and Children's Sleep

THE MISMATCH BETWEEN WESTERN LIFESTYLES AND SLEEP PHYSIOLOGY

Caroline H.D. Jones[1] and Helen L. Ball

5.1. Introduction

As a fundamental biological process, sleep is shared by every human on the planet, yet sleep patterns vary dramatically – both cross-culturally and through the life course – and are likely to have been fluid during evolutionary history. The importance of sleep is revealed in the numerous adverse consequences of insufficient or problematic sleep. However, the biological necessity of achieving sufficient sleep conflicts with twenty-first century western lifestyles, which promote a '24/7' culture in which sleep is perceived as a hindrance, something to be minimized in favour of other pursuits perceived as more worthwhile or entertaining.

As described elsewhere in this book, sleep is influenced by a complex array of biological and sociocultural factors, which interact to determine the patterning and amount of sleep of individuals and populations. Medical anthropology considers how social and cultural issues interact with biological factors to influence health and well-being, and how ill health is determined and experienced. With regard to sleep, it takes an evolutionary and cross-cultural approach to understanding sleep behaviour and sleep-related ill health. In this chapter, then, culturally determined expectations and behaviours regarding sleep (particularly infant and child sleep) are considered in the context of evolution.

The contemporary patterning, amount and functions of human sleep have been shaped biologically over two million years of evolutionary history. Consequently, human biological make-up reflects long-term adaptation to a very different way of life from that experienced in contemporary industrialized societies. As with many aspects of human biology, our post-space-age lifestyles push our stone-age bodies to the limits of physiological expectations and beyond, as we attempt to mould our sleep behaviours to fit historically novel expectations of how, when and where we should sleep. The relationship between human biological adaptation and environments experienced today (under the umbrella of 'evolutionary medicine') has been the focus of research into nutrition, activity and chronic modern-day health problems (see Trevathan, Smith and McKenna 2008). By comparison, the evolutionary context of sleep has received little attention, but investigating how sleep in contemporary western societies differs from that anticipated by evolved human biology can enhance our understanding of current sleep patterns, experience of sleep disorders and sleep-related ill health. Throughout this chapter our focus is on this discrepancy between the evolved biology and contemporary experience of sleep in post-industrial western societies, with a particular emphasis on children.

After presenting an overview of the evolutionary context of human sleep, we draw on research conducted at Durham University's Anthropology Sleep Laboratory. First, expectations for infant sleep and night-time care are examined; expectations for preschool children's sleep, and the influence of parents' attitudes and practices, are then explored; finally, the view that cultural discordance with sleep biology creates perceived sleep disorders is discussed.

5.2. The evolutionary context of sleep

Drawing on knowledge of sleep biology, and on observations in non-industrialized societies today, a picture has been compiled of the likely sleep practices of our remote ancestors – and it is very different from what we see in modern western society. Wehr and colleagues (1993) conducted a landmark study, exposing 15 volunteers to daily 14-hour 'night' periods of darkness. By the end of the month-long study, participants slept on average for eight hours per night, in two distinct periods separated by a period of wakefulness. The authors concluded that this segmented sleep was representative of ancestral human sleeping patterns. This was supported by a sociohistorical examination of sleep in England by Ekirch (2001), who posited that until the close of the early modern era, western European sleep was characterized by two distinct periods of sleep, either side of an hour or more of quiet wakefulness. He further proposed that in pre-industrial England, sleep onset occurred at dusk, and lasted until dawn (though this long period of sleep opportunity was vulnerable to intermittent disruption due to threat, discomfort and illness).

In contemporary non-industrialized societies, regular periods of darkness and daily cycles of activity provide regular and predictable night-time sleep periods, and sleep patterns during daylight periods are fluid and unbounded. Sleep occurs when needed and opportunistically; people are able to drift in and out of sleep throughout the day as well as at night, and are unlikely to experience restriction of sleep time (Worthman and Melby 2002). In non-western societies, and in our own societies in the recent historical past, sleep typically unfolds in shared spaces that feature constant background noise emanating from other sleepers, various domestic animals, fires maintained for warmth and protection from predators, and other people's night-time activities (Bower 1999). Adult sleepers in traditional societies recline on skins, mats, wooden platforms, the ground, or just about anything except a thick, springy mattress. Pillows or head supports are rare, and people doze in whatever they happen to be wearing. Individuals tend to slip in and out of slumber several times during the night (Worthman 2008).

By contrast, in modern industrial and post-industrial societies, technological advances, beginning with long-lasting artificial light, have gradually eroded the night-time period, and with it, sleep opportunity (Ekirch 2005). Highly scheduled and organized daytime periods, aided by mechanized devices for waking as well as artificial light, have led to maximization of active time and restriction of sleep time (indeed, in adults, too little time for sleep is a self-reported cause of insufficient sleep – see Broman, Lundh and Hetta 1996). Society demands conformity with standardized schedules and expects people to be available and functional at specific times of the day. All-night entertainment such as television has also contributed to restriction of night-time sleep. As noted in Chapter 4, in some countries, the acceptability of daytime napping in all sectors has been diminished by governmental legal decree, which demonstrates the restriction of daytime sleep opportunity as a consequence of globalization and '24/7' economies (Jenni and O'Connor 2005).

Ancestral sleep patterns have therefore been overridden by artificial light and pressures for productivity in contemporary industrialized societies (Wehr *et al.* 1993). Sleep patterns are no longer fluid and unbounded – instead, sleep is restricted to pre-defined, culturally appropriate periods, which are regulated and limited by scheduling constraints (Worthman and Melby 2002). Today, a western perception of 'good' sleep is independent sleep, in a dark, quiet location, in a consolidated night-time bout, with rapid sleep onset at the start of the sleep period, and minimized wakings during the night. As the remainder of this chapter will illustrate, these expectations are not biologically based, and attempting to force conformity to these expectations may result in negative consequences for the well-being of babies, children and adults.

5.3. How and where babies 'should' sleep

Infant sleep is a good example of how biological and cultural expectations have become mismatched. Sleep is a developmental process, and our needs for sleep change throughout the lifetime. Babies' sleep patterns mature over the first few years of life, and the sleep architecture* of newborns is very different from that of adults. Newborns sleep for most of the day, but only for two to three hours at a time. During the first year, overall sleep duration falls, and the majority of sleep becomes consolidated during night-time as circadian rhythms develop (Parmelee, Wenner and Schulz 1964).

The sleep cycle* of newborns is shorter than the adult sleep cycle. Adults typically drop quickly into non-rapid eye movement (NREM) at sleep onset, and the initial sleep cycles mostly comprise deep sleep with little REM sleep. As the night progresses, REM sleep begins to take over, with most REM sleep occurring towards the morning. The adult pattern of 15–20 per cent of sleep time consisting of REM sleep is not achieved until puberty (Peireno, Algarin and Uauy 2003).

Babies' brains grow rapidly throughout the first year of life, and the process of forming neural connections happens during sleep. REM sleep dominates newborn infant sleep cycles, although since babies do not move their eyes in sleep for a few months it is not known as REM sleep, but as 'active' sleep. From birth to three months most of a baby's sleep time is made up of active sleep, and when they fall asleep they spend 20 minutes or so in active sleep before dropping into NREM sleep. During active sleep babies wake easily whilst NREM sleep is often characterized as the 'floppy baby' stage of sleep when they can be easily moved without waking.

Babies, then, sleep very differently from their parents: they sleep throughout the day and night yet they do not sleep the whole night; they fall asleep differently, have shorter sleep cycles and experience much more active sleep. However, parents in clock-driven cultures, with rigid work schedules, are often poorly informed about, and ill-prepared to cope with, normal infant sleep habits. As a consequence this situation makes parents susceptible to claims about infant sleep training that promise them an infant who sleeps 'through the night' from an extremely early age. Sadly, such 'training' encourages parents to employ techniques that do not take an infant's developmental trajectory into consideration. Whilst one can train a young infant to remain quiet at night for long periods, and even to sleep for extended periods with strictly scheduled feeds and routines, the biological consequences of doing so are rarely considered. This approach unfortunately prioritizes parental social needs above infant developmental and biological needs.

Settling is the term used to describe the phase when a baby begins to fall quickly into deep sleep, and to stay asleep for prolonged periods of time (typically from 12 a.m. to 5 a.m.). Encouragement of early settling has only been considered a desirable parenting goal for the past 50 years. In the late 1950s sleep researchers reported that 70 per cent of the 160 babies they studied began settling by three months of age (Moore and Ucko 1957). The three-month goal became enshrined in paediatric textbooks and has, in the minds of Anglo-American parents and health professionals, come to represent the age at which babies 'should' be sleeping through the night. In the UK infant night waking is one of the most common reasons for parents consulting a health professional (Polnay *et al.* 1999). However, these 'milestones' for infant sleep were established under particular historical and cultural conditions that influenced infant care and sleep behaviour, as discussed below (Ball and Klingaman 2008).

Settling, like many aspects of infant development, cannot be isolated from other aspects of infant care. It is now clear that not only do all infants begin to settle at different ages, but that there are big differences in settling behaviour between breastfed infants and those who are fed cow's milk formula. Unfortunately, much paediatric and popular knowledge about babies' sleep maturation and regulation is based upon studies of formula-fed infants sleeping in isolation. Several research studies have now shown that breastfeeding is associated with a later onset of sleeping through the night, and with more frequent night waking, indicating that the 'established norms' for infant sleep do not apply to infants who are fed in the physiologically normal way, that is, breastfed (Elias *et al.* 1986). In fact, in societies where all babies are breastfed, 'settling' is an unknown concept and infant night waking is expected throughout the first year of life and beyond (Ball 2006).

Western parents often desire that their babies' sleep habits should match their own as early as possible. Because of the physiological characteristics of breastfed infants to wake and feed frequently throughout day and night, the desire for unbroken parental sleep is an impediment to breastfeeding in western societies; various studies report parents expressing their need for a satisfied baby that 'slept through the night' and did not feed too frequently (e.g. Marchand and Morrow 1994; Pinilla and Birch 1993). Parents often seem unprepared to discover that breastfed infants need to feed frequently during the night, and sometimes interpret this as a failure of breast milk to satisfy the baby – leading to early weaning, which can lead to a variety of negative health consequences during infancy, childhood and later life (e.g. infections, allergies, obesity); see Smith and Harvey (2010) for an overview of the consequences of premature weaning. Recent research has found that although breastfed infants may wake and feed more frequently in the night than artificially fed babies, the parents of breastfed infants obtain *greater* overall sleep duration (Doan *et al.* 2007; Montgomery-Downs, Clawges and Santy 2010). There is therefore a strong argument that the negative perceptions of breastfeeding and infant sleep need to be acknowledged and addressed.

Breastfed babies do wake and feed more frequently at night than those fed artificial formula, and this is the physiological norm for human infants. Babies generally double their birth weight by about six months of age, and grow their brains very rapidly, both of which require a large intake of calories. Newborns, however, have tiny stomachs (the size of a cherry, growing to the size of a ping-pong ball over the first week or so). Night feeding allows the baby to obtain sufficient nutrition (up to one third of daily calories), and as human milk is high in sugar, it provides easily mobilized calories for brain growth, but it is digested in about 90 minutes. Babies therefore feel hungry again after two or three hours. Experienced breastfeeding mothers are aware that minimizing the disruption of night-time breastfeeding is important in sustaining the breastfeeding relationship over many months. One way to accomplish this is for the mother and baby to sleep together, allowing the infant easy access to the mother's breasts, and requiring minimal sleep disturbance for the mother when her baby needs to feed. Numerous research studies in the past decade have shown a very strong and clear relationship between breastfeeding and bed sharing (Ball and Klingaman 2008). The relationship is an obvious one – and many mothers report that they generally do not notice feeding their babies in the night. Observations of bed-sharing breastfeeding infants show that they feed more frequently, and for longer periods than breastfeeding infants who do not sleep next to their mothers. Nonetheless, routinely bed-sharing mothers obtain as much or more sleep as those who sleep apart from their breastfed babies. Women who discover the ease with which they can nurse at night when bed sharing report that they continue breastfeeding for much longer than they would otherwise have done (Ball 2002, 2003). Whilst around 50 per cent of UK babies have slept with their parents at some point by the age of three months, over 70 per cent of breastfed babies have done so, compared with a third of babies who are not breastfed (Ball 2003; Blair and Ball 2004).

In non-western societies (and even some western ones with high breastfeeding rates), mother–infant sleep contact is highly prevalent –

the Euro-American custom of separating babies from their mothers for sleep is considered at best neglectful, and many non-westerners consider it tantamount to child abuse (e.g. Morelli *et al.* 1992). Notions regarding the desirability of independent infant sleep habits are historically novel, becoming fashionable in the 1920s and 1930s when 'scientific baby care' manuals written by infant care experts began to replace maternal instincts and confidence. Evolutionary biology indicates that 'normal sleep' for human infants involves close proximity to the caregiver, frequent breastfeeding throughout the night, and development of a mature diurnal rhythm by 9–12 months of age. Recent historical trends in infant care have promoted solitary sleep for lengthy periods from an early age, and have characterized infants who do not fit this pattern as 'problematic'. However, this recent history of infant sleep in the post-industrial West reflects the desires of society to have infant sleep patterns conform to contemporary parental needs regarding working schedules, rather than to reflect infant development. Whether the practices of encouraging early entrainment of diurnal rhythms and 'self-soothing' have long-term biological consequences affecting sleep behaviour in child or adulthood remains to be researched.

5.4. Children's sleep and parental expectations

In order to consider whether the mismatch between parental expectations and infant sleep biology continues into childhood, an understanding of biologically optimal sleeping patterns for children is needed. However, whilst it is established that sleep need decreases from infancy across childhood (Iglowstein *et al.* 2003), determining the amount of sleep that children need at different ages is difficult. Indeed, there are no *definitive* optimal sleep amounts for children. Various studies have aimed to determine sleep amounts in representative population samples in order to elucidate the typical duration of sleep in children at different ages. However, although examining the sleep duration of a population may help to determine the typical sleep patterns of children, this does not necessarily indicate sleep need or whether these sleep amounts are optimal for health and development (Wiggs 2007). Perhaps children 'get by' on less than optimal sleep in order to conform to societal norms, or are able to extend sleep further than they need. Typical sleep durations in a population may not reflect biologically optimal or adequate sleep amounts, but rather cultural norms and expectations regarding sleep amounts. When considering health-related outcomes in relation to sleep duration in order to determine optimal sleep amounts, there is some suggestion that a large proportion of children do not obtain adequate or optimal sleep (Hart and Jelalian 2008). This is supported by the increase in sleep duration when children are given the opportunity at weekends, for example (see Snell, Adlam and Duncan 2007), and by the high prevalence of sleepiness; for example, Amschler and McKenzie (2005) reported that over 80 per cent of 199 school children felt sleepy on two or more days a week. A particular difficulty in establishing sleep need is the large individual difference in sleep amounts within age groups and populations; this indicates that sleep need is not uniform for the entire population of children of any given age group (see Iglowstein *et al.* 2003).

Further to variation in sleep within populations, children's sleep varies cross-culturally, including differences in patterning of sleep throughout the day as well as overall daily sleep duration. For example, Mindell *et al.* (2010) found that young children from birth to three years from predominantly Caucasian countries had significantly earlier bedtimes and longer sleep compared to those from predominantly Asian countries. Crosby, LeBourgeois and Harsh (2005) reported black American children to nap more frequently and have shorter night-time sleep compared to white American children: although sleep was patterned differently throughout the day, black and white children slept for similar amounts in a 24-hour period.

The concept that population-level sleep duration has decreased over recent decades across different age groups provides further problems for determining normative sleep amounts. The proportion of young Americans reporting less than seven hours of sleep per night rose from 15.6 per cent in 1960 to 37.1 per cent in 2002 (National Sleep Foundation 2002). Dollman *et al.* (2007) reported that Australian children aged 10–15 had a reduction in time in bed of 30 minutes between 1985 and 2004; and Iglowstein *et al.* (2003) reported that between 1974–78 and 1986–93, daily sleep duration in Swiss children aged between six months and 14 years decreased by 20–40 minutes. Inconsistencies in definitions and measurements of sleep prevent definitive conclusions, but the data suggest that daily sleep duration has been decreasing, and that longer sleep is closer to biological need.

Like infants' sleep, children's sleep is not only determined by biological requirements and developmental physiology, but also by social and cultural context and, in particular, parents' attitudes and behaviours. Short sleep is largely attributable to late bedtimes (Mindell *et al.* 2009; Olds *et al.* 2010). Iglowstein *et al.* (2003) proposed that more liberal parental attitudes towards their children's bedtimes are responsible for the decline in children's sleep duration over recent years. Indeed, changes in parents' lifestyles, attitudes and expectations regarding children's sleep have occurred over several decades in western society (see Stearns, Rowland and Giarnella 1996). In the nineteenth century, children's sleep was considered to be self-regulating, requiring no medical or parental attention. It was in the early twentieth century that concerns about the adequacy of children's sleep emerged. Children were claimed to need an increasing amount of sleep, parental responsibility for adequate children's sleep increased, and – coinciding with the growing cultural desirability for independence and self-control in children – an impulse developed to impose regular schedules to which children could adhere without parental presence (Jenni and O'Connor 2005).

Parents are able to exert a positive influence over their children's sleep duration by promoting sleep hygiene* behaviours, including regular sleep schedules, bedtime routines with appropriately early bedtimes and lack of television and caffeine in the evening. There is empirical data linking these sleep hygiene practices to longer children's sleep (Mindell *et al.* 2009), but studies indicate that many parents do not adopt these measures, and consequently many children have 'bad sleep hygiene' habits and short sleep. In a survey of 184 American parents of children aged three months to 12 years, 42 per cent of children did not have a consistent bedtime, 43 per cent had a bedtime later than 9 p.m., 76 per cent had a television in their bedroom and 20 per cent consumed caffeine daily (Owens and Jones 2011). Furthermore, 76 per cent of parents underestimated their children's sleep need compared to USA National Sleep Foundation recommendations. A similar survey with a sample of 253 American parents found that recommended sleep habits were clustered together: parents who employed one 'bad sleep hygiene' habit were also more likely to employ others, and their children were more likely to obtain insufficient sleep for their age (Owens, Jones and Nash 2011).

Sleep choices made by parents (e.g. bedtime practices and sleep location) are often governed by environmental factors such as household size and space and climatic conditions (Owens 2004). However, cultural norms are also important: sleep choices are entrenched in a set of childrearing behaviours that reflect parents' values of 'good parenting' (Wolf *et al.* 1996). In western societies regulation of sleep, and independent sleeping, reflect how sleep is closely tied to a moral framework which dictates that 'good' sleep for children is independent, consolidated sleep, and that this is an indication of 'good' parenting and 'good', well-regulated children. Parents are responsible for training their children to sleep independently, which they achieve by setting regular sleep schedules, with children sleeping in a room of their own with limited or no parental interaction through the night.[2] The moral attributes assigned to children's sleep regulation exert social pressure on parents, who must conform to these cultural norms in order to be 'good' parents (Jenni and O'Connor 2005).

Cross-cultural comparisons of parenting and children's sleep shed light on the interaction between parents' expectations and children's sleep. Parents' expectations and priorities for children's sleep vary dramatically, even amongst westernized societies. For example, Super *et al.* (1996) described how Dutch parenting is organized around 'the three Rs': *Rust, Regelmaat* and *Reinheid* – translated as rest, regularity and cleanliness – and is fundamentally different from American parenting. The authors hypothesized that these cultural differences were expressed in parents' daily caretaking behaviours, which may have developmental consequences for children – specifically sleep duration, which was longer for Dutch than for American children. In Germany, the expectations of parents for young children to initiate and maintain sleep without their presence reflect parental desires to raise children who are self-reliant (Valentin 2005). Alternatively, where regulation and independence are not prioritized, regular bedtimes and sleep routines are not prominent; for example, Italian children share in adults' activities and fall asleep in the evening when they are tired rather than at scheduled times, since participation in family events is prioritized over regulation of sleep (Ottaviano *et al.* 1996). Thus children's sleep patterns and their regulation respond to wider cultural values, including the value placed on independence and self-regulation, and idealized family structures and behaviours (Jenni and O'Connor 2005).

Led by Caroline Jones, the authors recently conducted a study of 108 three-year-old children and their parents in Stockton-on-Tees, North East England; they explored children's sleep patterns (through parental diary report over four days and five nights) and parents' attitudes and perceptions regarding their children's sleep (through semi-structured interviews). Variation existed in parents' expectations regarding what role – if any – they should play in regulating their children's sleep. Some parents promoted regular bedtimes and bedtime routines, whilst others allowed their children to fall asleep when and where they wanted. For example, 76 per cent of parents described setting regular bedtimes for their children, and 60 per cent maintained a bedtime routine, including reading to their children. In contrast, almost a quarter of parents did not set a regular bedtime, and 24 per cent of children were able to fall asleep on the sofa at night whenever they were tired. Importantly, parents' attitudes and behaviours were associated with children's sleep outcomes: children whose parents promoted regulation and routine had significantly longer sleep compared to those who were self-governing with regard to sleep, with no parental regulation (Jones 2011).

The impact of parents' decisions regarding scheduling and regulation of sleep was particularly marked for daytime napping. Napping generally was negatively perceived by parents, and was not thought of as a strategy that could be employed to lengthen sleep duration or ensure adequate sleep for their children. Only nine parents reported encouraging their children to nap, whereas 35 spontaneously commented that they tried to prevent their children from napping. A main reason for prevention was the perception that if they napped, children would not go to sleep until later at night. Parents described various methods to prevent their children from napping, including engaging them in other activities, and providing them with sweets. Routine napping was not evident in this sample. Rather, when napping did occur, it was mainly opportunistic and unscheduled, and occurred in non-typical sleep locations such as on the sofa or in the car (rather than the bed they sleep in at night). Although around half of the children had at least one daytime nap during the four-day diary period, these were mostly short and sporadic. This may explain the relatively short overall daily sleep duration in this sample. Although a third of parents tried to prevent naps in order to prioritize night-time sleep, longer night-time sleep was generally not achieved. Perhaps an increase in napping, either opportunistic when children wanted, or scheduled and routine, could help to lengthen sleep in this population.

Thus cultural expectations for children to be awake during the day and to have only consolidated night-time sleep influence sleep opportunity and their sleep duration. Yet the expectation that children should sleep only at night contrasts with an evolutionary model, and with cross-cultural comparisons of sleep habits of children around the world. Combined night-time sleep and daytime napping is more consistent with children's evolved sleep biology. In the absence of sufficient night-time sleep, in order to align children's sleep experiences with their biological needs, we may need to challenge cultural attitudes such as those found in the Stockton-on-Tees study, and allow children to sleep more opportunistically, when needed, including substantial daytime naps.

5.5. The construction of sleep problems

The previous sections have referred to sleep in general (non-sleep-disordered) populations, but cultural expectations are also responsible for the construction of problematic sleep and sleep disorders. Sleep behaviours, related to parental regulation and limit setting, which do not fit well with societal norms and expectations, are considered abnormal and are medicalized.* Accordingly, 'limit setting sleep disorder' and 'sleep onset association disorder' are listed in the *International Classification of Sleep Disorders* (American Academy of Sleep Medicine 2001; see also Thorpy 2011). Both of these childhood sleep disorders are said to stem from a lack of consistency and appropriate regulation by parents at bedtime and throughout the night.

In the case of limit setting sleep disorder, parents demonstrate difficulties in adequately enforcing bedtime limits, for example displaying inconsistent or inappropriate bedtimes, which results in delayed sleep onset and reduced sleep duration and quality (Mindell *et al.* 2006). Sleep onset association disorder involves children relying on unsuitable and unsustainable sleep onset associations such as parental presence to fall asleep at bedtime; when children are unable to recreate these sleep associations they are then unable to sleep, and require parental assistance. The concept of sleep requiring bedtime limits, and certain sleep onset associations being unsuitable, is socially constructed. Parents' behaviours define their child's disorder. The reason why certain behaviours have become medicalized is that in the current western milieu, with restricted socially accepted sleep periods, regulation and limit setting have become necessary components of parenting to ensure sufficient child sleep. This explains the findings in the Stockton-on-Tees sample (above): current western lifestyles do not permit children to sleep as and when they need, and so children whose parents were regulatory and routine-driven achieved longer sleep compared with those whose parents did not promote regulation and routines.

Around a quarter of parents believe that their child has a sleep problem – a consistently reported rate across cultures (Owens 2005) – and difficulty falling asleep is a particular cause of concern in western societies. As described above, in non-western populations, as through evolutionary history, sleep occurs in shared spaces, with constant background noise and stimulation, and individuals fall in and out of sleep fluidly. In post-industrial western homes, individuals who are accustomed to sleeping in still, silent spaces may not learn to ground their sleeping and waking cycles in a flow of sensations. In fact, being forced to bounce back and forth between the sensory overload of the waking world and the sensory barrenness of dark, quiet bedrooms may make it difficult to relax, switch off and fall asleep as desired (Bower 1999). An anthropological perspective would therefore suggest that what many people consider as sleep onset insomnia is in fact an artificial disorder, created by our expectations for rapid transition from wakefulness to sleep.

Insomnia is another largely culturally defined sleep problem. Because of cultural expectations for consolidated night-time sleep, deviations from this pattern are thought to be pathological. It comes as a surprise to many people to learn that we routinely wake in the night as part of natural sleep: physiologically, in fact, it is normal for humans to wake several times a night between sleep cycles, but only for a brief length of time (see Chapter 2). A period of wakefulness in the middle of the night is often thought to be indicative of insomnia by parents whose children experience this, and by adults experiencing such wakefulness themselves. This promotes anxiety, and, particularly for adults, use of medication. However, the notion that it is normal for humans to sleep for a single unbroken stretch is a historically recent phenomenon.

Surveys indicate a high prevalence of reported sleep problems in adults as well as children. For example, in a survey by Leger *et al.* (2000) involving 12,778 French adults, 73 per cent of respondents indicated that they had suffered a nocturnal sleep problem during the preceding month, including difficulties initiating sleep, and night awakenings. Such surveys have led to sleep problems being characterized as a 'silent epidemic of staggering proportions' – a quote attributed to the USA National Commission on Sleep Disorders Research by Jacobs, Benson and Friedman (1996). Recommendations are made to alleviate sleep problems by improving 'sleep hygiene' through behavioural measures. Some of these recommendations are based on eliminating factors that interfere with sleep physiology, including daytime energy drinks and coffee, computer and television-induced hyper-stimulation and artificial light exposure. These aspects of twenty-first century lifestyles disrupt circadian rhythms and override our evolved physiological response to *zeitgebers** (external cues that entrain biological rhythms). However, other recommended 'sleep hygiene' behaviours are not based on limiting the mismatch between physiological expectations versus experiences, and are, in fact, behavioural entrainment issues. For example, recommendations include sleeping in a quiet dark room, free from distractions. Electronics such as televisions, computers and mobile phones negatively impact sleep due to the bright light that they provide, and because they prevent the sleep environment from being associated with the expectation of sleep. However, background sounds are not necessarily biologically problematic: indeed, humans around the world sleep in noisy environments. Whilst light is a natural *zeitgeber*, noise and silence are not, and preferring silence for sleep is based in cultural expectations and norms rather than biological need.

5.6. Conclusion

This chapter has explored expectations and perceptions of 'normal' or desired sleep patterns in contemporary western society, with a focus on infants and children. Parents routinely expect children to sleep in a consolidated night-time bout, from an early age, with rapid sleep onset and without night awakenings, in a dark, quiet, independent space. Indeed, independent sleep from an early age, in regular consolidated night-time bouts, is a sign of 'good' sleep, 'good' children, and 'good' parenting. However, whilst our cultural norms and expectations have changed rapidly in evolutionary terms, sleep biology has not. The mismatch between cultural expectations and human sleep physiology contributes to many problematic issues regarding sleep; these include infants sleeping independently and the impact on breastfeeding; children being unable to sleep opportunistically, which may impact on their daily sleep duration and the construction of sleep problems such as insomnia. We need to challenge cultural attitudes and expectations about sleep that are not biologically based, and return to a concept of 'normal' sleep that is in keeping with sleep biology.

Notes

1. Caroline H.D. Jones completed this chapter while she was at the Parent–Infant Sleep Lab, Department of Anthropology, Durham University.
2. Worthman, speaking at a presentation at the Congress of the International Pediatric Sleep Association in Rome on 5 December 2010.

References

American Academy of Sleep Medicine (2001) *The International Classification of Sleep Disorders, Revised: Diagnostic and Coding Manual*. Available at www.esst.org/adds/ICSD.pdf, accessed on 9 August 2011.

Amschler, D.H. and McKenzie, J.F. (2005) 'Elementary students' sleep habits and teacher observations of sleep-related problems.' *Journal of School Health 75*, 2, 50–56.

Ball, H.L. (2002) 'Reasons to bed-share: why parents sleep with their infants.' *Journal of Reproductive and Infant Psychology 20*, 4, 207–222.

Ball, H.L. (2003) 'Breastfeeding, bed-sharing and infant sleep.' *Birth 30*, 3, 181–188.

Ball, H.L. (2006) 'Night-time Infant Care: Cultural Practice, Evolution, and Infant Development.' In P. Liamputtong (ed.) *Childrearing and Infant Care Issues: A Cross-cultural Perspective*. Melbourne: Nova Science.

Ball, H.L. and Klingaman, K.P. (2008) 'Breastfeeding and mother–infant sleep proximity: implications for infant care.' In W. Trevathan, E.O. Smith and J.J. McKenna (eds) *Evolutionary Medicine and Health: New Perspectives*. New York, NY: Oxford University Press.

Blair, P.S. and Ball, H.L. (2004) 'The prevalence and characteristics associated with parent–infant bed-sharing in England.' *Archives of Disease in Childhood 89*, 12, 1106–1110.

Bower, B. (1999) 'Slumber's unexplored landscape.' *Science News 13*, 156, 205.

Broman, J.E., Lundh, L.G. and Hetta, J. (1996) 'Insufficient sleep in the general population.' *Neurophysiologie Clinique 26*, 1, 30–39.

Crosby, B., LeBourgeois, M.K. and Harsh, J. (2005) 'Racial differences in reported napping and nocturnal sleep in 2- to 8-year-old children.' *Pediatrics 115*, 1, 225–232.

Doan, T., Gardiner, A., Gay, C.L. and Lee, K.A. (2007) 'Breast-feeding increases sleep duration of new parents.' *Journal of Perinatal and Neonatal Nursing 21*, 3, 200–206.

Dollman, J., Ridley, K., Olds, T. and Lowe, E. (2007) 'Trends in the duration of school-day sleep among 10- to 15-year-old South Australians between 1985 and 2004.' *Acta Paediatrica 96*, 7, 1011–1014.

Ekirch, A.R. (2001) 'Sleep we have lost: pre-industrial slumber in the British Isles.' *American Historical Review 106*, 2, 343–386.

Ekirch, A.R. (2005) *At Day's Close: A History of Night-time.* London: Weidenfeld & Nicolson.

Elias, M.F., Nicolson, N.A., Bora, C. and Johnston, J. (1986) 'Sleep/wake patterns of breast-fed infants in the first 2 years of life.' *Pediatrics 77*, 3, 322–329.

Hart, C.N. and Jelalian, E. (2008) 'Shortened sleep duration is associated with pediatric overweight.' *Behavioral Sleep Medicine 6*, 4, 251–267.

Iglowstein, I., Jenni, O.G., Molinari, L. and Largo, R.H. (2003) 'Sleep duration from infancy to adolescence: reference values and generational trends.' *Pediatrics 111*, 2, 302–307.

Jacobs, G.D., Benson, H. and Friedman, F. (1996) 'Perceived benefits in a clinical behavioural-medicine insomnia program: a clinical report.' *American Journal of Medicine 100*, 2, 212–216.

Jenni, O.G. and O'Connor, B.B. (2005) 'Children's sleep: an interplay between culture and biology.' *Pediatrics 115*, Suppl. 1, 204–216.

Jones, C.H.D. (2011) 'Exploring the short-sleep obesity association in young children.' Doctoral thesis, Durham University. Available at: http://etheses.dur.ac.uk/856/, accessed on 20 February 2012.

Leger, D., Guilleminault, C., Dreyfus, J.P., Delahaye, C. and Paillard, M. (2000) 'Prevalence of insomnia in a survey of 12,778 adults in France.' *Journal of Sleep Research 9*, 1, 35–42.

Marchand, L. and Morrow, M.H. (1994) 'Infant feeding practices: understanding the decision-making process.' *Clinical Research and Methods 26*, 5, 319–324.

Mindell, J.A., Kuhn, B., Lewin, D.S., Meltzer, L.J. and Sadeh, A. (2006) 'Behavioral treatment of bedtime problems and night wakings in infants and young children.' *Sleep 29*, 10, 1263–1276.

Mindell, J.A., Meltzer, L.J., Carskadon, M.A. and Chervin, R.D. (2009) 'Developmental aspects of sleep hygiene: findings from the 2004 National Sleep Foundation *Sleep in America Poll.*' *Sleep Medicine 10*, 7, 771–779.

Mindell, J.A., Sadeh, A., Wiegane, B., How, T.H. and Goh, D.Y.T. (2010) 'Cross-cultural differences in infant and toddler sleep.' *Sleep Medicine 11*, 3, 274–280.

Montgomery-Downs, H.E., Clawges, H.M. and Santy, E.E. (2010) 'Infant feeding methods and maternal sleep and daytime functioning.' *Pediatrics 126*, 6, e1562–e1568.

Moore, T. and Ucko, C. (1957) 'Night waking in early infancy: part 1.' *Archives of Disease in Childhood 32*, 164, 333–342.

Morelli, G.A., Rogoff, B., Oppenheim, D. and Goldsmith, D. (1992) 'Cultural variations in infants' sleeping arrangements: questions of independence.' *Developmental Psychology 28*, 4, 604–613.

National Sleep Foundation (2002) *Sleep in America Poll.* Washington, DC: National Sleep Foundation.

Olds, T., Blunden, S., Dollman, J. and Maher, C.A. (2010) 'Day type and the relationship between weight status and sleep duration in children and adolescents.' *Australian and New Zealand Journal of Public Health 34*, 2, 165–171.

Ottaviano, S., Giannotti, F., Cortesi, F., Bruni, O. and Ottaviano, C. (1996) 'Sleep characteristics in healthy children from birth to 6 years of age in the urban area of Rome.' *Sleep 19*, 1, 1–3.

Owens, J.A. (2004) 'Sleep in children: cross-cultural perspectives.' *Sleep and Biological Rhythms 2*, 3, 165–173.

Owens, J.A. (2005) 'Introduction: culture and sleep in children.' *Pediatrics 115*, 1, 201–203.

Owens, J.A. and Jones, C.H.D. (2011) 'Parental knowledge of healthy sleep in young children: results of a primary care clinic survey.' *Journal of Developmental and Behavioral Pediatrics 32*, 6, 447–453.

Owens, J.A., Jones, C.H.D. and Nash, R. (2011) 'Caregivers' knowledge, behaviour, and attitudes regarding healthy sleep in young children.' *Journal of Clinical Sleep Medicine 7*, 4, 345–350.

Parmelee, A.H., Wenner, W.H. and Schulz, H.R. (1964) 'Infant sleep patterns: from birth to 16 weeks of age.' *Journal of Pediatrics 65*, 4, 576–582.

Peireno, P., Algarin, C. and Uauy, R. (2003) 'Sleep-wake states and their regulatory mechanisms throughout early human development.' *Journal of Pediatrics 143*, 4, 70–79.

Pinilla, T. and Birch, L.L. (1993) 'Help me make it through the night: behavioral entrainment of breast-fed infants' sleep patterns.' *Pediatrics 91*, 2, 436–444.

Polnay, L., Blair, M., Horn, N. and Nathan, D. (1999) *Manual of Community Paediatrics.* Edinburgh: Churchill Livingstone.

Smith, J.P. and Harvey, P.J. (2010) 'Chronic disease and infant nutrition: is it significant to public health?' *Public Health Nutrition 14*, 2, 279–289.

Snell, E.K., Adam, E.K. and Duncan, G.J. (2007) 'Sleep and the body mass index and overweight status of children and adolescents.' *Child Development 78*, 1, 309–323.

Stearns, P.N., Rowland, P. and Giarnella, L. (1996) 'Children's sleep: sketching historical change.' *Journal of Social History 30*, 2, 345–366.

Super, C.M., Harkness, S., van Tijen, N., van der Vlugt, E., Dykstra, J. and Fintelman, M. (1996) 'The Three R's of Dutch Child Rearing and the Socialization of Infant Arousal.' In S. Harkness and C.M. Super (eds) *Parents' Cultural Belief Systems: Their Origins, Expressions, and Consequences.* New York, NY: Guilford Press.

Thorpy, M.J. (2011) 'Classification of Sleep Disorders.' In M.H. Kryger, T. Roth and W.C. Dement (eds) *Principles and Practice of Sleep Medicine*, 5th edn. St Louis, MO: Elsevier Saunders.

Trevathan, W.R., Smith, E.O. and McKenna, J.J. (eds) (2008) *Evolutionary Medicine and Health: New Perspectives.* Oxford: Oxford University Press.

Valentin, S.R. (2005) 'Commentary: Sleep in German infants – the "cult" of independence.' *Pediatrics 115*, Suppl. 1, 269–271.

Wehr, T.A., Moul, D.E., Barbato, G., Giesen, H.A. *et al.* (1993) 'Conservation of photoperiod-responsive mechanisms in humans.' *American Journal of Regulatory, Integrative and Comparative Physiology 265*, 4, 846–857.

Wiggs, L. (2007) 'Are children getting enough sleep? Implications for parents.' *Sociological Research Online 12*, 5, 13. Available at www.socresonline.org.uk/12/5/13.html, accessed on 30 March 2011.

Wolf, A.W., Lozoff, B., Latz, S. and Paludetto, R. (1996) 'Parental Theories in the Management of Children's Sleep in Japan, Italy and the United States.' In S. Harkness and C.M. Super (eds) *Parents' Cultural Belief Systems: Their Origins, Expressions, and Consequences.* New York, NY: Guilford Press.

Worthman, C.M. (2008) 'After Dark: The Evolutionary Ecology of Human Sleep.' In W.R. Trevathan, E.O. Smith and J.J. McKenna (eds) *Evolutionary Medicine and Health: New Perspectives.* Oxford: Oxford University Press.

Worthman, C.M. and Melby, M.K. (2002) 'Toward a Comparative Developmental Ecology of Human Sleep.' In M.A. Carskadon (ed.) *Adolescent Sleep Patterns: Biological, Social, and Psychological Influences.* Cambridge: Cambridge University Press.

Further reading

National Sleep Foundation (n.d.) *How Much Sleep Do We Really Need?* Available at www.sleepfoundation.org/article/how-sleep-works/how-much-sleep-do-we-really-need, accessed on 20 July 2010.

6

Beyond 'Death's Counterfeit'

THE SOCIOLOGICAL ASPECTS OF SLEEP

Robert Meadows

6.1. Introduction

Adding to the arguments put forward in other chapters, that sleep and its disorders are historically and culturally divergent, this chapter illustrates that *how, when* and *where* we sleep (and *with whom*) are all sociocultural matters. Sleep is a temporally bounded phenomenon that we 'live through'; a phenomenon 'irreducible to any one domain or discourse, *arising* or *emerging* through the interplay of biological and psychological processes, environmental and structural circumstances (i.e. facilitators and constraints), and socio-cultural *elaboration*, conceived in temporal/spatially bounded and embodied terms' (Williams 2002, p.178; original emphasis). Sleep is not, as common sense would have us believe, a 'perceptual hole in time' (Dement and Vaughan 1999, p.14) or 'death's counterfeit' (*Macbeth*, II. iii. 74); sleep is both a shared human biological universal and a time of social interaction (Aubert and White 1959a, 1959b; Meadows 2005).

The chapter begins by suggesting that sleep is reached via an interaction between biology, individual understandings and attitudes and the impact of 'others'. It is then argued that the form and content of these interactions are affected by the rules and norms surrounding sleep and by 'status differentials' (Brunt and Steger 2008, p.18), such as gender and age. Finally, the chapter reflects on the fact that much of the recent sociological research on sleep has focused on normal, everyday sleep and less work has been done on sleep disorders. Using the exemplar of cessation of breathing during sleep it is suggested that sociology is well placed to do this. The focus throughout the chapter is on adult sleep within contemporary western societies.

6.2. Sleep as a time of interaction and negotiation

Sleep is driven by both biology and the social context in which it occurs. This is most apparent in cases where the sleeping environment is shared and where (at least) two sets of understandings, expectations and attitudes are brought to bear on one another to decide such things as:

> ...bedtime and wake up times; which side of the bed to sleep on; whether to have the windows open or closed; whether to have the heating on; what type of mattress and pillows to have; whether to read in bed or not; whether to sleep cuddled up or apart. (Hislop 2007)

Yet, this is not to suggest that people have to be physically present to be implicated in the social context and interactions surrounding sleep. Family members and previous partners may be the most salient reference points available for individuals when gauging notions of normality in relation to their own sleeping behaviours (Meadows *et al.* 2008a). As Crossley suggested,[1] individual understandings, expectations and attitudes toward sleep are often influenced by close, virtual, networks. He observed that when we tell ourselves that we need to sleep we take on the role of our own parent and that we may attempt to lull our self to sleep in ways first taught us by our parents.

The impact of bed partners and others can also continue when they are no longer there. Drawing on data from Italian women aged between 40 and 80, Bianchera and Arber (2007) explore how sleep is affected when caring for children, grandchildren, adult children and elderly family members. Sleep, the authors argue, can be disrupted by having to perform direct care (involving getting up at night), the anticipation of having to perform care and worries relating to the caregiving role. Significantly, they also note that when caring involves looking after a frail or sick relative or loved one, long-term consequences can continue to exist, even after the individual being cared for has died. As the authors state, 'women reported that the habit of light sleep, listening out, and sudden awakenings in the night endured for a long period of time, and altered their sleep patterns beyond the caring period' (Bianchera and Arber 2007).

'Others' (absent or present) are not just those 'intimate' 'family' members with whom we might share a bedroom or a house. Even when we sleep alone, our success in fulfilling our expectations about sleep quantity and quality are still dependent on others. On a simplistic level this is evidenced by the fact that, as Martin (2002, p.5) argues, our daily cycles of sleep and wake are no longer driven by dawn and dusk but by electric lighting, clocks and work schedules. These mechanisms involve 'choices', which are made as a result of a negotiation between individual expectations, desires and social roles and those of 'others', such as employers. Taking this wider still, Williams and Crossley (2008) suggest that our capacity to sleep requires the co-operation of others. This is not only because we make ourselves vulnerable to others when asleep (see Lowe, Humphries and Williams 2007), but also because others must:

> ...respect our right to sleep and refrain from interfering with it, directly or indirectly. This may be granted automatically but it may have to be fought for. Neighbours and, indeed, children of shift workers may have to be persuaded to keep noise at low levels, for example. (Williams and Crossley 2008, pp.4–5)

In essence, then, *no one sleeps alone*. How, where, when (and with whom) we sleep are all achieved via other people. 'Other people' includes those who share the sleeping environment (intimate, family and friends), others who are absent but whose legacy remains, and individuals from the wider community in which we live. These interactions and negotiations are not benign. As discussed below, the form and content they take are influenced by the rules and norms that surround sleep.

6.3. Rules and norms surrounding sleep

Within any given society, at any given time, normative rules and conventions exist which 'protect' sleep as an important form of periodic remission (Schwartz 1970) and which render it 'more or less legitimate depending on the circumstances and context in question' (Williams 2007, p.324). For example, Williams and Bendelow (1998) suggest that within contemporary western societies normative conventions require us: 'to sleep at night and therefore to conform to the general pattern of sleep time, unless legitimate social circumstances, such as work arrangements, dictate otherwise'; and, 'to sleep in a bed, or similar device, in a private place, away from public view, in proper attire (i.e. pyjamas, nightdress etc.)' (Williams and Bendelow 1998, pp.182–183). More 'mundane' conventions and rules tell us that we must not yawn when someone is talking to us and, if adults, we must not wet the bed. Social consequences, ranging from criminalization to embarrassment, are 'attached to those who, for whatever reason, breach or flout these conventions' (Williams 2007, p.324).

These normative conventions are situated alongside prevailing cultural and political attitudes towards sleep. 'Sleep', for example, is now everywhere within society. On 12 July 2009, Laura Porter posted the following on the London Travel Blog:

> To help tired parents, Pampers are touring the UK with the Golden Sleep Train, kitted out with easy to follow information and sleep experts on hand to provide one-on-one advice to parents. Mums and dads can learn how to establish a good bedtime routine to help babies sleep through the night in a fun and interactive way, whilst babies and kids can also enjoy touching, feeling and playing with all the low level toys on the train. (Porter 2009)

Around the same time as the Golden Sleep Train hit the tracks, Pampers (a brand of babies' nappies, or diapers) released a television advert which suggested that their product enables babies to obtain 12 hours of *golden* sleep a night. The designate 'golden' is used because sleep, they argue, helps babies memorize the faces of loved ones. There exists now an abundance of sleep-related information that can be consumed. A cursory glance in any shopping centre will illustrate the multitude of products which are now being promoted and sold in terms of how well they aid sleep (including iPhone™ applications on 'sleep hygiene'). Even the leisure and entertainment industries are in on the act, whether this be through books such as *Armadillo* (Boyd 1998), *The House of Sleep* (Coe 1998) (see Chapter 14) or *Asleep* (Yoshimoto 2000), films such as *Nightmare on Elm Street*, programmes based around sleep-deprived contestants (such as the UK Channel 4 series *Shattered*) or documentaries depicting the plight of those suffering from sleep disorders. As Williams and Boden (2004, para.3.21) succinctly put it, there is now 'big business' surrounding sleep.

We also now live in a society where the term 'sleep medicine' has gained currency and where each night thousands of patients stay in sleep laboratories (Kroker 2007). According to Dement (2005), 'premonitions' of sleep medicine can be found in the 1960s. During this decade sleep-onset REM periods★ were noted, sleep apnoea was 'discovered' (see Williams 2005, p.147 for discussion), benzodiazepines (see Chapter 11) were introduced and several symposia were organized which looked at 'abnormal' sleep (Dement 2005). Yet it was not until 1972, when the first sleep centre performing polysomnography (PSG)★ opened at Stanford University, that sleep medicine was said to be born (Todman 2008).

Discursive shifts have also seen sleep become construed as 'the ultimate performance and productivity enhancer for workers and/or the perfect antidote to the speeding up and urgency of everyday life' (Boden *et al.* 2008, pp.551–552). Within the UK, for example, the University of Warwick has recently installed 'energy pods' on campus. It is claimed that these pods allow for effective napping and may promote greater awareness of when you are most effective at particular tasks. Whilst sleep may not necessarily be *idealized*, especially in the same way that 'thin' bodies are, it would appear that 'sleepiness' is now *vilified*. Sleepy drivers, Williams (2008) notes, can now be prosecuted, 'drawing a moral and legal parallel between drowsiness and drunkenness behind the wheel' (p.649).

Yet, at the same time as sleep medicine develops, big business continues growing around sleep and sleepiness becomes vilified, discourses also suggest that sleep is a neglected, health-related, matter. We are told that there exists a 'macho culture of sleeplessness' (Appleyard 2002) and that we live 'in an incessant or unremitting society, which has steadily "colonized" night in a variety of ways, from the humble electric light bulb to shift-work, night-clubs to 24-hour television and convenience stores' (Williams and Boden 2004). Allison Pugh (2000), for example, suggests that 'negating' sleep forms the bedrock mythology of the information technology (IT) revolution because sleep is seen as 'unsalvageable time' and a 'waste of time' because it cannot be devoted to work. Further to this, modafinil,* a 'wake-promoting' pharmaceutical, may embody the Protestant work ethic (cf. Williams *et al.* 2008), providing individuals with a means to stay alert and productive in a time when capitalism has sped up and our means of escaping it (via sleep) are being reduced. This, in itself, opens up new debates and controversies. As one UK newspaper reported on 21 February 2010:

> Universities must investigate measures, including random dope testing, to tackle the increasing use of cognitive enhancement drugs by students for exams, a leading behavioral neuroscientist warns. Student use of drugs, such as Ritalin and modafinil, available over the internet and used to increase the brain's alertness, had 'enormous implications for universities', said Barbara Sahakian, a professor of clinical neuropsychology at Cambridge University's psychiatry department. (Davies 2010)

Therefore, the normative aspects of sleep are situated alongside complex cultural and political attitudes towards sleep, medication and work. The norms, rules and discourses both influence the form and content of interactions surrounding sleep, and are themselves influenced by 'status differentials', such as gender and age. These are discussed further below.

6.4. The form and content of interactions: gender

Throughout history, women have needed to be alert at night. As Klug (2008) illustrates, the 'brave knight' found within German language literature protects his lady during the day and his lady keeps watch over him whilst he sleeps at night. Nowadays, women need to be alert at night because of their caring roles for children and other family members. Drawing on data from interviews and focus groups with mid-life women, Hislop and Arber (2003a) suggest that the interaction of the physical and emotional labour involved in caring for family members, and the worries and concerns associated with work and family responsibilities, compromise women's access to quality sleep. Somewhat similarly, Venn *et al.* (2008) use qualitative interview data from 26 healthy, heterosexual couples to illustrate how nocturnal care for young children is largely provided by women. Large-scale quantitative studies of women's sleep also lend support to these arguments. Arber *et al.* (2007), for example, indicate that women's subjective sleep quality is most influenced by how their partners slept, how their children slept and their own worries.

This body of research also suggests that there is very little discussion within families about who should undertake physical and emotional care. Women's compromised access to sleep quality is, therefore, often the result of 'unspoken', implicit decision-making and non-negotiation. Several reasons are offered as to *why* this situation occurs. For example, it is suggested that women subjugate their own sleep needs to those of their male partner because social norms and rules dictate that it is appropriate for women to undertake the supportive and protective role (Venn 2007). Paid employment is also implicated here. As Venn *et al.* (2008) suggest:

> ...non-working mothers perceived it as reasonable to argue that they are better suited to getting up in the night, if their partners have to go to work. However, on returning to work, there was seldom ever a re-negotiation of night-time responsibilities by the women. (Venn *et al.* 2008, p.95)

Many of these conclusions concerning women's sleep are reached via a comparison with men's discussions of sleep. For example, whereas women are found to be embarrassed by issues to do with snoring, men are said to talk about their bodies in a very matter-of-fact way and *emphasize* their unconsciousness and lack of control whilst asleep (Venn 2007). Similarly, Venn (2007) suggests that strategies for dealing with a snoring partner differ between men and women. Men tend to wake their snoring partner abruptly and forcefully whilst women employ strategies which actually disrupt their own sleep; for example, prodding (but not waking) their male snoring partner, laying still and listening, and/or moving out of the bedroom to sleep elsewhere.

None of this is meant to suggest that men never experience or complain of poor sleep. Whereas women's subjective reports of sleep quality are embedded within narratives of childcare and partners, men tend to stress the impact that paid employment has on their sleep. Lengthy work hours and work stresses were all implicated in men's discussion of their poor sleep quality (Meadows 2008). Assuming that this is more than simply rhetoric, it would seem that whilst men's sleep is afforded higher priority because of their role as the primary/ dominant earner, they are required to deny and distort their sleep needs in order to conform to work demands (see also Chatzitheochari and Arber 2009; Henry *et al.* 2008).

It is also not intended to imply that these findings are particular to heterosexual relationships. In a recent study in New Zealand, Kirkman (2010) conducted interviews with 20 women and men, aged between 45 and 65, in same-sex couple relationships. Whilst important evidence of blurring of the boundaries between men and women was found, Kirkman (2010) also observed how some of her findings reflected earlier work on heterosexual couples. The women in Kirkman's study demonstrated how they were involved in caring for their partner, which, the author noted, could be seen as a reflection of the way in which women, generally, are socialized to be nurturant and caring. Similarly, male discussions of sleep disruption often focused on how they could prevent their sleep being disrupted rather than how they could avoid disturbing their partner's sleep (Kirkman 2010).

More work is needed here. Whereas gender is undoubtedly an important factor within the ways in which we interact around sleep, research has yet to explore fully the relationship between results from subjective, qualitative enquiry and those from more 'objective' measures, such as actigraphy* and EEG.* Research is also needed on a more diverse range of 'couples' – including those from different socioeconomic backgrounds. A nascent body of research has suggested that socioeconomic status impacts upon subjective sleep quality. Taylor (1993) has argued that those who see sleep as a leisure pursuit are liable to have attained a certain socioeconomic status, but 'hard-working peasantry' are more likely to view sleep as respite from labour (Taylor 1993, p.468). Quantitative research carried out by Arber, Bote and Meadows (2009) indicates that a major reason for women's greater sleep problems relate to their more disadvantaged socioeconomic circumstances.

6.5. The form and content of interactions: age

Along with gender, age has also been shown to impact on individual understandings, expectations and attitudes, as well as the power one has within any interactions surrounding sleep. Studies illustrate how young children find it difficult to articulate feelings and attitudes towards sleep (Williams, Lowe and Griffiths 2007), and that their nights are populated by a range of actors, presences and activities, such as parents, siblings and soft toys (Moran-Ellis and Venn 2007). With teenagers, the situation becomes more complex – not least because they are afforded the means (mobile phones, etc.) to continue interactions long into the night.

At the other end of the age continuum, the biomedical literature contains a 'narrative of decline', stating that as we age the amount of time spent in deep, slow-wave sleep (SWS)* diminishes, as does rapid eye movement (REM)* (dreaming) sleep, whilst the time spent in lighter, stage 1 and stage 2 (S1 and S2) sleep increases (see Chapter 2). Older people may find it takes longer to get to sleep, have more fragmented sleep and wake up earlier (Bliwise 2005). There is also an ongoing debate about whether the change in night-time sleep experienced by older people leads to a propensity for daytime napping (Münch, Cajochen and Wirz-Justice 2005), or has no effect on whether older people sleep during the day or not (Klerman and Dijk 2008).

This 'narrative of decline' finds its way into younger men's understandings of how sleep changes with age (Meadows *et al.* 2008b). For example, a 54-year-old male interviewee in their study suggested:

> There is such a huge variability between people and also over the course of our lives. I mean it depends on how old you are. Quite clearly elderly people sleep very much more. It is a lot of dozing sleep and so on and babies sleep a tremendous amount more so I find that a very absurd statement [that everybody needs seven hours sleep]. (Meadows *et al.* 2008b, pp.702–703)

However, studies of older people's attitudes and understandings suggest that they themselves pay little attention to this 'narrative of decline'. In their study of older women, Davis, Moore and Bruck (2007), for example, found that both 'good' and 'poor' sleepers reported significant sleep disruption. Using data collected from the Pittsburgh Sleep Quality Index (PSQI),* several psychosocial measures, and in-depth interviews with 18 of these participants, Davis *et al.* (2007) illustrated that the key factor in distinguishing the 'good' and 'poor' sleepers was 'the way that they thought about their own sleep quality, in the wider context of their construction of normal sleep, which was often based on their engagement with comparison strategies' (Davis *et al.* 2007). As one of their elderly respondents stated, illustrating the use of 'others' to gauge *normality* and sleep quality: 'I do have a lot of sleep. Much more than a lot of the other girls around there' (Davis *et al.* 2007).

Taylor (1993) offers an argument which links the two ends of the age spectrum. He suggests that, *normatively*, sleep becomes more private as we grow older. We move from infancy, where sleep is monitored through such means as the baby intercom, to adulthood where we attain the right to be left alone whilst asleep and to sleep at a time of our own choosing. The prevalence of observed sleep within hospitals and prisons, and especially residential care homes, could be seen as reverting the adult to childhood. Moran-Ellis and Venn (2007) state that adults attempt to order children's sleep through surveillance and monitoring, whilst research into residential care homes has shown that residents may lack power in negotiations over their own sleep. Within care settings, staffing levels are the strongest predictor of time spent in bed (Bates-Jenson *et al.* 2004), and the nocturnal checks and repositioning carried out by staff result in institutional care residents experiencing large periods of wake after sleep onset (Schnelle *et al.* 1993; see also Meadows *et al.* 2010).

In reality, the impacts of age and gender intermingle. For example, age brings with it a greater risk of declining health, and couples are often left in a situation where one partner is caring for their spouse with a chronic illness or dementia: this impacts upon the sleep of both parties. The one receiving care may be considered vulnerable or a danger to themselves at night, and require the caregiver to be involved in surveillance, monitoring or maintaining night-time vigilance (Martin and Bartlett 2007). Reflecting discussions of childcare above, extensive research has shown that family (or informal) caregivers are more likely to be women than men (Arber and Ginn 1991). Whilst similar proportions of men and women carry out informal care for their spouse, women carry out the major share of 'intergenerational kith and kin care' (Arber, Davidson and Ginn 2003, p.5). Women's sleep at any

stage of the lifecourse is therefore more likely to be adversely affected
by direct care provision at night.

6.6. Considering obstructive sleep apnoea

One thing apparent from the discussion above is that the majority of
sociological research on sleep has focused on 'normal' 'everyday' sleep.
This is not to suggest that it offers no insight into sleep medicine,
or into sleep disorders such as obstructive sleep apnoea (OSA).
OSA was 'the first condition to be developed under the jurisdiction
of sleep medicine and is nowadays the most commonly diagnosed
"sleep disorder"' (Moreira 2006, p.55); recent years have witnessed a
growing number of people who are 'self-diagnosing' and seeking help
for snoring and OSA via non-traditional routes. Yet, at one and the
same time, it is said to remain largely undiagnosed, unrecognized and
untreated (Young, Peppard and Gottlieb 2002). Individuals are not
recognizing and engaging with risk factors (such as obesity); they are
not engaging with symptoms (such as snoring); medical education is
said to fall short; and, once OSA is diagnosed, there is poor compliance
with treatment – known as continuous positive airway pressure (CPAP);
see Chapter 9.

The discussion throughout this chapter highlights how sociology
has (at least) two things to offer our understanding of OSA. First, the
sociological emphasis on the 'lived experience' of embodied action
offers a useful framework for understanding how an individual becomes
reflexive about their OSA, how they decide on which treatment options
to engage with and how they experience treatment. For example,
theories of the 'lived experience' of embodiment highlight how the
body is 'absent' and how, because of this, it is difficult to directly
audit our sleep quality or quantity (Leder 1990, p.58). Instead we
infer the quality and quantity of our sleep or we learn of it indirectly
from others. These theories also tell us that the frame of reference
through which our bodies are known to us is personal and subjective
(Hughes 2000); yet we live in a society where we are all expected to
assume the role of 'informed patient' or 'consumer' (Cant and Calnan
1992; Lupton 1997), and to 'self-examine' and apply a clinical frame
of reference to our bodies (Hughes 2000, p.25). Moreira's (2006,
2008) recent research, using posts by CPAP users on internet message

boards, brings these points into relief. He highlights how CPAP users share their experiences, creating a form of 'collective expertise' that is recursively used and which adapts as new questions or challenges are posted. Moreira (2008) also sheds light on how the incorporation of CPAP machines into people's homes can entail using the body to gauge how well the machine 'fits'. Individuals also have to re-engineer aspects of their everyday/night lives (such as intimacy, changing beds), 'normalize' the presence of the CPAP machine and reframe and reform (expert) identities as their knowledge of the machine changes.

The second thing sociology has to offer our understanding of OSA relates to 'wider contexts'. As noted throughout this chapter, sociology places great emphasis on the fact that sleep, and our 'lived experience' of sleep, is embedded within society. At one level, this can relate to household dynamics. For example, OSA has been shown to negatively affect bed partners (Parish and Lyng 2003) whilst, at the same time, bed partners are said to assist in the identification of 'symptoms' (snoring) and treatment compliance (Cartwright 2008; see also authors such as Kloesch and Dittami 2008; Meadows *et al.* 2009; Pankhurst and Horne 1994; Troxel *et al.* 2010). At another level, this can relate to the 'normativity', 'rules' and cultural attitudes that surround sleep. For example, women's reluctance to acknowledge publicly their snoring may be a reflection of ideals surrounding 'femininity' (Venn 2007) and may play some role in the under-reporting of OSA. Similarly, the trend towards self-diagnosis may be linked to wider, cultural shifts that have seen the traditional doctor–patient relationship being somewhat usurped by the media (see Kroll-Smith 2003 for an interesting discussion of this in relation to insomnia).

There is currently much debate within sociology over whether or not sleep (and therefore OSA) has become 'medicalized' – 'defining a [social] problem in medical terms, using medical language to describe the problem, adopting a medical framework to understand a problem, or using medical intervention to "treat" it' (Conrad 1992, p.211). Put somewhat differently, the question, according to Kroll-Smith and Gunter (2005, p.346), becomes: how was 'a private, routinely occurring state of partial consciousness de-privatized, linked to public health vernaculars, and transformed into a reprobate condition'? For Wolf-Meyer (2008) the answer can be found in the way that, for sleep medicine to develop, sleep had to shift from being a 'matter of fact' to become a 'matter of concern', and new conceptions of 'normal' and 'pathological' were required (Wolf-Meyer 2008). When these shifts occurred, histories were (re)written to make them seem the consequence of a heightened, more accurate, state of scientific awareness whilst divergences and disagreements are ignored.

The main protagonists in the 'medicalization'* of sleep debate have been Williams (with others) and Hislop and Arber. Whilst tending to err on the 'side' of medicalization, Williams *et al.* (2008) suggest that issues surrounding medicalization may differ depending on the sleep disorder under study. In their examination of media constructions of insomnia and snoring, they illustrate how insomnia is portrayed through a 'psychologized' discourse that draws upon notions of stress and anxiety. These discourses also stress personal responsibility: people with insomnia are often portrayed as their own worst enemy and are seen as individuals who exaggerate their plight, which, in turn, exacerbates their sleeping problems. Snoring provides a different picture. Media coverage frequently includes members of the sleep medicine community, alerting people to the links between snoring and sleep apnoea and emphasizing the public health risks that this entails. The ways in which this all translates to 'individual experiences' is debated within sociological circles. Hislop and Arber (2003b), for example, suggest that medicalization only plays a small role in mid-life women's sleep management. Rather than resort to medication and doctors, mid-life women, it is argued, 'have developed a range of personalized strategies over time to manage their sleep without recourse either to externally invoked healthy lifestyle practices or medical intervention' (Hislop and Arber 2003b, p.822). These personalized techniques include such things as consuming hot milky drinks and reading. Critiquing this, Seale *et al.* (2007, p.429) suggest that many of the personalized strategies employed by mid-life women are 'discussed and debated in the popular public forum of the *Daily Mail* [one of the UK newspapers Seale and colleagues investigated], so they are far from being wholly private (or personalised) solutions'.

6.7. Summary

This chapter has sought to illustrate that *how, when* and *where* we sleep are all social variables. At the core of the argument is the idea that sleep is achieved through interaction and is 'negotiated', with 'self' and 'others'. Individuals have their own particular understandings, expectations and attitudes toward sleep that are then brought to bear on others' understandings, expectations and attitudes. This is most notable when the sleeping environment is shared, but extends to all sleeping situations. William C. Dement, a founding father of sleep medicine, noted this in 1972 when he suggested that the 'anthropological and sociological implications of sleep are vast and complex' (1972, p.2). Clearly, he was right.

Acknowledgements

The author would like to thank Professor Sara Arber and Dr Brigitte Steger, who both commented on early drafts of this chapter. The editors also offered interesting and salient comments.

This chapter was completed in July 2010.

Note

1. Speaking at the Sleep and Society Seminar at Warwick University on 3 December 2004.

References

Appleyard, B. (2002) 'Night waves.' *New Statesman*, 8 July. Available at www.newstatesman.com/node/143377/23, accessed on 12 April 2012.

Arber, S. and Ginn, J. (1991) *Gender and Later Life*. London: Sage Publications.

Arber, S., Bote, M. and Meadows, R. (2009) 'Understanding how socio-economic status, gender and marital status influence self-reported sleep problems in Britain.' *Social Science & Medicine 68*, 2, 281–289.

Arber, S., Davidson, K. and Ginn, J. (2003) 'Changing Approaches to Gender and Later Life.' In S. Arber, K. Davison and J. Ginn (eds) *Gender and Ageing: Changing Roles and Relationships*. Buckingham: Open University Press.

Arber, S., Hislop, J., Bote, M. and Meadows, R. (2007) 'Gender roles and women's sleep in mid and later life: a quantitative approach.' *Sociological Research Online 12*, 5, 3. Available at www.socresonline.org.uk/12/5/3.html, accessed on 27 July 2010.

Aubert, V. and White, H. (1959a) 'Sleep: a sociological interpretation I.' *Acta Sociologica 4*, 2, 46–54.

Aubert, V. and White, H. (1959b) 'Sleep: a sociological interpretation II.' *Acta Sociologica 4*, 3, 1–16.

Bates-Jensen, B.M., Schnelle, J.F., Alessi, C.A., Al-Samarrai, N.R. and Levy-Storms, L. (2004) 'The effects of staffing on in-bed times of nursing home residents.' *Journal of the American Geriatrics Society 52*, 6, 931–938.

Bianchera, E. and Arber, S. (2007) 'Caring and sleep disruption among women in Italy.' *Sociological Research Online 12*, 5, 4. Available at www.socresonline.org.uk/12/5/4.html, accessed on 27 July 2010.

Bliwise, D.L. (2005) 'Normal Aging.' In M.H. Kryger, T. Roth and W.C. Dement (eds) *Principles and Practice of Sleep Medicine*, 4th edn. Philadelphia, PA: Elsevier Saunders.

Boden, S., Williams, S.J., Seale, C., Lowe, P. and Steinberg, D.L. (2008) 'The social construction of sleep and work in the British print news media.' *Sociology 42*, 3, 541–558.

Boyd, W. (1998) *Armadillo*. London: Hamish Hamilton.

Brunt, L. and Steger, B. (2008) 'Introduction.' In L. Brunt and B. Steger (eds) *Worlds of Sleep*. Berlin: Frank & Timme.

Cant, S. and Calnan, M. (1992) 'Using private health insurance: a study of lay decisions to seek professional medical help.' *Sociology of Health and Illness 14*, 1, 39–57.

Cartwright, R. (2008) 'Sleeping together: a pilot study of the effects of shared sleeping on adherence to CPAP treatment in obstructive sleep apnea.' *Journal of Clinical Sleep Medicine 4*, 2, 123–127.

Chatzitheochari, S. and Arber, S. (2009) 'Lack of sleep, work and the long hours culture: evidence from the UK time use survey.' *Work, Employment and Society 23*, 1, 30–48.

Coe, J. (1998) *The House of Sleep*. London: Penguin.

Conrad, P. (1992) 'Medicalization and social control.' *Annual Review of Sociology 18*, 209–232.

Davies, C. (2010) 'Universities told to consider dope tests as student use of "smart drugs" sours.' *The Observer Online*, 21 February. Available at www.guardian.co.uk/society/2010/feb/21/smart-drugs-students-universities, accessed on 27 August 2010.

Davis, B., Moore, B. and Bruck, D. (2007) 'The meanings of sleep: stories from older women in care.' *Sociological Research Online 12*, 5, 7. Available at www.socresonline.org.uk/12/5/7.html, accessed on 27 July 2010.

Dement, W.C. (1972) *Some Must Watch Whilst Others Sleep*. Stanford, CA: Freeman.

Dement, W.C. (2005) 'History of Sleep Physiology and Medicine.' In M.H. Kryger, T. Roth and W.C. Dement (eds) *Principles and Practice of Sleep Medicine*, 4th edn. Philadelphia, PA: Elsevier Saunders.

Dement, W.C. and Vaughan, C. (1999) *The Promise of Sleep*. London: Macmillan.

Henry, D., McClellen, D., Rosenthal, L., Dedrick, D. and Gosdin, M. (2008) 'Is sleep really for sissies? Understanding the role of work in insomnia in the US.' *Social Science & Medicine 66*, 3, 715–726.

Hislop, J. (2007) 'A bed of roses or a bed of thorns? Negotiating the couple relationship through sleep.' *Sociological Research Online 12*, 5, 2. Available at www.socresonline.org.uk/12/5/2.html, accessed on 27 July 2010.

Hislop, J. and Arber, S. (2003a) 'Sleepers wake! The gendered nature of sleep disruption among mid-life women.' *Sociology 37*, 4, 695–711.

Hislop, J. and Arber, S. (2003b) 'Understanding women's sleep management: beyond medicalization-healthicization?' *Sociology of Health and Illness 25*, 7, 815–837.

Hughes, B. (2000) 'Medicalized Bodies.' In P. Hancock, B. Hughes, E. Jagger, K. Paterson *et al.* (eds) *The Body, Culture and Society*. Maidenhead: Open University Press.

Kirkman, A. (2010) '"My bed or our bed?": gendered negotiations in the sleep of same-sex couples.' *Sociological Research Online 15*, 2, 5. Available at www.socresonline.org.uk/15/2/5.html, accessed on 27 July 2010.

Klerman, E.B. and Dijk, D.-J. (2008) 'Age-related reduction in the maximal capacity for sleep – implications for insomnia.' *Current Biology 18*, 15, 1118–1123.

Kloesch, G. and Dittami, J.P. (2008) 'A Bed for Two? Gender Difference in the Reactions to Pair-sleep'. In L. Brunt and B. Steger (eds) *Worlds of Sleep*. Berlin: Frank & Timme.

Klug, G. (2008) 'Dangerous Doze: Sleep and Vulnerability in Medieval German Literature.' In L. Brunt and B. Steger (eds) *Worlds of Sleep*. Berlin: Frank & Timme.

Kroker, K. (2007) *The Sleep of Others and the Transformations of Sleep Research*. Toronto: University of Toronto Press.

Kroll-Smith, S. (2003) 'Popular media and "excessive daytime sleepiness": a study of rhetorical authority in medical sociology.' *Sociology of Health and Illness 25*, 6, 625–643.

Kroll-Smith, S. and Gunter, V. (2005) 'Governing sleepiness: somnolent bodies, discourse, and liquid modernity.' *Sociological Inquiry 75*, 3, 346–371.

Leder, D. (1990) *The Absent Body*. Chicago, IL: Chicago University Press.

Lowe, P., Humphries, C. and Williams, S.J. (2007) 'Night terrors: women's experiences of (not) sleeping where there is domestic violence.' *Violence Against Women 13*, 6, 549–561.

Lupton, D. (1997) 'Consumerism, reflexivity and the medical encounter.' *Social Science & Medicine 45*, 3, 373–381.

Martin, P. (2002) *Counting Sheep: The Science and Pleasures of Sleep and Dreams*. London: HarperCollins.

Martin, W. and Bartlett, H. (2007) 'The social significance of sleep for older people with dementia in the context of care.' *Sociological Research Online 12*, 5, 11. Available at www.socresonline.org.uk/12/5/11.html, accessed on 27 July 2010.

Meadows, R. (2005) 'The "negotiated night": an embodied conceptual framework for the sociological study of sleep.' *The Sociological Review 53*, 2, 240–254.

Meadows, R. (2008) 'Sociological Exploration into Sleep: Couples and Men.' Unpublished PhD Thesis, University of Surrey.

Meadows, R., Arber, S., Venn, S. and Hislop, J. (2008a) 'Unruly bodies and couples' sleep.' *Body & Society 14*, 4, 75–92.

Meadows, R., Arber, S., Venn, S. and Hislop, J. (2008b) 'Engaging with sleep: male definitions, understandings and attitudes.' *Sociology of Health and Illness 30*, 5, 696–710.

Meadows, R., Arber, S., Venn, S., Hislop, J. and Stanley, N. (2009) 'Exploring the interdependence of couples' rest-wake cycles: an actigraphic study.' *Chronobiology International 26*, 1, 80–92.

Meadows, R., Luff, R., Eyers, I., Cope, E., Venn, S. and Arber, S. (2010) 'An actigraphic study comparing community dwelling poor sleepers with non-demented care home residents.' *Chronobiology International 27*, 4, 1–13.

Moran-Ellis, J. and Venn, S. (2007) 'The sleeping lives of children and teenagers: night-worlds and arenas of action.' *Sociological Research Online 12*, 5, 9. Available at www.socresonline.org.uk/12/5/9.html, accessed on 27 July 2010.

Moreira, T. (2006) 'Sleep, health and the dynamics of biomedicine.' *Social Science & Medicine 63*, 1, 54–63.

Moreira, T. (2008) 'Continuous positive airway pressure machines and the work of coordinating technologies at home.' *Chronic Illness 4*, 2, 102–109.

Münch, M., Cajochen, C. and Wirz-Justice, A. (2005) 'Sleep and circadian rhythms in ageing.' *Zeitschrift für Gerontologie und Geriatrie 38*, Suppl. 1, 121–123.

Pankhurst, F.P. and Horne, J.A. (1994) 'The influence of bed partners on movement during sleep.' *Sleep 17*, 4, 308–315.

Parish, J.M. and Lyng, P.J. (2003) 'Quality of life in bed partners of patients with obstructive sleep apnea or hypopnea after treatment with continuous positive airway pressure.' *Chest 124*, 3, 942–947.

Porter, L. (2009) 'Pampers Golden Sleep Train.' Laura's London Sleep Blog. Available at http://golondon.about.com/b/2009/07/12/pampers-golden-sleep-train.htm, accessed on 27 July 2010.

Pugh, A. (2000) 'Sleep in a Sleepless Age: A Sociology of Sleep, Work and Family.' In E. Balka and R. Smith (eds) *Women, Work and Computerization: Charting a Course to the Future.* Boston, MA: Kluwer Academic Publishers.

Schnelle, J.F., Ouslander, J.G., Simmons, S.F., Alessi, C.A. and Gravel, M.D. (1993) 'The nighttime environment, incontinence care, and sleep disruption in nursing homes.' *Journal of the American Geriatrics Society 41*, 9, 910–914.

Schwartz, B. (1970) 'Notes on the sociology of sleep.' *The Sociological Quarterly 11*, 4, 485–499.

Seale, C., Boden, S., Williams, S., Lowe, P. and Steinberg, D. (2007) 'Media constructions of sleep and sleep disorders: a study of UK national newspapers.' *Social Science & Medicine 65*, 3, 418–430.

Taylor, B. (1993) 'Unconsciousness and society: the sociology of sleep.' *International Journal of Politics, Culture and Society 6*, 3, 463–471.

Todman, D. (2008) 'A history of sleep medicine.' *The Internet Journal of Neurology 9*, 2. Available at www.ispub.com/journal/the_internet_journal_of_neurology/volume_9_number_2_5/article/a_history_of_sleep_medicine.html, accessed on 10 July 2010.

Troxel, W.M., Buysse, D.J., Matthews, K.A., Kravitz, H.M. *et al.* (2010) 'Marital/cohabitation status and history in relation to sleep in midlife women.' *Sleep 33*, 7, 973–981.

Venn, S. (2007) '"It's okay for a man to snore": the influence of gender in addressing sleep disruption in couples.' *Sociological Research Online 12*, 5, 11. Available at www.socresonline.org.uk/12/5/11.html, accessed on 27 July 2010.

Venn, S., Arber, S., Meadows, R. and Hislop, J. (2008) 'The fourth shift: exploring the gendered nature of sleep disruption in couples with children.' *British Journal of Sociology 59*, 1, 79–97.

Williams, S.J. (2002) 'Sleep and health: sociological reflections on the dormant society.' *Health: An Interdisciplinary Journal for the Social Study of Health, Illness and Medicine 6*, 2, 173–200.

Williams, S.J. (2005) *Sleep and Society: Sociological Ventures into the (Un)Known.* London: Routledge.

Williams, S.J. (2007) 'The social etiquette of sleep: some sociological reflections and observations.' *Sociology 41*, 2, 313–328.

Williams, S.J. (2008) 'The sociological significance of sleep: progress, problems and prospects.' *Sociology Compass 2*, 2, 639–653.

Williams, S.J. and Bendelow, G. (1998) *The Lived Body: Sociological Themes, Embodied Issues.* London: Routledge.

Williams, S.J. and Boden, S. (2004) 'Consumed with sleep? Dormant bodies in consumer culture.' *Sociological Research Online 9*, 2. Available at www.socresonline.org.uk/9/2/williams.html, accessed on 27 July 2010.

Williams, S.J. and Crossley, N. (2008) 'Introduction: sleeping bodies.' *Body & Society 14*, 4, 1–13.

Williams, S.J., Lowe, P. and Griffiths, F. (2007) 'Embodying and embedding children's sleep: some sociological comments and observations.' *Sociological Research Online 12*, 5, 6. Available at www.socresonline.org.uk/12/5/6.html, accessed on 27 July 2010.

Williams, S.J., Seale, C., Boden, S., Lowe, P. and Steinberg, D.L. (2008) 'Waking up to sleepiness: Modafinil, the media and the pharmaceuticalisation of everyday/night life.' *Sociology of Health and Illness 30*, 6, 839–855.

Wolf-Meyer, M. (2008) 'Sleep, signification and the abstract body of allopathic medicine.' *Body & Society 14*, 4, 93–114.

Yoshimoto, B. (2000) *Asleep.* London: Faber & Faber.

Young, T.P., Peppard, E. and Gottlieb, D.J. (2002) 'Epidemiology of obstructive sleep apnea: a population health perspective.' *American Journal of Respiratory and Critical Care Medicine 165*, 9, 1217–1239.

7

A Question of Balance

THE RELATIONSHIP BETWEEN DAILY
OCCUPATION AND SLEEP

Andrew Green

7.1. Introduction

Sleep occupies more of our time than any other activity and is the single most important natural act around which we structure our everyday occupation. The insomniac Wordsworth described it as the 'blessed barrier between day and day' (1801, p.563), and it is difficult to imagine a life without sleep and with continuous consciousness (although J.G. Ballard had a stab at it[1]). Sleep remains an essential punctuation of time but, as other chapters show, it does not simply fill the space between each day's activities: it is closely interrelated with them. Sleep influences the performance of activities but, conversely, our daily activities influence sleep. As suggested by Green *et al.* (2005), the two-way relationship between sleep and activity, or the 'reciprocal relationship between biological rhythms and social occupations' (Matuska and Christiansen 2008, p.15), should be of greater interest to occupational therapists than it appears to be.

'Occupational therapy is a client-centred health profession concerned with promoting health and well being through occupation.

[Its] primary goal…is to enable people to participate in the activities of everyday life' (World Federation of Occupational Therapists 2010). There has been much debate over the years about the definition of 'occupation' (and its theoretical distinction from 'activity'[2]) but that is a question that has been addressed elsewhere (Green 2008), and the matter has been best summed up thus: 'However we define and differentiate occupations, they are concerned with people's *use of time*' (Finlay 2004, p.42; original emphasis). If that is so, it seems illogical for sleep to be overlooked by occupational therapists, since we spend so much of our time asleep.

This chapter therefore aims to investigate the relevance of sleep to occupational therapy and after a brief look at how sleep *has* been addressed in occupational therapy so far, it examines the extent to which we choose how much we sleep, and when. The chapter then explores the reciprocal relationship between sleep and activity, first, by looking at how sleep, or lack of it, can affect performance of activity and second, by examining how daytime activity might affect sleep.

7.2. Sleep and occupational therapy

Sleep was accorded a place in the 'big four' of Adolf Meyer, a neuropsychiatrist and advocate of occupational therapy early in the twentieth century who emphasized the importance of balance between work, play, rest and sleep for good health (Meyer 1977, first published in 1922). Meyer has been widely quoted in subsequent decades by occupational therapists and his common-sense assertion appears to have been accepted as if an article of faith. Only more recently has there been analysis of the concept of balance (Christiansen and Matuska 2006; Matuska and Christiansen 2008; Westhorp 2003), and whilst occupational therapists have focused on work and recreation in particular, they have still paid little attention to sleep. A review by Green (2008) found that discussion of sleep in the literature of occupational therapy was neither consistent nor comprehensive. For example, Kielhofner, prominent in occupational therapy since the 1980s, scarcely mentioned sleep except in discussing habits, stating that: 'while the adult generally has habits organized around requirements for productivity, habits must also allow time for rest, play and sleep'

(Kielhofner and Burke 1985, p.29). There was no significant discussion of sleep then, or in his subsequent work (e.g. Kielhofner 2002), the importance of habits for maintaining good sleep notwithstanding. However, late in 2008 the American Occupational Therapy Association published a revised practice framework and a significant change was the inclusion of sleep as an 'area of occupation' (AOTA 2008, p.630). The document illustrates that maintaining routines and preparing for sleep are not simple matters.[3]

A possible reason for the previous neglect of sleep by occupational therapists, suggested by Howell and Pierce (2000), is that sleep is regarded as unproductive in western society (see also Chapter 13), and that occupational therapy has been shaped by society's values. However, occupational *science* has recognized the importance of sleep as part of the rest/activity cycle. The discipline of occupational science emerged in the early 1990s and, as explained by the founders, Clark *et al.* (1991), one of its purposes was to 'organize and transmit the interdisciplinary knowledge that supports [the] practice' (p.307) of occupational therapy, in the way that anatomy and physiology support medicine. They ambitiously stated that 'occupational science...attempts theoretically to address the entire range of phenomena surrounding human occupation' (p.304). The extent to which this has been achieved is open to question, but the research and reflection that have been stimulated are welcome nonetheless. Two influential writers who have taken an interest in sleep are Wilcock in Australia (Wilcock 2003, 2006) and, writing with various co-authors, Christiansen in the USA (Christiansen 1996; Christiansen and Baum 2005; Christiansen and Matuska 2006; Christiansen and Townsend 2004).

Having explored sleep science, Wilcock (2006) concluded that human systems are flexible and capable of being overridden, thereby facilitating 'occupational flexibility' (p.82). This flexibility is important since, as Matuska and Christiansen (2008) have observed, there is an increasing perception that the demands of modern life exceed the time available for them; people have 'insufficient time to rest or participate in discretionary pursuits or to accomplish work-related tasks at desired performance levels' (p.14). Whether this perception is valid, and whether there is a sleep debt, are debatable (see below), but time allowed for sleep is often (and has long been) one of the first things to suffer at times of other pressure – hence the expressions 'burning the midnight oil' and 'burning the candle at both ends of the day'. Everybody will have limited their sleep at some time to meet an important deadline – whether wrapping birthday presents, completing an assignment or catching an early train. There can be little doubt that it is necessary to be able to overrule the sleep/wake cycle occasionally, but most people would probably agree that it would be unhealthy if curtailing sleep were a persistent habit. This prompts the question: how do we allocate time for sleep?

7.3. Sleep and time use

The literature of occupational therapy and occupational science tells us little about how we choose when to sleep in normal circumstances. Some work (described below) has been done amongst people with mental health problems, although such studies tend to be small. To ascertain how much sleep people normally take it is helpful to turn to time-use surveys and the kind of data gathered by government agencies. Such studies often involve large samples but unfortunately, there are still several difficulties in calculating sleep time. Measurement of sleep depends on self-report, involving the individual estimating when consciousness is lost. Furthermore, Tang and Harvey (2005) have shown that people generally tend to overestimate time, including time awake at night, and therefore might underestimate sleep. An average figure also has to be viewed with some caution when there is a lot of variation; for example, an average work time of about three hours (Lader, Short and Gershuny 2006) is relatively meaningless because so many people do no paid work at all, whereas full-time workers typically do seven or eight hours of work on five days, and none on two days. Finally, a particular problem in estimating sleep time in time-use studies is defining the activity. It is necessary to differentiate between the hours spent sleeping and time spent in bed awake, perhaps in the hope of sleeping. There is also the matter of categorizing daytime sleep: it could also be counted as 'rest' or be included under 'watching television' by someone who dozes off whilst watching a film (which could be described as *polychronic* sleep: see Chapter 4).

The difficulty of classification of sleep time is exemplified by Soupourmas (2005) who observed that Australian adolescents (aged 15–19) were apparently sleeping longer in 1997 compared to 1990 (about 20 minutes longer on school days and almost an hour longer on non-school days). However, in the 1997 survey, 'lying in bed awake' was counted with 'sleep', but not in 1990, when it was 'resting' (Soupourmas 2005, p.578). A large UK survey reported by Lader *et al.* (2006) had a similar problem if 2005 data were compared with data from 2000 (see below). Basner *et al.* (2007) described a large USA study where respondents were asked to record 'sleeplessness' ('tossing and turning, lying awake, counting sheep') but then for the most part they included this with 'sleep time' to cover all sleep periods in the 24-hour period, as well as transitions into or out of sleep.

Despite the data-coding problems, time-use studies still reveal some interesting insights. For example, the 2005 UK study (Lader *et al.* 2006) showed that 90 per cent of people took their sleep between the hours of 9 p.m. and 9 a.m. whilst 50 per cent had retired to bed by 11 p.m. and 50 per cent had risen by 7 a.m. (see Figure 7.1a and b). Sleep was the only daily activity reported by 100 per cent of participants; even eating and drinking were reported by only 97 per cent of respondents. The study found that men slept for a little over eight hours (484 minutes) per day, and women for about eight-and-a-quarter hours (498 minutes). This was an apparent decline since 2000 of 19 and 15 minutes respectively, although it was probably accounted for by the reported similar increase in rest time. (Table 7.1 summarizes details from this and all the time-use studies cited here.) The figures are comparable with the larger and more detailed time-use study in the USA in which Basner *et al.* (2007) reported that the average working day sleep time varied from just under eight hours (472 minutes) in the 45–54 age group, to almost nine hours (539 minutes) for the over-75 age group.

Table 7.1. Summary of time-use studies

Author	Country	Respondents					Sleep time (minutes)	Rest time (minutes)	Sleep + rest (minutes)
		Status	Number	Sex	Age				
Soupourmas (2005)[1] Reporting Australian Bureau of Statistics data (1997)	Australia	Adolescents	862	M & F	15–19		528	5	533
Soupourmas (2005) Reporting Australian Bureau of Statistics data (1992)	Australia	Adolescents	1,210	M & F	15–19		507	20	527
Lader et al. (2006)[2] UK Time-use survey (2005)	UK	General population	4,941	M & F	≥16		491	46	537
Lader et al. (2006) UK Time-use survey (2000)	UK	General population	16,566	M & F	≥16		508	22	530
Basner et al. (2007)[3] US Time-use survey (2003–2005)	USA	General population	47,731	M & F	≥15		472–539	–	–

Farnworth et al. (2004)[4]	Australia	Patients with severe mental illness in a secure unit	8	M	24–48	–	–	640
Stewart and Craik (2007)[5]	UK	Patients with schizophrenia in a secure unit	5	M & F	20–50	561	216	777
Shimitras et al. (2003)[6]	UK	People with schizophrenia living in the community	228	M & F	Mean: 46 (19–89)	580	–	–
Aubin et al. (1999)[7]	Canada	People with severe mental illness living in the community	45	M & F	Mean: 39 (26–58)	544	120–150	658–700

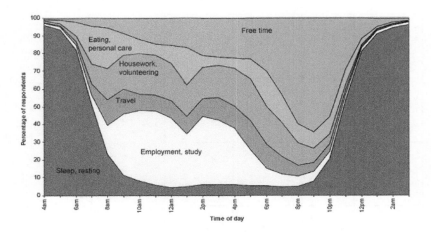

Figure 7.1a. The distribution of activities on weekdays
From Lader *et al.* (2006). Crown copyright: Office for National Statistics.

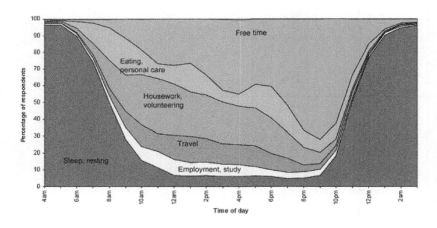

Figure 7.1b. The distribution of activities on weekends
From Lader *et al.* (2006). Crown copyright: Office for National Statistics.

In examining the relationship between work and sleep more closely, Basner *et al.* (2007) found work to be the activity that was most commonly exchanged for sleep. Those sleeping for less than 4½ hours worked an average of 93 minutes more on weekdays compared with the average sleeper; those sleeping for more than 11½ hours worked an average of 143 minutes less than the average sleeper. That is, sleep time decreased as work time increased – a finding echoed by Swanson *et al.* (2011). From the perspective of economics, Biddle and Hamermesh (1990) reviewed data from studies in various countries and calculated that for each additional hour of work the cost was roughly ten minutes of sleep; employed people slept about an hour less than those who did not work. Furthermore, they found that sleep time was inversely related both to wage and to time spent working, and suggested that as income increases, the price of time increases and so the demand for sleep decreases. They suggested: 'In short, sleep is subject to consumer choice and is affected by the same economic variables that affect choices about other uses of time', and concluded that 'at least part of sleep time is a reserve on which people can draw when economic circumstances make other uses of time more attractive' (Biddle and Hamermesh 1990, p.941). As Gunderson (2001, p.432) put it: 'people with a high opportunity cost of time sleep less'.[4]

However, for considerations based in economics to apply to time use there needs to be a free market, or freedom of choice. Studies involving people in more restricted circumstances where there are fewer choices have indicated longer sleep times – for example, people detained in forensic psychiatry units. (The studies also illustrate the difficulties in classifying activity, mentioned above, although it should be stressed that the occupational therapist researchers were not focusing on sleep.) In a study involving eight inpatients in an Australian secure unit, Farnworth, Nikitin and Fossey (2004) counted sleep as part of 'personal care' that took up 50 per cent of the respondents' time on weekdays, compared with 46 per cent within the general Australian population. Eighty-nine per cent of that personal care time was spent sleeping – suggesting sleep duration of 10 hours and 41 minutes – possibly even longer at weekends when 55 per cent of time was spent in personal care. In another small study in a similar setting, in the UK, Stewart and Craik (2007) found that respondents slept on average for 4 per cent of the 'daytime' but for 39 per cent (9 hours 20 minutes) of the 24-hour period; they rested for an additional 15 per cent of the time (3 hours 36 minutes). Given the small sample sizes, and the difficulty in distinguishing sleep from rest, it is hard to draw conclusions from these two studies in secure units, except that detainees probably do sleep for longer than the average person. There is, however, an interesting parallel in the animal kingdom where captive animals have been found to sleep for extended periods (see Box 7.1).

Box 7.1. The sleep of captive and free sloths

The three-toed sloth is renowned for its sleep and an average of 15 hours and 51 minutes of daily sleep has been measured in captive animals. Using modern techniques of radiotelemetry (involving monitors attached to the animals' heads to transmit data by radio), Rattenborg et al. (2008) recorded the sleep of three adult female sloths in the wild (in Panama) for a total of nearly 13 days between them. It was found that the sloths slept for an average of only 9 hours and 40 minutes per day. Even allowing for the inclusion of juveniles in the captive sample (which is likely to have raised their average sleep time) it is a substantial difference when compared with sleep of the animals in the natural setting. It suggests that the wild animals have increased ecological demands – such as foraging and looking out for predators – and therefore take the minimum necessary sleep, whilst captive animals, whose food is provided, sleep as if to pass the time.

Further possible explanations of the forensic patients' apparent long sleep are their mental illness[5] or side effects of medication. It is helpful therefore to compare with community studies. Shimitras, Fossey and Harvey (2003) found that respondents with a diagnosis of schizophrenia in London slept for an average of 9 hours and 40 minutes a day. This is in line with the forensic inpatients' sleep (and, coincidentally, exactly the same as the sloths' in the forest); it is rather longer, however, than was found in an earlier smaller community-based study involving 45 people with a similar diagnosis. In that Canadian study Aubin, Hachey and Mercier (1999) found that respondents slept for 9 hours and 4 minutes (38% of the 24 hours). Sleep was, however, differentiated from daytime rest (in which respondents spent between about 2 and 2½ hours). These studies demonstrate again the difficulty in categorizing sleep, but they also confirm a tendency for people with a chronic mental illness to sleep longer than average, and to be less active than others. It remains uncertain whether they sleep as a consequence of their illness – or as a side effect of treatment – or whether they sleep as a substitute for another activity, which, as a result of the illness, they may lack the motivation to carry out. In any event there would appear to be a strong case, at least to an occupational therapist, for encouraging the re-engagement in activity.

That last point is emphasized by an additional finding of Aubin *et al.* (1999) – that sleeping was 'especially meaningful in the participants' daily life, since it obtained the highest rating regarding perceived competence and pleasure and the second highest rating for importance' (p.58); the authors commented that these findings could appear disconcerting. Whilst it is appropriate to rate sleep as important, and it is reasonable to enjoy sleep, it is a little worrying that anyone could rate sleep as the thing at which they are *most competent*. Of course, it might indicate that the respondents had no problem in sleeping (and therefore considered they were good at it), but it probably tells us more about their overall quality of life and their non-participation in other activities. (It could also be that it was unwise in the first place to rate sleep alongside other activities – as if comparing apples and cats.)

Some indication of the extent to which sleep is valued by people generally has also been provided by Biddle and Hamermesh (1990) who cited a survey where people in the USA were asked what two or three activities they would do if there were an additional four hours in a day. Sleeping was only the seventh most frequently cited activity by the 776 respondents. This could suggest that sleep is undervalued by respondents, but maybe with an additional four hours people would feel that they had enough time to do the things they needed to (or wanted to) and would not then need to curtail time for sleep – or perhaps they just felt they already had enough sleep. Similarly, in an interactive web survey (in conjunction with a television programme), Anderson and Horne (2008) asked people about a notional extra hour a day. They found that, despite an apparent sleep deficit of 25–30 minutes amongst almost half of respondents, only 19 per cent of men and 23.4 per cent of women said they would actually use the hour for additional sleep.

Horne (2006, p.204) cites this research (before its publication) in opposing the idea of sleep debt, or the suggestion that, as a society, we have insufficient sleep. Martin (2002) has argued the case *for* sleep debt. He notes the widespread sleepiness felt by people when they are awake, and findings that people spend less than eight hours asleep – considerably less than our ancestors who did not have the modern pressures of work and round-the-clock leisure opportunities. Sleep debt would be the consequence if there were no reserve to draw on, as suggested by Biddle and Hamermesh (1990). Horne's (2006) contention, however, is that we eat and drink for pleasure, rather than only for physiological need, and likewise, we can take longer sleep for pleasure. Horne explains his theory that we need 'core sleep' (between six and seven hours) and can also take 'optional sleep' (pp.204–205). He argues that extra sleep is unnecessary for health and that it might actually be more beneficial to use the time for exercise instead. This is a particularly pertinent observation, since, as the next section shows, there is evidence that exercise itself is good for sleep.

7.4. The relationship between sleep and daily activity

It has been noted already that there is a reciprocal relationship between sleep and activity. For example, there is an extensive literature on the effects of shift patterns on work performance and driver safety, and on the importance of sleep for memory and learning. It is not possible to look at more than a fraction of it here – a review could fill a chapter on its own. Therefore, the remainder of this chapter takes a brief look at some of the main issues, before moving on to examine the ways that daily activity patterns might affect sleep.

The importance of sleep for the performance of activities

We know that sleep affects performance of daily activity, and we know it from personal experience: at the simplest level, after sleep loss it can be difficult just to stay awake but most people will also have experienced difficulty concentrating, for example. The catalogue of major incidents that have occurred at night when, biologically, workers would otherwise be asleep, and are therefore sleep-deprived, is often cited as evidence of the problem, and is well known: Three Mile Island,[6] Bhopal, Exxon Valdez, to name three – although Philip and Åkerstedt (2006) note that these events provide only circumstantial or anecdotal evidence of any link between sleep loss and accidents. In the UK there have been prominent examples of serious accidents caused by drivers apparently falling asleep at the wheel – notably the Selby rail crash in 2001 (see Chapter 15) and the M40 minibus crash in 1993 (MacKinnon 1994).[7]

Alhola and Polo-Kantola (2007) provide a review of the impact of sleep deprivation, noting that 'people who are exposed to sleep loss usually experience a decline in cognitive performance and changes in mood' (p.554). They suggest a two-way classification of theories to explain the decline in performance. First, effects on alertness and attention can be attributed to microsleeps[8] where the homeostatic pressure to sleep (see Chapter 2) becomes too much to maintain full wakefulness, whilst the effort involved in continuing a task prevents the individual falling into sleep: this is the state instability hypothesis (Doran, van Dongen and Dinges 2001). Second, it is suggested that sleep deprivation has selective effects on certain areas of the brain – the sleep-based neuropsychological perspective (see Babkoff et al. 2005; Harrison and Horne 2000). This can affect many areas of performance, but one that is important for many people and is relatively easily measured – often using reaction time measures – is driving.

Evidence that sleepiness is linked with risk on the road is offered by Connor et al. (2002) who analysed data from over 600 road traffic accidents in New Zealand and compared the drivers with a control group. They found a strong association between acute sleepiness in drivers (interviewed after the incident) and the risk of a crash involving injury or fatality: this was unrelated to acute alcohol consumption or other major confounding factors. 'There was an eightfold increased risk of accident if drivers reported sleepiness and almost a threefold risk for drivers who were driving after five hours of sleep or less' (Connor et al. 2002, p.4).

Investigating naturally occurring sleep deprivation, Altena et al. (2008) performed vigilance tests on a group of people with a diagnosis of primary insomnia and a similar group of good sleepers (average age: 60). It was found that participants with insomnia performed faster on a straightforward vigilance task, whereas they performed more slowly on a relatively complex task involving a decision before the motor response. Reassuringly, it was found that following sleep therapy, their performance matched that of the controls. The researchers suggested that the better performance of the participants with poor sleep was consistent with a state of high arousal associated with insomnia (see Chapter 9). The findings also seem to accord with everyday experience where we might feel able to cope with routine tasks after a poor night's sleep but struggle with more complex issues that involve thinking. It is possible, however, that because we can manage simple tasks we might overestimate performance when sleep-deprived – assuming, of course, that we are aware how sleep-deprived we are: there is evidence that we may not be.

In a widely cited study conducted in the USA involving 48 adults (aged 21–38), van Dongen *et al.* (2003) randomly assigned volunteers, in carefully controlled laboratory conditions, to periods of eight hours, six hours or four hours of sleep for two weeks; a fourth group had no sleep at all for three days. It was found that having only four or six hours of nightly sleep progressively eroded performance in a neurobehavioural test battery measuring vigilance, working memory and cognitive throughput (using a serial addition/subtraction task). The findings therefore did not support claims that humans adapt to chronic sleep restriction in a few days (which shorter-lasting studies might indicate), since chronic sleep restriction to four or six hours produced deficits at 14 days comparable to those found with total deprivation of one to two days. The researchers concluded that 'even relatively moderate sleep restriction – if sustained night after night – can seriously impair waking neurobehavioral functioning in healthy young adults' (van Dongen *et al.* 2003, p.124). Even more disturbingly, subjective sleepiness did not match levels of actual sleep deprivation (except in the case of total sleep deprivation). It is suggested that once sleep loss becomes chronic, people are less aware of the need for sleep – as long as they have at least four hours' sleep a night, they believe that they have adapted to short sleep because they are not sleepy. This leads to an unsettling conclusion that there are people on the roads convinced that they manage on minimal sleep, but reacting as if they are totally sleep-deprived (see also Philip and Åkerstedt 2006).

In another study that manipulated sleep schedules Cohen *et al.* (2010) monitored reaction times of volunteers whose sleep/wake times were desynchronized over the course of three weeks. They found that chronic sleep loss resulted in increased deterioration of performance during wakefulness, especially during the circadian night – hence the apparent association with major incidents at that time. Furthermore, they found that individuals could develop a chronic sleep debt in the face of apparent full recovery from acute sleep loss. A chronically sleep-restricted individual may therefore have a false sense of recovery from their prior sleep debt as a result of performing well for the first several hours of a usual waking day. The researchers remind us that acute sleep loss is hazardous:

> 19 hours of sustained wakefulness from 8am to 3am is associated with performance deficits equivalent to a blood alcohol concentration of 0.05%, and after 24 hours of sustained wakefulness the performance deficit is equivalent to an alcohol concentration of 0.10%. (Cohen *et al.* 2010, p.5)

Cohen and colleagues might have also pointed out that the 'drink-drive' limit in the UK and USA is 0.08 per cent (or 80mg of alcohol per 100ml of blood) and that it is lower (0.05% or even 0.02%) in many European countries. A majority of drivers would probably not take to the road knowing they were over the blood alcohol limit, whilst they are unaware of the risks they are running in driving without adequate sleep. However, there is some evidence that sleep deprivation is associated with increased risk taking – albeit in extreme circumstances. Killgore, Kamimori and Balkin (2011), observing that sleep deprivation is linked with decreased metabolic activity in parts of the brain involved in judgement and impulse control, conducted laboratory tests involving a risk-taking exercise and a self-report measure of risk-taking propensity. It was found that after three nights of total sleep deprivation there was an increase in risk-taking behaviour, but without corresponding changes in self-reported risk propensity. (They found, incidentally, that two-hourly 200mg dosing of caffeine during the nights reduced the behavioural and self-reported risk propensity.) Whilst this is hardly applicable in daily life, it nevertheless reinforces the importance of regulations for professional drivers – and explains military interest in drugs like modafinil (see Kim 2007, and Chapter 15).

Many of the studies cited here relate to the homeostatic pressure to sleep, whereas the sleep-based neuropsychological perspective also offers an explanation for the decline in performance; it is suggested that sleep deprivation affects functioning of certain areas of the brain. Horne (1993), for example, argues that sleep deprivation affects functions dependent on the prefrontal cortex – such as language, executive functions and creativity – and suggests that the prefrontal cortex 'obtains particular benefit from sleep' (p.485). He cites his own studies where, after 36 hours of total sleep deprivation impairments were found in tests of word fluency, non-verbal planning, creativity and originality – all related to the prefrontal cortex. Impairment was only partly reversed by increased effort – in contrast to reversal found in tasks not involving the prefrontal cortex. Perseveration was commonly found in divergent thinking tests whereas convergent thinking was unimpaired.

Much research has been done on the relationship of sleep and memory; memory is a complex phenomenon and to help make sense of it, Stickgold (2005) offers a simple classification. Declarative memories can be called to mind – for example, the capital of France (semantic memory) or last night's dinner (episodic memory) – whereas non-declarative memories are used without conscious recollection –for example, 'how to ride a bicycle or how to talk your way out of a parking ticket' (Stickgold 2005, p.1272). Research has also attempted to establish the role of different stages of sleep in the memory process.

Stickgold (2005) reported on three studies where volunteers took part in different tasks involving procedural memory (a subcategory of non-declarative memory). It was shown that participants' performance in learning simple tasks (e.g. a motor sequence task) improved after a period of sleep, but not after a similar interval of wakefulness. He inferred from this that sleep contributes to memory consolidation, but it was not possible to specify that any particular stage of sleep was responsible and it was concluded that each stage of sleep contributes differently to the processes. He therefore suggests that 'the multiplicity of sleep stages has evolved, in part, to provide optimal brain states for a range of distinct memory consolidation processes' (Stickgold 2005, p.1273).

However, there is some evidence of involvement of different stages of sleep in certain circumstances. Wagner, Gais and Born (2001) compared memory retention of emotional text and neutral text across a three-hour period of sleep in which either slow-wave sleep (SWS) or rapid eye movement (REM) sleep was predominant. It was found that memory of emotional material was improved after a period of sleep where REM predominated, thereby suggesting that REM sleep has a key role in the formation of emotional memories. Schabus *et al.* (2004) demonstrated the involvement of sleep spindle activity (during stage 2 [S2] sleep: see Chapter 8) in memory consolidation in a declarative memory task (learning word pairs) although the relationships are not straightforward. They also cite evidence of links between sleep architecture* and spatial memory, motor skill learning and implicit perceptual memory.

Sleep is further involved in other more diffuse cognitive processes. For example, Wagner *et al.* (2004) showed that sleep is instrumental in the process of gaining insight, which they defined as a 'mental restructuring that leads to a sudden gain of explicit knowledge allowing qualitatively changed behaviour' (p.352). The experimental task involved a mathematical puzzle where the object is to turn a sequence of eight digits into a new sequence using two simple rules. However, there was a third hidden rule, not mentioned in the training, which, after discovery, meant that participants could solve the puzzle more quickly; the point at which they gained insight could then be ascertained. The training period was followed by an eight-hour interval in which groups of participants had eight hours of nocturnal sleep, nocturnal wakefulness or daytime wakefulness. It was found that sleep more than doubled the probability of gaining insight into the rule. It was concluded that sleep 'not only strengthens memory traces quantitatively, but can also "catalyse" mental restructuring' (Wagner *et al.* 2004, p.354).

Research into the effects of sleep loss continues (e.g. Balkin *et al.* 2008; Swanson *et al.* 2011; Tucker *et al.* 2010) but, whilst it may need a psychologist to interpret such findings fully, there is sufficient evidence that sleep contributes to a range of cognitive functions that we depend on for the performance of daily activity. As noted earlier, the evidence supports our everyday experience (that is, what we know without being told by scientists), but it also suggests that we underestimate the importance of sleep. What is less well established, however, is the way that activity affects sleep.

The potential effects of daily activity on sleep

Chapter 3 explains the importance of circadian rhythms and how *zeitgebers** (environmental cues or timekeepers) keep the body clock in synchrony. Light is the most powerful of these, and seeing daylight on rising is one reason why it is important for an individual to keep regular hours, but amongst other *zeitgebers* is activity. There is little hard evidence to be found in the literature of occupational therapy or occupational science on the benefits of activity for health, never mind for sleep and, once again, it is necessary to turn to other disciplines for clues.

Exercise is a particularly quantifiable activity: distance covered, number of repetitions, weights lifted (as well as physiological responses) can all be measured, and a great deal of research has been done in relation to exercise and its effect on sleep and circadian rhythms (e.g. Driver and Taylor 2000). There is also some evidence from studies that have attempted to look at *activity*, despite the difficulty of measurement (e.g. how do you quantify or measure the level of a person's participation in 'church activities'?). This evidence comes from two sources: small experimental or correlational studies, and large surveys carried out by epidemiologists. The problem with the first is that numbers are insufficient to draw firm conclusions and with the second, that sleep may be only one of many factors under investigation and causal connections cannot be made. However, despite these problems, some innovative research has been carried out, and some interesting findings have been made.

Shapiro *et al.* (1981) showed a clear link between exercise and sleep architecture. They found that participants in an 'extreme event' (a 92km road race) not only had more sleep than usual for two nights afterwards but they also had more deep sleep and less REM* sleep. In fact, they slept for longer on the second night than the first night, which may have been disturbed by muscle and blister pains. There is more recent evidence that regular but less extreme exercise can aid the sleep of adolescents. In a Swiss study, Brand *et al.* (2009) compared the sleep of 36 male 'chronic and intense' footballers with 34 matched controls – all aged 15. When the data from sleep diaries and questionnaires were compared it was found that the footballers slept sooner and longer, with fewer awakenings and had higher sleep quality scores. There was also an improvement in self-reported levels of concentration and tiredness. The reasons for improvement are not clear and, as ever, many factors may be involved. Does the effect of exercise on the body, and enhanced fitness, influence sleep? Does the sense of well-being, satisfaction and enjoyment that can result from training and from being in the team lead to reduced levels of anxiety and depression? Do the increased levels of self-discipline (and/or parental discipline or influence) that go with team membership affect adherence to good routines? A particular difficulty in answering such questions and interpreting the findings of these studies is that it was not recorded whether any participants actually complained of poor sleep or whether improvement was necessary.

In a questionnaire survey, Sherrill, Kotychou and Quan (1998) asked more than 700 'middle-aged to elderly' respondents, aged over 40, about sleep problems and exercise levels. Regular exercise was associated with a lower prevalence of sleep symptoms; this included, amongst women (but not men, where there were insufficient data), a reduced risk of nightmares. This was an unexpected finding but something that might result from a reduction in stress. In discussing the physiological mechanism whereby exercise could promote sleep, the researchers observed that exercise might enhance sleep architecture by increasing central nervous system temperature (although exercise close to bedtime is known to disrupt sleep). As in the other exercise studies, Sherrill *et al.* (1998) also appear not to take account of the possibility that people who sleep well might be more inclined to exercise. A way to investigate causal relationships is in experimental studies where there is more control over variables.

One such study was by King *et al.* (1997) who conducted an experiment where 20 volunteers (aged between 50 and 76) with moderate sleep complaints completed a 16-week exercise programme whilst 23 controls remained on a waiting list. The 30–40-minute exercise sessions were held four times a week and included aerobics and brisk walking. At the end of the programme the exercisers showed an increase in subjective sleep quality, measured on the Pittsburgh Sleep Quality Index (PSQI).* Total sleep time increased by over 40 minutes whilst sleep onset latency (time taken to get to sleep) halved. These measures differed significantly from the control group's measures after 16 weeks, but not at 8 weeks. This suggests that it is important to persist with exercise, although a further study by King *et al.* (2008)[9] yielded only modest improvements in sleep over 12 months.

Li *et al.* (2004) showed that Tai Chi could act as an alternative form of exercise to improve the sleep of older people. In a study involving adults aged between 60 and 92 randomly assigned to a 24-week Tai Chi programme (one hour three times a week) or to low impact exercise classes (mainly seated, with stretching and controlled breathing), they compared the effects of each on participants' perceived sleep quality. After the programme, the Tai Chi group members' sleep was improved: sleep onset latency decreased by an average of 18 minutes and participants' average sleep duration increased by 48 minutes. In contrast there were no improvements for the control group. The findings were comparable with those of King *et al.* (1997), apparently supporting the importance of physical activity for sleep, although the more meditative aspect of Tai Chi cannot be discounted as a reason for improved sleep.

Although it is difficult to measure general activity, some studies have attempted to assess its consequences. Observing how we can feel sleepy after a day's sightseeing and travelling in a new environment (acknowledging different levels of physical exertion), Horne and Minard (1985) carried out an elegant small experiment with nine female graduate students in their twenties. Participants believed that they were to spend a day doing psychological tests as part a trial involving three other, uneventful, days on campus and five nights in a sleep laboratory. They were in fact treated to a surprise long day out, including visits to a shopping centre, zoo and amusement park and cinema. It was found that the participants were markedly sleepier at the end of that day and duly went to sleep in eight minutes – half the time taken previously. Whilst they slept for no longer overall, they had more deep sleep – even on the second night – than at baseline: REM sleep was unaffected. Despite various uncontrolled factors, the inference was that it was the novel experience that was tiring.

Despite noteworthy findings amongst younger people in such studies, as in the case of exercise, the clinical importance of the relationship between activity and sleep is greater amongst older people, whose circadian systems become less well synchronized (Van Someren and Riemersma-van der Lek 2007). In a telephone survey involving over 13,000 people in the UK, Italy and Germany, Ohayon *et al.*

(2001) found that 'activity status' (essentially, whether the person was working or not) and satisfaction with social life had a greater influence on the sleep habits of older people than aging alone. The authors suggested that the relationship between insomnia and increasing age could be explained by such factors, and they observed that healthy older people (with neither physical nor mental illness) had a prevalence of insomnia symptoms similar to rates in younger people. They added, however, that being active and leading a satisfying social life could protect against insomnia at any age.

The association between social activity and sleep has also been demonstrated by Nasermoaddeli *et al.* (2005) who analysed data from various questionnaires completed by civil servants in the UK (6873 respondents, aged 40 and over) and in Japan (1628 respondents across the working age range). Respondents completed measures of sleep quality as well as a questionnaire about leisure activities. The latter were classified according to the extent to which they involved engagement with others. It was found that increased social leisure activities were linked with decreased sleep problems. It was stressed that it was *social* activity – not necessarily associated with physical activity – that was related to sleep quality. However, it was also acknowledged that, conversely, poor sleep could lead to low mood and, in turn, to less participation in social activities – again raising doubts about which causes the other.

Other studies have supported the findings of Ohayon *et al.* (2001) with regard to older people. In one (Habte-Gabr *et al.* 1991), social activities such as membership of a club, having a close friend and involvement in religious activities were found to be related to better sleep quality. Another study, using polysomnography (PSG)* (Hoch *et al.* 1987), compared the sleep of a group of elderly nuns, who had remained engaged in their vocations and who restricted their time in bed, with a matched group of healthy retired women who had no religious affiliation. The nuns spent about an hour less in bed each night but fell asleep more quickly and slept for longer, with less early morning wakening than the controls. It is not clear whether the nuns' continued activity and security were important, or whether it was their highly entrained routine that was the key factor behind their better sleep. Perhaps it was all of these. Ohayon *et al.* (2001) note that some retired people might overlook the need to keep regular hours in the absence of the constraints that would normally regulate sleep/wake patterns (such as work and other people's needs). They conclude that continuing engagement in life and curtailing time in bed preserve sleep quality and they suggest that it is important not to dismiss an elderly person's sleep problem as just something to be expected with age.

The studies by Ohayon *et al.* (2001) and Nasermoaddeli *et al.* (2005), although large, only compared data cross-sectionally, whereas a small pilot study by Benloucif *et al.* (2004) observed experimentally changed behaviour. They found that a daily social and physical activity programme for 12 older adults (aged between 67 and 86) improved not only their subjective sleep quality (measured by the PSQI), but also their performance in a neuropsychological test battery (by 4–6%). Participants took part in 90-minute activity sessions involving two 30-minute sessions of mild to moderate physical activity separated by 30 minutes of social activity (talking and playing cards or board games). The sessions were held either at 9 a.m. or 7 p.m. for 14 consecutive days. Despite the reported subjective improvement in sleep, there were no objective changes (measured by actigraphy* or PSG) but the perceived improvement in sleep occurred after the activity programme, whether it was the morning or evening session. With regard to the neuropsychological improvement, the researchers observed cryptically: 'regular activity at any time of day would be preferable to irregular activity at a specified time of day' (Benloucif *et al.* 2004, p.1549).

The importance of regularity of activity for sleep has been shown by Monk *et al.* (2003) who demonstrated a potential link between lifestyle regularity and sleep quality. In a study involving 100 adults (aged between 19 and 49), regularity was measured using a diary in which respondents recorded the time at which 17 daily events occurred (e.g. getting up, starting work, mealtimes, etc.) over the course of two weeks; from this a 'regularity' score was computed. Subjective sleep quality was measured using the PSQI. When the two scores were compared it was found that participants with a sleep quality score above a level normally associated with sleep difficulty had significantly lower scores on the regularity measure. The result therefore supported the hypothesis that regular rhythms are related to better sleep. However, as seen before, Monk and colleagues were unable to state which factor caused the other: does good sleep permit regular activity or does regularity promote good sleep?

Recent research at Durham University[10] (see also Chapter 5) suggests that it could be routine that leads to greater sleep duration, at least in children, since small children do not decide about what to do, or when, on the basis of the amount of sleep they have had. Researchers studied the sleep of three-year-old children and found that those with routine-led sleep (regular bedtime with a bedtime story, in bed, as opposed to being allowed to fall sleep on the sofa) slept on average for about 20 minutes longer than children without such routines. Furthermore, it was found that more controlled routines in eating and other activities – such as watching television – were also linked with better sleep (and with lower rates of obesity). There is therefore increasing evidence – albeit tentative – that routines are good for sleep. Indeed, it may be supposed that the routine of the lives of prisoners, mentioned in the previous section, could be another factor explaining their extra sleep.

7.5. Conclusion

This chapter set out to highlight the relevance of sleep to occupational therapy. First, it has been suggested that we are able to exert a significant degree of choice over when and how much we sleep. One of the chief determinants of sleep timing and duration is work: the more hours we work, the fewer hours we tend to sleep. Second, the relationship between daily activity and sleep has been explored. The importance of sleep for performance seems undeniable but it has also been shown that activity, physical and social, can affect subjective sleep and in some cases can affect the structure of sleep (or the relative proportion of deep sleep and REM sleep). It seems especially relevant for older people to maintain activity levels, and for both the elderly and the very young to keep to routines in order to promote good sleep.

The evidence, however, is still not conclusive, and the direction of causality remains uncertain. This highlights the need for research by occupational therapists, occupational scientists and others to investigate further the relationship between occupation and sleep. Since sleep can be considered important for health, demonstrating a relationship between occupation and sleep could be one way to explore the relationships between occupation and health and to test Meyer's contention about the importance of balance.

Acknowledgement

Thanks are due to Dr Cary Brown of the University of Alberta for her helpful comments on an earlier draft.

This chapter was completed in the summer of 2010, with the exception of the first part of Section 7.4, which was added in the autumn of 2011 along with some other amendments.

Notes

1. In his short story *Manhole 69*, first published in 1957, Ballard (2006) imagined experimental surgical 'narcotomy'. The experiment is not a success. The more doubtful of the researchers observes: 'Maybe you need eight hours off a day just to get over the shock of being yourself' (p.69). In a similar way, Schwartz (1970, p.497) argues that sleep provides periodic remission 'from the demands and irritations of social life'.

2. It has been observed (Golledge 1998, p.101) that it is difficult to define 'occupation' without using the word 'activity'. For the purpose of discussion here, no distinction is made, and the words are used without any specialized meaning.

3. In the table of changes to the framework it is noted that the category 'rest and sleep' is no longer considered as an 'activity of daily living' but is an 'area of occupation' because of the importance of rest and sleep in supporting other areas of occupation. The rationale for the change is explained thus:

    > Rest and sleep are two of the four main categories of occupation discussed by Adolf Meyer (1977). Unlike any other area of occupation, all people rest as a result of engaging in occupations and engage in sleep for multiple hours per day throughout their lifespan. Within the occupation of rest and sleep are activities such as preparing the self and environment for sleep, interactions with others who share the sleeping space, reading or listening to music to fall asleep, napping, dreaming, night-time care of toileting needs, night-time caregiving duties, and ensuring safety. Sleep significantly affects all other areas of occupation. [It is] suggested that providing sleep prominence in the framework as an area of occupation will promote the consideration of lifestyle choices as an important aspect of participation and health. (AOTA 2008, p.665)

4. Opportunity cost 'is a measure of costs expressed as alternatives given up, rather than in terms of money... For any...resource constraint if you want more of one thing you have to give up something else' (Lipsey and Chrystal 2007, p.5).

5. In a small six-week actigraphy study, Wulff *et al.* (2012) found that participants with schizophrenia had more sleep disruption, including circadian misalignment and excessive sleep, when compared to matched unemployed controls. Occupational therapists are also referred to Bromundt *et al.* (2011) for evidence of the importance of well-defined daytime activity as part of rehabilitative process in schizophrenia.

6.   Yaniv (2004) cites evidence that the Three Mile Island incident was subsequently associated with severe insomnia amongst nearby residents; sleep deprivation was therefore potentially both a causal factor and an effect of the incident.

7.   Twelve children died in the crash in November 1993 when the minibus, driven by their teacher, hit a stationary maintenance lorry on the hard shoulder of the motorway. The driver had been awake for 18 hours when the accident occurred just after midnight on the return journey from London to Worcestershire. At the inquest, expert witness, Professor Jim Horne, said it appeared to be a 'classic case of falling asleep at the wheel'.

8.   A microsleep is a brief episode of sleep that may last for less than a second or up to half a minute, often a consequence of sleep deprivation. The individual is usually unaware.

9.   A 12-month study involving adults over 55 using home PSG to compare the effects of an exercise programme with a health education control programme.

References

Alhola, P. and Polo-Kantola, P. (2007) 'Sleep deprivation: impact on cognitive performance.' *Neuropsychiatric Disease and Treatment 3*, 5, 553–567.

Altena, E., van der Werf, Y.D., Strijers, R.L.M. and Van Someren, E.J.W. (2008) 'Sleep loss affects vigilance: effects of chronic insomnia and sleep therapy.' *Journal of Sleep Research 17*, 3, 335–343.

Anderson, C. and Horne, J.A. (2008) 'Do we really want more sleep? A population-based study evaluating the strength of desire for more sleep.' *Sleep Medicine 9*, 2, 184–187.

AOTA (American Occupational Therapy Association) (2008) 'Occupational therapy practice framework: domain and process, 2nd edition.' *American Journal of Occupational Therapy 62*, 6, 625–683.

Aubin, G., Hachey, R. and Mercier, C. (1999) 'Meaning of daily activities and subjective quality of life in people with severe mental illness.' *Scandinavian Journal of Occupational Therapy 6*, 2, 53–62.

Babkoff, H., Zukerman, G., Fostick, L. and Ben-Artzi, E. (2005) 'Effect of the diurnal rhythm and 24 h of sleep deprivation on dichotic temporal order judgment.' *Journal of Sleep Research 14*, 1, 7–15.

Balkin, T.J., Rupp, T., Picchioni, D. and Wesensten, N.J. (2008) 'Sleep loss and sleepiness: current issues.' *Chest 134*, 3, 653–660.

Ballard, J.G. (2006) *The Complete Short Stories*, Vol 1. London: Harper Perennial.

Basner, M., Fomberstein, K.M., Razavi, F.M., Banks, S. *et al.* (2007) 'American time use survey: sleep time and its relationship to waking activities.' *Sleep 30*, 9, 1085–1095.

Benloucif, S., Orbeta, L., Oritz, R., Janssen, I. *et al.* (2004) 'Morning or evening activity improves neuropsychological performance and subjective sleep quality in older adults.' *Sleep 27*, 8, 1542–1551.

Biddle, J.E. and Hamermesh, D.S. (1990) 'Sleep and the allocation of time.' *Journal of Political Economy 98*, 5, pt 1, 922–943.

Brand, S., Beck, J., Gerber, M., Hatzinger, M. and Holsboer-Trachsler, E. (2009) '"Football is good for your sleep": favourable sleep patterns and psychological functioning of adolescent male intense football players compared to controls.' *Journal of Health Psychology 14*, 8, 1144–1155.

Bromundt, V., Köster, M., Georgiev-Kill, A., Opwis, K. *et al.* (2011) 'Sleep-wake cycles and cognitive functioning in schizophrenia.' *British Journal of Psychiatry 198*, 269–276.

Christiansen, C.H. (1996) 'Three Perspectives on Balance in Occupation.' In R. Zemke and F. Clark (eds) *Occupational Science: The Evolving Discipline.* Philadelphia, PA: F.A. Davis.

Christiansen, C.H. and Baum, C.M. (2005) 'The Complexity of Human Occupation.' In C.H. Christiansen, C.M. Baum and J. Bass-Haugen (eds) *Occupational Therapy: Performance, Participation and Well-Being*, 3rd edn. Thorofare, NJ: Slack.

Christiansen, C.H. and Matuska, K.M. (2006) 'Lifestyle balance: a review of concepts and research.' *Journal of Occupational Science 13*, 1, 49–61.

Christiansen, C.H. and Townsend, E.A. (2004) 'An Introduction to Occupation.' In C.H. Christiansen and E.A. Townsend (eds) *An Introduction to Occupation: the Art and Science of Living.* Upper Saddle River, NJ: Prentice Hall.

Clark, E.A., Parham, D., Carlson, M.E., Frank, G. *et al.* (1991) 'Occupational science: academic innovation in the service of occupational therapy's future.' *American Journal of Occupational Therapy 45*, 4, 300–310.

Cohen, D.A., Wang, W., Wyatt, J.K., Kronauer, R.E. *et al.* (2010) 'Uncovering residual effects of chronic sleep loss on human performance.' *Science Translational Medicine 2*, 14, 14ra3.

Connor, J., Norton, R., Ameratunga, S., Robinson, E. *et al.* (2002) 'Driver sleepiness and risk of serious injury to car occupants: population based case control study.' *British Medical Journal 324*, 7346, 1125. Available at www.ncbi.nlm.nih.gov/pmc/articles/PMC107904/, accessed on 25 October 2011.

Doran, S.M., van Dongen, H.P.A. and Dinges, D.F. (2001) 'Sustained attention performance during sleep deprivation: evidence of state instability.' *Archives Italiennes de Biologie 139*, 3, 253–267.

Driver, H.S. and Taylor, S.R. (2000) 'Exercise and sleep.' *Sleep Medicine Reviews 4*, 4, 387–402.

Farnworth, L., Nikitin, L. and Fossey, E. (2004) 'Being in a secure forensic psychiatric unit: every day is the same, killing time or making the most of it.' *British Journal of Occupational Therapy 67*, 10, 430–438.

Finlay, L. (2004) *The Practice of Psychosocial Occupational Therapy*, 3rd edn. Cheltenham: Nelson Thornes.

Golledge, J. (1998) 'Distinguishing between occupation, purposeful activity and activity, part 1: review and explanation.' *British Journal of Occupational Therapy 61*, 3, 100–105.

Green, A. (2008) 'Sleep, occupation and the passage of time.' *British Journal of Occupational Therapy 71*, 8, 339–347.

Green, A., Hicks, J., Weekes, R. and Wilson, S. (2005) 'A cognitive-behavioural group intervention for people with chronic insomnia: an initial evaluation.' *British Journal of Occupational Therapy 68*, 11, 518–522.

Gunderson, M. (2001) 'Economics of personnel and human resource management.' *Human Resource Management Review 11*, 4, 431–452.

Habte-Gabr, E., Wallace, R.B., Colsher, P.L., Hulbert, J.R., White, L.R. and Smith, I.M. (1991) 'Sleep patterns in rural elders: demographic, health, and psychobehavioral correlates.' *Journal of Clinical Epidemiology 44*, 1, 5–13.

Harrison, Y. and Horne, J.A. (2000) 'The impact of sleep deprivation on decision making: a review.' *Journal of Experimental Psychology: Applied 6*, 3, 236–249.

Hoch, C.H., Reynolds, C.F., Kupfer, D.J., Houck, P.R., Berman, S.R. and Stack, J.A. (1987) 'The superior sleep of elderly nuns.' *International Journal of Aging and Human Development 25*, 1, 1–9.

Horne, J.A. (1993) 'Human sleep, sleep loss and behaviour: implications for the prefrontal cortex and psychiatric disorder.' *British Journal of Psychiatry 162*, 413–419.

Horne, J.A. (2006) *Sleepfaring.* Oxford: Oxford University Press.

Horne, J.A. and Minard, A. (1985) 'Sleep and sleepiness following a behaviourally "active" day.' *Ergonomics 28*, 3, 567–575.

Howell, D. and Pierce, D. (2000) 'Exploring the forgotten restorative dimension of occupation: quilting and quilt use.' *Journal of Occupational Science 7*, 2, 68–72.

Kielhofner, G. (2002) 'Habituation: Patterns of Daily Occupation.' In G. Kielhofner (ed.) *A Model of Human Occupation: Theory and Application*, 3rd edn. Baltimore, MD: Lippincott Williams & Wilkins.

Kielhofner, G. and Burke, J.P. (1985) 'Components and Determinants of Human Occupation.' In G. Kielhofner (ed.) *A Model of Human Occupation: Theory and Application.* Baltimore, MD: Williams & Wilkins.

Killgore, W.D.S., Kamimori, G.H. and Balkin, T.J. (2011) 'Caffeine protects against risk-taking propensity during severe sleep deprivation.' *Journal of Sleep Research 20*, 3, 395–403.

Kim, D.Y. (2007) 'Modafinil: the journey to promoting vigilance and its consideration by the military in sustaining alertness.' Available at www.docstoc.com/docs/76136036/Modafinil-the-military%E2%80%A6.rtf, accessed on 31 March 2012.

King, A.C., Orman, R.F., Brassington, G.S., Bliwise, D.L. and Haskell, W.L. (1997) 'Moderate-intensity exercise and self-rated quality of sleep in older adults: a randomized controlled trial.' *Journal of the American Medical Association 277*, 1, 32–37.

King, A.C., Pruitt, L.A., Woo, S., Castro, C.M. *et al.* (2008) 'Effects of moderate-intensity exercise on polysomnographic and subjective sleep quality in older adults with mild to moderate sleep complaints.' *Journals of Gerontology: Medical Sciences 63A*, 9, 997–1004.

Lader, D., Short, S. and Gershuny, J. (2006) *The Time Use Survey, 2005. How We Spend Our Time.* London: Office for National Statistics. Available at www.timeuse.org/files/cckpub/lader_short_and_gershuny_2005_kight_diary.pdf, accessed on 12 June 2012.

Li, F., Fisher, K.J., Harmer, P., Irbe, D., Tearse, R.G. and Weimer, C. (2004) 'Tai chi and self-rated quality of sleep and daytime sleepiness in older adults: a randomized controlled trial.' *Journal of the American Geriatrics Society 52*, 6, 892–900.

Lipsey, R. and Chrystal, A. (2007) *Economics*, 11th edn. Oxford: Oxford University Press.

MacKinnon, I. (1994) 'M40 crash driver "probably fell asleep".' *The Independent*, 30 June. Available at www.independent.co.uk/news/uk/m40-crash-driver-probably-fell-asleep-1425967.html, accessed on 8 October 2011.

Martin, P. (2002) *Counting Sheep: The Science and Pleasures of Sleep and Dreams.* London: HarperCollins.

Matuska, K.M. and Christiansen, C.H. (2008) 'A proposed model of lifestyle balance.' *Journal of Occupational Science 15*, 1, 9–19.

Meyer, A. (1977) 'The philosophy of occupational therapy.' *American Journal of Occupational Therapy 31*, 10, 639–642. (Original work published in 1922.)

Monk, T.H., Reynolds, C.F., Buysse, D.J., DeGrazia, J.M. and Kupfer, D.J. (2003) 'The relationship between lifestyle regularity and subjective sleep quality.' *Chronobiology International 20*, 1, 97–107.

Nasermoaddeli, A., Sekine, M., Kumari, M., Chandola, T., Marmot, M. and Kagamimori, S. (2005) 'Association of sleep quality and free time leisure activities in Japanese and British civil servants.' *Journal of Occupational Health 47*, 5, 384–390.

Ohayon, M.M., Zulley, J., Guilleminault, C., Smirne, S. and Priest, R.G. (2001) 'How age and daytime activities are related to insomnia in the general population: consequences for older people.' *Journal of the American Geriatrics Society 49*, 4, 360–366.

Philip, P. and Åkerstedt, T. (2006) 'Transport and industry safety: how are they affected by sleepiness and sleep restriction?' *Sleep Medicine Reviews 10*, 5, 347–356.

Rattenborg, N.C., Voirin, B., Vyssotski, A.L., Kays, R.W. *et al.* (2008) 'Sleeping outside the box: electroencephalographic measures of sleep in sloths inhabiting a rainforest.' *Biology Letters 4*, 4, 402–405.

Schabus, M., Gruber, G., Parapatics, S., Sauter, C. *et al.* (2004) 'Sleep spindles and their significance for declarative memory consolidation.' *Sleep 27*, 8, 1479–1485.

Schwartz, B. (1970) 'Notes on the sociology of sleep.' *The Sociological Quarterly 11*, 4, 485–499.

Shapiro, C.M., Bortz, R., Mitchell, D., Bartel, P. and Jooste, P. (1981) 'Slow-wave sleep: a recovery period after exercise.' *Science 214*, 4526, 1253–1254.

Sherrill, D.L., Kotchou, K. and Quan, S.F. (1998) 'Association of physical activity and human sleep disorders.' *Archives of Internal Medicine 158*, 17, 1894–1898.

Shimitras, L., Fossey, E. and Harvey, C. (2003) 'Time use of people living with schizophrenia living in a North London catchment area.' *British Journal of Occupational Therapy 66*, 2, 46–54.

Soupourmas, F. (2005) 'Work, rest and leisure – trends in late adolescent time use in Australia in the 1990s.' *Society and Leisure 28*, 2, 571–589.

Stewart, P. and Craik, C. (2007) 'Occupation, mental illness and medium security: exploring time-use in forensic regional secure units.' *British Journal of Occupational Therapy 70*, 10, 416–425.

Stickgold, R. (2005) 'Sleep-dependent memory consolidation.' *Nature 437*, 7063, 1272–1278.

Swanson, L.M., Arendt, J.T., Rosekind, M.R., Belenky, G., Balkin, T.J. and Drake, C. (2011) 'Sleep disorders and work performance: findings from the 2008 National Sleep Foundation Sleep in America poll.' *Journal of Sleep Research 20*, 3, 487–494.

Tang, N.K. and Harvey, A.G. (2005) 'Time estimation ability and distorted perception of sleep in insomnia'. *Behavioral Sleep Medicine 3*, 3, 134–150.

Tucker, A.M., Whitney, P., Belenky, G., Hinson, J.M. and van Dongen, H.P.A. (2010) 'Effects of sleep deprivation on dissociated components of executive functioning.' *Sleep 33*, 1, 47–57.

van Dongen, H.P.A., Maislin, G., Mullington, J.M. and Dinges, D.F. (2003) 'The cumulative cost of additional wakefulness: dose-response effects on neurobehavioral functions and sleep physiology from chronic sleep restriction and total sleep deprivation.' *Sleep 26*, 2, 117–126.

Van Someren, E.J.W. and Riemersma-van der Lek, R.F. (2007) 'Live to the rhythm, slave to the rhythm.' *Sleep Medicine Reviews 11*, 6, 465–484.

Wagner, U., Gais, S. and Born, J. (2001) 'Emotional memory formation is enhanced across sleep intervals with high amounts of rapid eye movement sleep.' *Learning and Memory 8*, 2, 112–119.

Wagner, U., Gais, S., Haider, H., Verlager, R. and Born, J. (2004) 'Sleep inspires insight.' *Nature 427*, 6972, 352–355.

Westhorp, P. (2003) 'Exploring balance as a concept in occupational science.' *Journal of Occupational Science 10*, 2, 99–106.

Wilcock, A.A. (2003) 'Occupational Science: the Study of Humans as Occupational Beings.' In P. Kramer, J. Hinjosa and C.B. Royeen (eds) *Perspectives in Human Occupation: Participation in Life.* Philadelphia, PA: Lippincott Williams & Wilkins.

Wilcock, A.A. (2006) *An Occupational Perspective of Health*, 2nd edn. Thorofare, NJ: Slack.

Wordsworth, W. (1801) 'To Sleep.' In J.O. Hayden (ed.) (1977) *William Wordsworth: The Poems*, Vol. 1. Harmondsworth: Penguin.

World Federation of Occupational Therapists (2010) Statement on Occupational Therapy. Available at www.wfot.org/Portals/0/PDF/Statement_on_Occupational_Therapy.pdf, accessed on 22 May 2012.

Wulff, K.L., Dijk, D.-J., Middleton, B., Foster, R.G. and Joyce, E. (2012) 'Sleep and circadian rhythm disruption in schizophrenia patients.' *British Journal of Psychiatry 200*, 4, 308–316.

Yaniv, G. (2004) 'Insomnia, biological clock, and the bedtime decision: an economic perspective.' *Health Economics 13*, 1, 1–8.

8

Recording and Quantifying Sleep

Nigel Hudson

8.1. Introduction

Several mentions of PSG and EEG are made in other chapters of this book: this chapter explains what they are. PSG is the short term for polysomnography, a recording of multiple physiological variables during overnight sleep. EEG, the abbreviation used for electroencephalogram,[1] is the most important of the various physiological parameters that make up the PSG. The abbreviations EEG and PSG are used throughout this chapter.

PSG is one of the steps in the diagnostic pathway for a number of sleep disorders, which are discussed in more detail in Chapter 9. Problems occurring in sleep may be categorized simply as follows:

- hypersomnias: being more sleepy than normal, characterized by falling asleep during the daytime and in inappropriate situations such as when driving or even when standing up

- hyposomnias or insomnias: not sleeping enough, or at all

- parasomnias: abnormal events during sleep, such as sleepwalking or other more bizarre behaviours

- circadian rhythm disorders: having one's body clock out of synchronization with the diurnal cycle

- nocturnal seizure events and epileptic events.

PSG may be helpful in any of the above conditions but will not be necessary in many cases which may be diagnosed by less expensive investigations such as oxygen saturation monitoring.

During PSG a minimum number of EEG channels (a channel being the waveform representing the voltage difference between two electrodes) must be recorded, as well as blood oxygen saturation, respiratory effort, oro-nasal airflow, the electrocardiogram (ECG), movement and sound. The respiratory parameters are measured to differentiate between various sleep-related breathing disorders such as obstructive sleep apnoea (OSA), central sleep apnoea and upper airway resistance syndrome.

This chapter focuses first on the EEG and how it came to be used to investigate the brain; how the EEG changed brain research; and how it advanced our understanding of sleep. It then describes each of the other variables, how they are measured and how they contribute to the assessment of sleep-related disorders.

8.2. Development of the EEG

The EEG is a recording of the tiny electrical potentials generated by neurons in the brain. In truth, recording the EEG seems intuitively not to be a very scientific endeavour: the technique may be likened to trying to investigate how a computer works by using a stethoscope to listen to noises inside it. A number of silver discs are applied to the scalp and connected to sensitive physiological amplifiers so that the fluctuations in electrical potential between pairs of electrodes are amplified and then displayed. The resulting squiggly lines on the computer screen are far removed from what is happening at the cellular level, but it turns out that they are a reliable means of non-invasively investigating the function of the brain. It is endlessly fascinating for those of us bitten by the bug, and it has never failed to amaze me that, when I apply the electrodes to a person's head and connect them to a recording instrument, I can watch the ever-changing patterns of oscillating waves that comprise the EEG. Over the years of the development of the

EEG, the careful application of scientific principles has resulted in the discipline of clinical neurophysiology.

The term 'electroencephalogram' is derived from the Greek word *encephalon*, meaning head, so, literally, it is a graph of the electrical activity of the head. Brain electrical activity is very small, and measured in microvolts, and it is very difficult to record because it is so easily obscured by various types of interference, such as 50Hz frequency from mains cables or appliances near the recording subject. Indeed, it is hard to imagine how it ever came to be used as the clinical tool it has become today, and looking back to the discovery of the EEG one wonders how and why Richard Caton, the Liverpool-based physician, managed to record brain activity at all.

Caton was working with the exposed brain of rabbits and cats rather than recording through the intact scalp but even so, the signals he was attempting to record were still very small. His recording instrument was a reflecting galvanometer which worked by the minute electrical currents causing movement of a small mirror which in turn deflected a spot of light projected onto a screen – an early form of amplification. In 1875 he recorded single channel EEG signals and the significance of this was that he recognized the dynamic nature of the EEG. He realized that the EEG recording changed when the brain was stimulated and therefore that brain activity reflected consciousness in a measurable way (Caton 1875).

It was not until 1924 that Hans Berger, a German psychiatrist, recorded the first human EEG, this time recording from beneath the scalp through burr holes in the skull. He had chosen subjects with skull defects in order to measure the pulsation of the brain caused by blood pressure changes during the cardiac cycle, and was the first to describe the alpha rhythm, the fundamental electrical oscillation of the waking brain (see below). It was discovered subsequently that the alpha rhythm is maximal when the brain is relaxed but alert. This property was exploited by manufacturers of 'alpha feedback' machines that were popular in the mid-1970s when transcendental meditation was in vogue. Meditation techniques were said to be enhanced by practising using the feedback machine, which used a few EEG electrodes placed on the scalp and which emitted a humming noise when maximum alpha activity was achieved. Alpha activity is attenuated, or diminished, by attention to visual or other stimuli or by concentration on something like mental arithmetic. It is also not seen during sleep and so its disappearance is an important marker of the onset of sleep.[2]

Berger did not manage to convince anyone that the EEG was a useful tool, but he sowed the seed, and subsequent scientists, notably Adrian and Matthews (1934), confirmed his findings and furthered the development of the EEG by making it a scientifically credible technique. Once it had been established that it was possible to record brain activity reliably, the way was open for the dynamic nature of the EEG to be exploited. Uniquely, the EEG could be shown to respond to various stimuli and the subsidiary technique of evoked potentials, where the brain's response to a specific stimulus is measured, was born. In 1937, William Grey Walter, working at the Burden Neurological Institute in Bristol, established that brain activity was also altered by brain pathology when he recorded the changes associated with a cerebral tumour (Grey Walter 1937). Whilst Berger (1929) was the first person to recognize spike and slow-wave activity during epileptic seizures using the EEG, during the 1930s in the USA Gibbs, Lennox and Gibbs showed inter-ictal (between-seizure) epileptic spikes to be an indicator of a liability to seizures (Gibbs, Lennox and Gibbs 1936).

For the purpose of description, the EEG signals are conventionally divided into frequency bands, similar to the division of radio frequencies into bands (both being arbitrary and for the purpose of convenience). The stages of sleep (N1–N3 – see Chapter 2) mentioned below will be described further below, but the bands are as follows.

Alpha rhythm: The first band to be discovered was the alpha rhythm and this is a rhythmic component which is of maximal amplitude over the posterior part of the scalp and between 8 and 13Hz in frequency. Amplitude is variable up to about 200 microvolts (a microvolt is a millionth of a volt usually abbreviated thus: μV) but it should be fairly symmetrical about the midline. As mentioned above, the alpha rhythm is normally reduced or abolished by visual attention (i.e. when the eyes are open); see Figure 8.1 on p157.

Beta activity: The next band to be described was, logically, named beta activity; this is the higher frequency, low amplitude activity, often diffusely distributed over the scalp at frequencies of above 13Hz up to about 30Hz. Again, this activity is seen in normal subjects where it should be symmetrical about the midline: it is not a significant feature of sleep.

Theta activity: This is the intermediate band between alpha and delta so this activity spans the range between 4 and 8Hz. It was named theta by Grey Walter due to his belief that it originated in the thalamus. This activity is mainly seen during light sleep (N1) where it gradually replaces the alpha rhythm; see Figure 8.2 on p.158.

Delta activity: This is the lowest frequency band and describes the slow waves below 4Hz. This activity is seen in deep sleep (N3) and there may be odd delta components during stage N2; see Figure 8.3 on p.158.

The bands are not therefore named in an apparently logical sequence but may be summarized thus:

- Delta = <4Hz
- Theta= 4–<8Hz
- Alpha = 8–13Hz
- Beta = >13–30Hz

A number of other sleep-related phenomena are recorded by the EEG. These are as follows.

Vertex sharp waves: As their name implies, these arise from the vertex area (the mid-central region, or topmost part of the skull); they are sharply contoured waves of relatively high amplitude. They are associated with arousal from sleep in response to stimuli, but are also seen spontaneously in stages N1 to N3; see Figure 8.2 on p.158.

K-complexes: These are a composite waveform comprising a vertex sharp wave, closely followed by a high amplitude slow (delta) wave also maximal at the vertex; when recorded in a bipolar montage[3] the sharp and slow wave complex forms a letter K; see Figure 8.3 on p.158.

Sigma activity: A rhythmic 12–14Hz component of sleep, usually occurring in brief bursts often referred to as *spindles* because of their characteristic outline. These are seen mainly in stages N2 and N3 sleep and often follow K-complexes; see Figure 8.3 on p.158.

Positive occipital sharp transients of sleep (POSTS): These are low amplitude, triangular waves recorded from the occipital region during stage N2 sleep, also referred to as lambdoid waves because of their similarity in waveform and distribution to the lambda waves seen during ocular movements in the waking EEG.

8.3. The EEG and sleep

The EEG has evolved from the single channel (single voltage/time curve) string galvanometer used in the 1920s by Berger, via multi-channel paper chart recorders, to the current standard of 32 channel digital recorders with simultaneous video recording and the even more advanced research systems with 128 or 256 channels. It has been instrumental in the development of our understanding of sleep.

In the 1930s it was thought that the brain in sleep was in a passive state and that it was awakened by sensory 'bombardment'. To test this hypothesis the Belgian neurophysiologist Frédéric Gaston Bremer performed experiments that cut the cat brain from its sensory inputs to see if the brain would then be asleep; the experiments cut the brain in different places. The so-called 'encephale isole' experiment sectioned the brain at the posterior medulla so that it still had sensory inputs from cranial nerves I, II, VI and VII (olfactory, visual, auditory/vestibular and facial senses). Following this operation the cortical EEG showed alternating cycles of sleep and waking, thus demonstrating that this lesion had not altered the ability to sleep and to awaken.

In the 'cerveau isole' preparation, the brain was sectioned just posterior to cranial nerve III, just anterior to the midbrain so that it still had sensory inputs only from cranial nerves I and II (olfactory and visual). Following this operation the cortical EEG showed only sleep EEG, so the ability to awaken had been destroyed.

Another transection lower in the brainstem had the effect of producing persistent insomnia – the Batani transection (Batini *et al.* 1959). This led to the notion that the cerveau isole cut the *output* of the ascending reticular activating system whilst the Batani transection, in the pons (part of the brainstem), cut the *input* to the ascending reticular activating system, leaving it permanently 'on' and the animal unable to go to sleep. The encephale isole, made at the junction of the brainstem and spinal cord, produced no effect because, in contrast to these other transactions, it had no effect on the ascending reticular activating system. These studies were valuable in showing that sleep was an active neural process dependent on brainstem mechanisms.

In 1953 Nathaniel Kleitman recognized the phenomenon of rapid eye movements (REM) in sleep and realized that subjects exhibiting these eye movements were easily aroused from sleep and that, when aroused, they were often able to recall dreams. Working with William Dement, Kleitman went on to use the EEG to help to define five stages of sleep (Dement and Kleitman 1957 and see below – and Chapter 2). Sleep staging has become the mainstay of sleep analysis and is the basis for the hypnogram – a graphical representation of the cyclical changes of sleep depth that occur normally throughout the night. Sleep staging came to be based on the work of Allan Rechtschaffen and Anthony Kales who refined the definitions and created a standardized method for staging sleep based on EEG activity, ocular movement and muscle activity (Rechtschaffen and Kales 1968). Sleep staging criteria were revised recently with the publication by the American Academy of Sleep Medicine of *The AASM Manual for the Scoring of Sleep and Associated Events* (Iber *et al.* 2007).[4] In 1960 Gerry Vogel reported that REM sleep begins near sleep onset in people with narcolepsy, rather than one to two hours later as in normal sleepers. This observation led to the development of the multiple sleep latency test (MSLT) for the diagnosis of narcolepsy (see below).

EEG hypnograms are now a familiar and very useful tool as they convey an impression of a night's sleep in an easily assimilated but informative way. It is thus possible, at a glance, to tell what sort of night a person has had. Unfortunately, arriving at the hypnogram is not so simple. It is usual to divide the overnight sleep EEG (of 7–9 hours) into epochs of 20 or 30 seconds and to score each epoch according to the AASM criteria. Traditionally, this has been carried out by the electroencephalographer 'eyeballing' each epoch and assigning a score. These days it is possible to let software do the scoring so that the hypnogram is available within seconds of the cessation of recording. However, experts differ in their estimations of how accurate software scoring is: estimates of accuracy range from about 50 to 90 per cent. In practice, most sleep experts do not entirely trust the output of automated scoring and insist on manual editing of the automated hypnogram. Once again, we are back to 'eyeballing' every epoch – although this is less daunting than it sounds as it is possible, with practice, to manually edit an automated hypnogram in a little over an hour.

There are, however, difficulties with sleep scoring using 30-second epochs in that it is possible to miss very brief changes of sleep stage. For instance, if an epoch begins with stage N3 sleep but after 20 seconds the subject awakens, that epoch is scored as stage N3; but, if the awakening occurs after 10 seconds, the epoch is scored as awake. There is obviously a trade-off between having a reasonable epoch to score, which does not take an excessive amount of time to analyse, and having a short epoch which captures very brief changes but which requires much more time to analyse. For clinical studies, 30 seconds appears to be fairly standard and the limitations are recognized but accepted.

Automatic sleep staging usually takes into account data from three to five channels of polygraphic data. However, to correct erroneously scored epochs more data may be recorded and may be used by the person reviewing the record:

- an EEG channel recording from the posterior part of the scalp to capture alpha rhythm
- an EEG channel recording near the vertex of the scalp to capture vertex sharp waves, K-complexes and sigma activity
- one or two electro-oculogram (EOG) channels, to capture rolling eye movements associated with drowsiness and rapid eye movements associated with REM sleep
- a sub-mental (under the chin) electromyography (EMG) channel to capture changes in, or loss of, muscle tone associated with REM sleep.

Scoring is relatively straightforward for the experienced polysomnographer. Various criteria are used in determining the stage of sleep that occupies at least 50 per cent of the epoch, and may be seen in Figures 8.1–8.5. The straightforward rules distinguish the various stages of sleep and lend themselves to automation but, as stated above, automated staging is not universally trusted as it can be shown to be inaccurate in some circumstances. Sleep staging is used to condense the information contained in an overnight EEG record to a single page of graphical information (see e.g. Figure 2.3 in Chapter 2).

Figures 8.1–8.5. Note

The letter and number combinations on the left of each image in Figures 8.1–8.5 refer to pairs of electrodes: each channel represents the ongoing voltage difference between the two electrodes. The electrodes are positioned according to the 10–20 international measurement system. The letters refer to the locations of the electrodes: C = central; F = frontal; O = occipital; T = temporal; A = mastoid; the numbers refer to which side of the head that they are on, with even numbers on the right side and odd numbers on the left: Z refers to the midline electrodes.

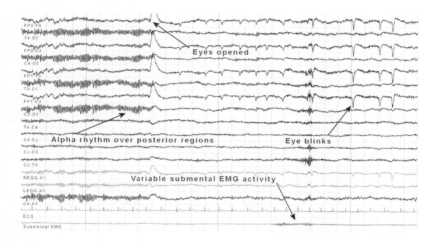

Figure 8.1. Awake: stage W

A 30-second epoch from a PSG recording showing wakefulness. A bilateral alpha rhythm is present over the posterior regions. When the patient opens their eyes the alpha rhythm blocks and eye blinks can then be seen over the anterior EEG channels as well as the EOG channels. Also note the presence of muscle activity which can often be seen on the EMG (electromyography) channel. Copyright © 2012 North Bristol NHS Trust.

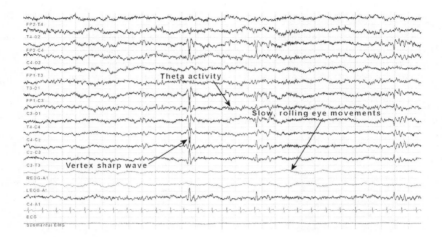

Figure 8.2. Stage N1 sleep

A 30-second epoch from a PSG recording showing stage 1 sleep. In order to score stage 1 sleep the alpha rhythm must not be present for >50% of the 30-second epoch and this figure shows that the alpha rhythm has disappeared and been replaced by low amplitude, mixed frequency activity, being predominantly 4–7Hz theta activity. A vertex sharp wave (which is not required to score stage 1 sleep) is also present along with slow eye movements which are often present during drowsiness and following sleep onset. Copyright © 2012 North Bristol NHS Trust.

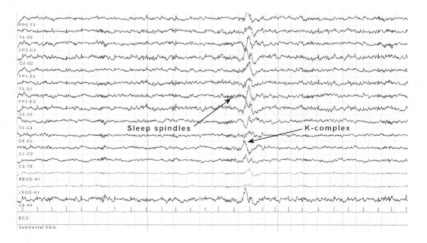

Figure 8.3. Stage N2 sleep

A 30-second epoch from a PSG recording showing stage 2 sleep. The onset of stage 2 sleep is determined by the appearance of sleep spindles or K-complexes. Vertex sharp waves can also be present. Copyright © 2012 North Bristol NHS Trust.

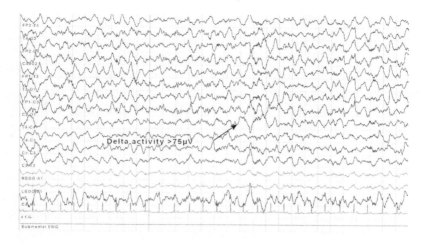

Figure 8.4. Stage N3 sleep – slow-wave sleep

A 30-second epoch from a PSG recording showing stage 3 sleep. Stage 3 sleep can be scored when >20% of a 30-second epoch comprises delta activity with frequencies of 0.5–2Hz and amplitudes of >75µV. Copyright © 2012 North Bristol NHS Trust.

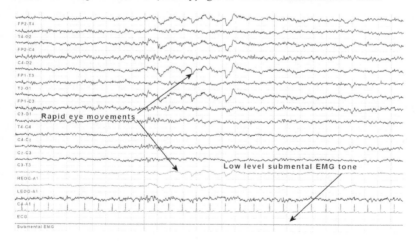

Figure 8.5. Rapid eye movement (REM) sleep

A 30-second epoch from a PSG recording showing REM sleep. During REM sleep the background of the EEG is similar to wake or stage 1 sleep with low amplitude, mixed frequency activity present. During REM sleep, rapid eye movements comprising of paroxysms of high amplitude activity with a relatively sharp outline occur over EOG, and often anterior EEG channels simultaneously. The submental EMG channel shows the lowest amplitude activity compared with all other stages. Copyright © 2012 North Bristol NHS Trust.

8.4. Diagnosing sleep disorders with EEG/PSG

Many people who carry out PSG prefer to use a full EEG montage rather than the minimal four or five channels required for sleep staging. The reason for this is that some nocturnal events, which may be assumed to be parasomnias of one kind or another, may in fact turn out to be epileptic seizures and need to be distinguished from them. If this is the case, it is much better to have a full head of electrodes so that seizure foci can be identified and the seizure type can be more reliably diagnosed.

Sleep is often regarded as an evocative technique in the study of epilepsy; that is to say that sleep is likely to increase the likelihood of capturing some abnormal activity. Many types of epilepsy exhibit more abnormal activity during sleep and there are some syndromes in which sleep recording is essential to the diagnosis. For example, conditions such as Tassinari Syndrome and Landau-Kleffner Syndrome show continuous epileptic spike activity during sleep.

Many focal epilepsies are more evident during sleep – notably, benign epilepsy with centro-temporal spikes. This condition causes nocturnal seizures in childhood but is a relatively innocuous condition characterized by prominent centro-temporal spikes in the waking EEG. Focal epilepsies of the frontal lobes are particularly likely to be more active during sleep and frontal lobe seizures are often confused with parasomnias due to their occasionally bizarre semiology. The notable thing about frontal lobe seizures is that there may be little or no electrographic evidence from the scalp EEG. This is where video EEG comes into its own: frontal lobe seizures exhibit some stereotypical clinical features that may be quite subtle. These, in association with the EEG (which often confirms that the seizure onset arises during slow-wave sleep [SWS]), may be the only clues to clinching the diagnosis and differentiating this condition from a parasomnia or an emotionally determined, behavioural disorder. On the other hand, sleep deprivation is known to increase the risk of seizures in some epileptic disorders.

8.5. Other aspects of polysomnography

As well as overnight EEG, a number of other measures are possible, according to the indications. The first of those mentioned here is very specific and usually carried out when narcolepsy is suspected, and much essential information for the diagnosis of sleep-related breathing disorders can be gained in respiratory metrics. It can also be important to record movement.

The *multiple sleep latency test* (MSLT)* that was devised by Carskadon and Dement (1977) enables the sleep latency to be measured accurately. Sleep latency is usually defined as time taken from 'lights out' to fall asleep with sleep onset defined as the first epoch of more than 15 seconds of cumulative sleep in a 30-second epoch. This is normally stage N1, but it can be any stage of sleep. In the MSLT a number of sleep opportunities are offered to the individual (usually four or five) at approximately two-hour intervals throughout the day.[5] The important metrics are the sleep latency, as defined above, and the REM latency, which is the time from sleep onset to the first two epochs of REM sleep. In normal sleep, individuals pass through stages N1 to N3 before entering REM sleep after about 90 minutes. However, people with narcolepsy may pass directly from waking to REM sleep; if a person enters REM sleep within 15 minutes of sleep onset this is called a sleep onset REM period (SOREMP), and if the person has two or more SOREMPs on more than two occasions during an MSLT, this is highly suggestive of narcolepsy. Care must be taken, however, as this criterion cannot be reliably applied if the individual is significantly sleep-deprived. Patients should have an overnight PSG to ensure that they are not sleep-deprived and that the MSLT can therefore give a valid result. The AASM guidelines for MSLT recommend a minimum of six hours of sleep during the night before (Littner *et al.* 2005).

Pulse oximetry detects the level of oxygen saturation in the blood and is thus able to indicate when ventilation becomes inadequate. The device used to measure this is a pulse oximeter that uses light absorption of two light sources at different wavelengths to compute the level of oxygenation of the blood haemoglobin (haemoglobin is the red pigment in blood and its colour ranges from a deep crimson to bright scarlet depending on the oxygen saturation level). Pulse oximeters, which clip on a finger or earlobe overnight, are non-invasive and relatively inexpensive. They provide a secondary function in that they also record the pulse wave that provides another useful measurement as pulse rate is another useful indicator of the level of arousal.

Respiratory effort sensors indicate whether ventilatory effort in the chest and abdomen is adequate and can therefore differentiate obstructive causes (collapsed airway) from central causes (lack of ventilatory drive). Respiratory effort sensors are usually bands made from elastic material that encircle the chest and abdomen. An oscillating current passing through a wire within the band is modulated by changes in the circumference of the band as the chest and abdomen expand and contract; consequent changes in the impedance of the wire, caused by the ventilatory movement, are the basis of the recording.

Oro-nasal airflow can be measured by the detection of changes of temperature associated with the cool inhaled air and the warm exhaled air at the mouth and nose. This is achieved with the aid of thermistors, or thermocouples, attached to the face near the mouth and nose. Alternatively, airflow can be measured with a pressure transducer attached to a nasal cannula.

The *electrocardiogram* (ECG) is also recorded because it relates to arousal, and a derivative measurement known as the pulse transit time (PTT) can be used to estimate blood pressure (BP), which can increase in sleep apnoea. PTT is derived from the ECG and the pulse wave from the pulse oximeter. It relies on the theory that, when blood vessels are non-compliant (i.e. the smooth muscles in the walls of arteries are contracted), BP increases. When the arteries are in this relatively inelastic state, the time taken between the contraction of the heart muscle (co-incident with the QRS complex of the ECG) and the arrival of the pulse wave at the extremities (usually the index finger) is reduced. The resulting metric (PTT) is inversely proportional to the BP, and there are algorithms that calculate the BP based on PTT which are said to be reasonably accurate, thereby obviating the need for intrusive measures involving periodic inflation of a cuff.

Movement can be measured using video recording and computer software that is able to log the number of pixel changes during each epoch of time. It is then possible to graphically represent movements so that periods of movement can be easily identified. This enables conditions such as periodic limb movements[6] of sleep to be diagnosed; it also enables movements associated with epilepsy and parasomnias, such as sleepwalking or REM sleep behaviour disorder, to be found quickly. The video recording can then be reviewed to ascertain the details of the movement event. Alternatively, limb movements can be measured using accelerometers as in actigraphy (below) or by recording EMG of moving muscles.

Actigraphy is often used in the investigation of circadian rhythms and their disorders. This uses an accelerometer, a movement sensor, usually worn on the wrist that detects whether the person is moving or still. The movements are logged over time so that it is possible to condense many hours or even days of continuous recording into a graph showing periods of activity and quiescence. It has been shown that periods of quiescence are strongly correlated with sleep, and so it is possible, without using the EEG, to get a fairly accurate assessment of the proportion of time spent asleep by an individual wearing an actigraph, coupled with his/her own activity log. Mounted on a wrist strap the device is quite unobtrusive and therefore does not affect the study; this is in contrast to the PSG that involves sleeping in a strange environment as well as being attached to electrodes and wires. Obviously, the wealth of information contained in the PSG is not available, but the very simple recording of activity enables some very useful information to be obtained in the investigation of, and research into, insomnia and circadian rhythm disorders; see Figure 8.6, for example.

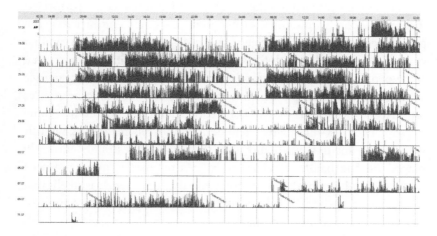

Figure 8.6. Actigraph analysis

The chart shows two days per row. The patient's sleep is fairly disrupted, with variations in sleep onset and awakenings. The patient consistently went to bed very late. On working days he woke between 7 a.m. and 8 a.m.: at weekends he went to bed slightly later and extended his time in bed until 10 a.m. or 12 noon. The actigraph clearly shows a delay in the major sleep period in relation to the patient's desired sleep and wake times. This sleep pattern suggests a circadian rhythm disorder of the delayed sleep type. Copyright © 2012 North Bristol NHS Trust.

8.6. Concluding comments

It is crucial to interpret a PSG, and all other data, in a holistic manner, taking all the parameters into account. It is easy to pounce on an obviously abnormal parameter and make a diagnosis based on this alone whilst missing other, perhaps more subtle, but no less significant, features. To adequately report a PSG, it is necessary to view it in several passes concentrating on one or a few channels at a time. Current technology makes it folly not to include video as one of the recordings; there are innumerable cases where confusing or ambiguous graphical data can be resolved quickly by viewing the video recording.

Diagnosis of many sleep disorders is aided by PSG but there are limits to its utility. For example, it has little to offer in the investigation of insomnia apart, perhaps, from exacerbating the problem by adding the discomfort of trying to sleep with a host of transducers attached. However, it is possible that some people complaining of insomnia benefit from having undergone PSG because it may demonstrate to them that their sleep is better than they think – if they subsequently worry less about their sleep.

The complexity of a full PSG means that it is usually only performed in hospitals or sleep clinics, rather than at home. The fact that the person being investigated is sleeping in a strange bed and an unfamiliar environment, coupled with the application of multiple transducers that some people find uncomfortable, means that people rarely experience a 'normal' night's sleep – at least not on the first night. Some centres routinely book subjects for two consecutive nights in order to overcome the so-called 'first-night effect' and obtain more reliable results, but this is by no means universal, and with the financial restraints currently placed on the health services, most centres use a single night of recording and accept the limitations that that imposes. It is likely that in the future, technological advances – increasing miniaturization of electronic components and innovative design of clinical systems – will enable full PSG to be offered to patients in their own homes. This would have huge advantages in both cost and effectiveness: first, it would virtually eliminate the first-night effect, and would improve the diagnostic accuracy of PSG; second, it would enormously reduce the cost of the procedure and make it more accessible to more people.

Acknowledgements

The editors are grateful to Kelly Blake and Peter Walsh of the Grey Walter Department of Neurophysiology at Frenchay Hospital, Bristol, for assistance in the final preparation of the typescript for this chapter and compiling the illustrations.

Notes

1. In the same way that PSG could also stand for polysomnography and polysomnogram, EEG also stands for electroencephalography: the distinction is usually clear from the context.

2. It might seem counterintuitive that alpha rhythm is weaker when concentrating on something, is strong when relaxed, and absent in sleep, since we need to relax for sleep. What happens is that as drowsiness builds, the alpha rhythm becomes intermittent and begins to wax and wane in amplitude. During the waning phases, it is replaced by intermittent theta. Gradually, the alpha periods become shorter, and the theta longer, until the alpha disappears altogether. This can happen over several minutes or within ten seconds.

3. The montage is the arrangement of pairs of electrodes on the head representing a series of channels.

4. Sleep stages were re-categorized to create stages N1–N3 in place of stages S1–4. See also Chapter 2.

5. Nap times vary depending on if and when the patient falls asleep. For clinical MSLTs the recording is continued for 15 minutes from the first epoch greater than 15 seconds of cumulative sleep (any stage of sleep) in a 30-second epoch, or for a maximum of 20 minutes if the patient does not sleep at all.

6. Periodic limb movements in sleep are repetitive leg movements; they are usually stereotyped and most often bilateral. 'In periodic limb movement disorder (PLMD), by definition, there needs to be a clinical consequence on sleep quality or daytime wakefulness caused by the leg movements' (Wetter 2010, p.87). It is commonly associated with restless legs syndrome (an urge to move the legs, often accompanied by unpleasant sensations) and can be categorized as a sleep-related movement disorder.

References

Adrian, E.D. and Matthews, B.H.C. (1934) 'The Berger Rhythm – potential changes from the occipital lobes in man.' *Brain 57*, 4, 355–384.

Batini, C., Moruzzi, G., Palestini, J., Rossi, G.F. and Zanchetti, A. (1959) 'Effects of complete pontine transaction on the sleep wakefulness rhythm: the mid-pontine pretrigeminal preparation.' *Archivio Italienne de Biologie 97*, 1–12.

Berger, H. (1929) 'Über das elektrenkephalogramm des Menschen.' *Archiv für Psychiatrie und Nervenkrankheiten 87*, 527–570.

Carskadon, M.A. and Dement, W.C. (1977) 'Sleep tendency: an objective measure of sleep loss.' *Sleep Research 6*, 200.

Caton, R. (1875) 'The electric currents of the brain.' *British Medical Journal 2*, 278.

Dement, W. and Kleitman, N. (1957) 'The relation of eye movements during sleep to dream activity: an objective method for the study of dreaming.' *Journal of Experimental Psychology 53*, 5, 339–346.

Gibbs, F.A., Lennox, W.G. and Gibbs, E.L. (1936) 'The electroencephalogram in diagnosis and in localization of epileptic seizures.' *Archives of Neurology and Psychiatry 36*, 1225–1235.

Grey Walter, W. (1937) 'The electroencephalogram in cases of cerebral tumour.' *Proceedings of the Royal Society of Medicine 30*, 5, 579–598.

Iber, C., Ancoli-Israel, S., Chesson, A. and Quan, S.F. (2007) *The AASM Manual for the Scoring of Sleep and Associated Events: Rules, Terminology and Technical Specification.* Westchester, IL: American Academy of Sleep Medicine.

Littner, M.R., Kushida, C., Wise, M., Davila, D.G. *et al.* (2005) 'Practice parameters for clinical use of the multiple sleep latency test and the maintenance of wakefulness test.' *Sleep 28*, 1, 113–121.

Rechtschaffen, A. and Kales, A. (1968) *A Manual of Standardised Terminology, Techniques and Scoring System for Sleep Stages in Normal Subjects.* Washington, DC: United States Department of Health and Welfare.

Wetter, T.C. (2010) 'Restless Legs Syndrome and Periodic Limb Movement Disorder.' In S. Overeem and P. Reading (eds) *Sleep Disorders in Neurology: A Practical Approach.* Chichester: Wiley-Blackwell.

Further reading

Kroker, K. (2007) *The Sleep of Others and the Transformations of Sleep Research.* Toronto: Toronto University Press.

Shneerson, J.M. (2005) *Sleep Medicine: A Guide to Sleep and its Disorders,* 2nd edn. Oxford: Blackwell Publishing.

Stradling, J.R. (1993) *Handbook of Sleep-related Breathing Disorders.* Oxford: Oxford University Press.

9

Broken Sleep

SLEEP DISORDERS

Jane Hicks and Andrew Green

9.1. Introduction

The importance of good sleep, which has been described in other chapters, is perhaps brought home to the individual when a sleep disorder develops and sleep is disrupted. Most people probably think of a sleep disorder as having too little sleep, but sleeping too much, or at the wrong time, can be equally disruptive to everyday life; and there are also problems, known as parasomnias, that occur during sleep.

Sleep disorders have received increasing publicity in the last 10–15 years. There is a large sleep medicine 'industry' in North America, where diagnosis and management of sleep disorders are widely covered by medical insurance, and where the number of clinics specializing in sleep tripled during the 1990s, whilst in the UK there is now a growing interest in the field. Sleep disorders are important because they can be associated with, or cause, other illness: some research even shows sleeping too little or too much can be associated with a shortened lifespan (Kripke *et al.* 1979). Recent research has demonstrated that lack of sleep could be a risk factor for obesity in children (Bell and Zimmerman 2010; Chaput *et al.* 2011). Other important sleep-related problems or hazards include the increased risk of hip fracture

in the elderly on sleeping pills (Vermeeren 2004)[1] and the greater
cardiovascular risks amongst sleep apnoea sufferers (Bradley and Floras
2009). The consequences of heightened sleepiness in people with sleep
apnoea or narcolepsy (Maclean, Davies and Thiele 2003; Mazza *et al.*
2006) pose further risks to individuals and to society at large.

Classification of sleep disorders can be difficult because, as in the case
of insomnia, terms can be used as a diagnosis, a symptom or a complaint,
but a particular problem is distinguishing between disorders of sleep *per
se* and disturbed sleep that is a feature of another disorder. The distinction
between primary and secondary insomnia is discussed below, but, for
example, sleep may be disturbed in people with dementia when there
have been degenerative changes in the biological clock with subsequent
disturbance of circadian rhythms. Conversely, sleep difficulties can cause
other problems: obstructive sleep apnoea is essentially a problem related
to breathing that disturbs sleep, but there is evidence that it is also
associated with changes in the brain that could cause motor dysfunction
and cognitive decline (Morrell *et al.* 2010). There is a close connection
between Parkinson's disease and sleep problems.[2] Furthermore, the same
symptom of sleep disorder can be caused by a number of processes; for
example, excessive daytime sleepiness can relate to a breathing difficulty
or a movement disorder that disturbs night-time sleep, or by a disruption
in the timing of sleep. However, such complications aside, sleep problems
may be classified as follows:

- insomnia – sleeping too little, interrupted sleep or unrefreshing
  sleep

- hypersomnia – excessive daytime sleepiness and sleeping too
  much

- parasomnia – unusual happenings in sleep such as sleepwalking
  and night terrors

- circadian rhythm disorders – sleeping at the wrong time.

It is not possible to cover comprehensively all sleep disorders here –
other books do that. For example, Wilson and Nutt (2008) provide an
accessible and concise summary and Kryger, Roth and Dement (2011)
an encyclopaedic guide. Instead, this chapter focuses on sleeping too
little (insomnia), the most common sleep complaint; two different
ways that people sleep too much or are sleepy by day (narcolepsy
and sleep apnoea); and on some of the problems that occur in sleep

(parasomnias). It also looks briefly at disrupted sleep patterns (circadian rhythm disorders).

9.2. Insomnia

Defined as 'complaints of disturbed sleep in the presence of adequate opportunity and circumstance for sleep' (NIH 2005, p.5), insomnia has been identified and discussed by the scientific community for over 2000 years, since Aristotle's monograph on sleeplessness was written in 350 BCE (see also Summers-Bremner 2008). History is strewn with creative and powerful people said to have suffered from insomnia: Charles Dickens, William Wordsworth, Thomas Edison, Groucho Marx, Sir Isaac Newton and Napoleon Bonaparte, for example, and several US presidents including Abraham Lincoln and Theodore Roosevelt. Winston Churchill's[3] poor sleep may well have been related to his recurrent depression and there are unverified suggestions that his successor Margaret Thatcher's[4] famously short sleep was actually the consequence of difficulty getting off to sleep. However, there is still no overall agreement between patients, healthcare professionals and sleep researchers on what exactly constitutes insomnia. This is partly because the term 'insomnia' is used as both a symptom and a diagnosis.

In a sleep clinic patients typically report one or more of the following:

- difficulty falling asleep (initial insomnia)
- difficulty in maintaining sleep (sleep maintenance insomnia)
- early morning wakening and difficulty returning to sleep.

Furthermore, to make a diagnosis – and to meet diagnostic criteria for research (Edinger *et al.* 2004) – there should be a complaint of daytime impairment because of poor sleep. This, perhaps, is something of a truism since without daytime consequences people are likely to assume that they simply need less sleep than others, or than they once did, and may be glad of the extra hours in the day. Many people report that they experience a reasonable period of sleep but do not feel refreshed on waking. Unrefreshing sleep, however, is no longer included in the definition of insomnia (NIH 2005, p.5), but it remains a common complaint in a sleep clinic and the consequences can be very disabling; it could be due to many things, including another sleep disorder or another medical condition entirely, and it is therefore important to investigate the causes. Insomnia has been considered to be 'chronic' after persisting for six months, or for as little as 30 days (NIH 2005, p.5).

Discussion about insomnia is made complicated by confusing differences between terms and the various mental health classifications – International Classification of Diseases (ICD-10),[5] Diagnostic and Statistical Manual of Mental Disorders (DSM-IV)[6] and the International Classification of Sleep Disorders (ICSD-2)[7] – and their revisions. For detailed discussion on classification see Buysse (2003) or Thorpy (2011), but for the purposes of this chapter it is sufficient to consider the term 'primary insomnia' and to differentiate it from other terms. The ICSD-2 lists a variety of types of primary insomnia, including psychophysiologic insomnia[8] (see Table 9.1), whereas DSM-IV simply lists primary insomnia. For everyday purposes the terms 'primary insomnia' and 'psychophysiological insomnia' are often used interchangeably in that they refer to insomnia that is not the result of any other condition, or a consequence of the behaviour of the individual.

Primary and psychophysiological insomnia have to be distinguished from secondary insomnia that, as implied, is secondary to something else. A consensus conference proposed that secondary insomnia be known as 'comorbid' insomnia because 'the direction of causality' (NIH 2005, p.6) cannot be determined with certainty: does the accompanying condition play a causal role in the insomnia? Is it the consequence of the insomnia? Is it incidental to the insomnia? It was also felt that the term 'secondary insomnia' could lead to under-treatment. Comorbid insomnia is therefore insomnia that occurs in the context of a known mental or physiological condition. However, Thorpy (2011) notes that 'secondary' is still an appropriate term 'when there is a clear development of insomnia related to the underlying medical or psychiatric disorder' as in pain disorders (p.688). In any case, there is a high prevalence of insomnia co-existing with one or more psychiatric or medical conditions, with particularly high rates seen in patients with depression, chronic pain, respiratory conditions and diabetes. It is important to treat insomnia and the comorbid condition simultaneously, as separate conditions: this may result in greater improvements in each than there would be if treating either condition alone. Table 9.1 summarizes the ICSD-2 classification of insomnia and some possible causes.

Table 9.1. ICSD-2 categories of insomnia

Primary insomnia	
Adjustment sleep disorder	Acute insomnia which is associated with particular stressful events or circumstances
Psychophysiological insomnia	Insomnia not resulting from the individual's behaviour or from any other condition
Paradoxical insomnia	Formerly known as sleep state misperception where the patient reports little sleep (or none) but has inconsistent daytime impairment. The patient copes better than would be expected on the small amount of sleep they believe they have had
Idiopathic insomnia	Long-standing insomnia that starts in childhood
Inadequate sleep hygiene	Insomnia resulting from activity that is not conducive to sleep, including irregular sleep/wake schedule
Behavioural insomnia of childhood	Lack of limit setting or dependence on inappropriate associations (see Chapter 5)
Secondary insomnia	
Insomnia due to a mental disorder	Possible causes: depressive disorders, bipolar disorders, psychotic disorders, anxiety disorders, eating disorders
Insomnia due to a drug or substance	Use or abuse of, or withdrawal from, psycho-active substances: alcohol, caffeine, hypnotics, anxiolytics, cocaine, amphetamines, opioids
Insomnia due to a medical condition	Possible causes: arthritis, heart disease, cerebrovascular disease, gastric ulcer, gastrointestinal disease, obesity, food allergy, migraine, menopause, head injury, epilepsy, Parkinson's disease, Huntington's disease

The difficulty in defining insomnia makes it hard to establish its prevalence although it has been attempted through questionnaire and interview surveys that ask about 'difficulty sleeping' (at least two sleep complaints on three nights a week) but without regard to clinical significance or causal factors. For example, a survey of the general population of five northern European countries estimated the prevalence of severe insomnia to be between 4 and 22 per cent (Chevalier *et al.* 1999).[9] It was higher in women than men but was not related to increasing age (although most studies do indicate that insomnia is more common amongst the elderly). According to Roth (2007), about a third of people will suffer with some symptoms of insomnia, whereas about a tenth meet diagnostic requirements if daytime impairment is included (see also LeBlanc *et al.* 2009).

In the survey described above (Chevalier *et al.* 1999), insomnia was found to have a negative impact on the quality of life of respondents and the degree of impairment was directly related to the severity of insomnia. People with severe insomnia also showed a higher level of healthcare consumption. Amongst the consequences of insomnia are susceptibility to accidents (including road traffic accidents), medical and psychiatric morbidity, poor performance at work, absenteeism and increased mortality (Chilcott and Shapiro 1996; Wilson *et al.* 2010). Daytime tiredness and functional impairment in the daytime are also often complained of, but there is less clear evidence from laboratory studies for a decrease in alertness or performance in people suffering from chronic insomnia. Also, people with insomnia typically observe that they cannot sleep during the day either. This suggests that high arousal levels could be the problem. Primary insomnia, as Horne puts it, is a '24 h disorder affecting both waking and sleeping life and is more a disorder of wakefulness that intrudes into sleep' and is 'secondary to a poor quality of waking life and persistent hyperarousal' (Horne 2010, p.6).

Insomnia sufferers have a higher prevalence of psychiatric disorder: amongst one sample of patients consulting their primary care doctor about insomnia, 53 per cent presented with psychiatric symptoms (Charon, Dramaix and Mendlewicz 1989). The risk of depression is probably four times higher in people with insomnia (Sandor and Shapiro 1994), whereas the complaint of insomnia may be an early marker for psychiatric disorders such as depression and anxiety (see Chapter 10). Some people use alcohol to help them get to sleep and there is an association between insomnia and alcohol abuse (Stein and Friedmann 2005); the rate of alcohol and other substance abuse is increased amongst people with insomnia compared to the rate in good sleepers.

But all the evidence of negative consequences of poor sleep does not adequately describe the experience of chronic insomnia. Everyone occasionally has a few bad nights' sleep, but the actual impact that insomnia has on people's lives has been demonstrated in two small focus group studies. Participants in a study in the USA by Carey *et al.* (2005) described the struggle to carry on with so little sleep, and complained of the lack of understanding from other people and the sense of isolation that might result from that. They also complained of the failure of doctors to understand their problems, and were particularly frustrated at being told they were depressed, whereas for them their low mood was the *consequence* of the poor sleep. In the UK Green, Hicks and Wilson (2008) made similar findings in a study involving six women, with an average age 50 (see Box 9.1).

Box 9.1. Experiences of insomnia

'It impacts on your *whole* life.'

'You go through your whole life under a blanket of tiredness and exhaustion.'

'It's affected my level of concentration and my level of safety.'

'It just means to me that I can't do what I want to do in the day because I've had such a bad night. That's one of the overwhelming things. [For example]…the garden needs doing badly and I just think: oh I can't face it.'

'I knew I wasn't safe to be in charge of a car and, because I knew that, I wasn't safe to be in charge [at work].'

'It's dominated and shaped my entire life… [For example,] it affects your sex life because no one will sleep with me because I can't go to sleep at night.'

'I'm very scared of not having the chance to do the things I wanted to do. If I was [like this] in 10 years' time I wouldn't dream of having children. I'm scared that I'm not going to be able to go back to my studies and go to university.'

Amongst people presenting to sleep clinics psychophysiological insomnia is most commonly seen in middle-aged women, usually starting during their thirties. Patients often describe themselves previously as light sleepers and present with a relatively long history of poor sleep, waxing and waning in severity, and precipitated perhaps by a bout of depressive illness.

Sometimes, insomnia develops by gradually 'feeding on itself', and a hallmark of psychophysiological insomnia is the particular focus of patients on their sleep problem whilst the same patients often minimize other mental or emotional concerns. A number of models, of varying complexity, have been devised to explain the way that insomnia develops (see Perlis *et al.* 2011). For example, in describing the 'attention–intention–effort pathway' to persistent insomnia, Espie *et al.* (2006) suggest that good sleepers approach sleep without thinking about it, without a plan, and probably could not explain how they sleep successfully. On the other hand, if someone in a period of acute insomnia begins to pay attention to the process of sleeping and pays selective attention to their internal environment (such as bodily sensations) and their external environment (e.g. by clock watching), they prevent the necessary disengagement that precedes sleep. Attention to a perceived threat spontaneously leads to action, and a specific intention to sleep develops, further inhibiting the natural decrease in arousal needed for sleep onset. Subsequent active effort to sleep compounds the problem. Espie *et al.* (2006) note that, in a similar way, 'paying attention to, and attempting to take control of, the actions of your feet as you run downstairs' (p.220) is likely to diminish performance. Models such as the 'attention–intention–effort pathway' underlie the rationale for cognitive behavioural therapy of insomnia (CBT-I) (see below).

The management of insomnia depends initially on taking a good history as it is important to treat potential causes of sleeplessness. This should include questions about psychiatric symptoms and previous medications as well as alcohol use. Sleep diaries may be useful and all patients should be advised about good sleep hygiene.* The duration and cause of the insomnia should be a guide to treatment with medication. If a patient has insomnia associated with depression, an antidepressant is a useful choice, particularly one with sedating properties. Sleep disturbances related to circadian rhythms, such as jet lag, shift work, delayed and advanced sleep phase syndrome, can be treated with medication such as melatonin. Recent guidelines on the treatment of insomnia in the UK and USA (NICE 2004; NIH 2005) recommend only short-term use of the most recently developed hypnotic medications (often known as the 'z-drugs': zopiclone, zolpidem and zaleplon). These might be used appropriately for the treatment of transient insomnia (e.g. because of stress over exams). Short-acting benzodiazepines such as temazepam can also be used. All these drugs tend to be absorbed quickly, have a minimal time to peak concentration and are eliminated swiftly with minimal hangover effects (see Chapter 11).

If further or longer-term treatment of insomnia is required, patients should have access to CBT-I (NICE 2004; NIH 2005). CBT-I consists of a variety of strategies (see Box 9.2).

Box 9.2. Cognitive behavioural strategies for managing insomnia

Stimulus control aims to strengthen the association between the bedroom and sleep by not staying in bed if not asleep – typically after 15 minutes. The bed is for sleep and sex only. The person should not go to bed unless sleepy and should avoid daytime naps.

Sleep restriction/sleep scheduling restricts time in bed to the person's usual average sleep time or six hours – whichever is the greater. The homeostatic drive to sleep should take over and allow the person to begin to consolidate sleep in the available time. The time in bed can then be gradually increased.

Cognitive therapy teaches the person to challenge the unhelpful and ill-informed beliefs about sleep and insomnia and its daytime consequences that perpetuate the vicious cycle of insomnia.

Paradoxical intent aims to alleviate anxiety about sleep in that the person tries to remain awake in bed with their eyes open.

Imagery is a technique of engaging the mind sufficiently to prevent anxiety-provoking thought by, typically, creating and rehearsing a detailed image of oneself in some pleasant place such as a beach or the countryside.

Relaxation is an essential part of 'winding down' for sleep, and some people benefit from formal training. Various methods exist to reduce muscle tension and physiological arousal but, like any skill, practice is needed over a period of weeks in order to be able to relax at will in bed.

This treatment can be given in an individual or group format (NIH 2005) or, for self-management of milder insomnia, a variety of self-help books is available (e.g. Espie 2006; Wiedman 1999). The limited availability of CBT-I is the main barrier to its use, even though its effectiveness has been shown to be equivalent to medication in the short term (Riemann and Perlis 2009; Smith *et al.* 2002), and even superior to medication up to 24 months after treatment (NIH 2005). Current research is therefore focused on ways of providing CBT-I in the most accessible and cost-effective ways (Espie 2009; Siriwardena *et al.* 2009).

9.3. Excessive daytime sleepiness

Two prominent causes of excessive daytime sleepiness (EDS) that are discussed here are obstructive sleep apnoea (OSA) and narcolepsy. Other causes are:

- insufficient opportunity for sleep at night: EDS is likely to improve with extended sleep (at weekends, or on holiday)

- circadian rhythm disorders (see below): for example, advanced and delayed sleep phase syndrome, shift work, jet lag

- idiopathic hypersomnolence (excessive sleeping for no known cause) – prolonged unrefreshing nocturnal sleep with long daytime naps: it is very rare

- sleep-related movement disorder (periodic limb movements or PLMs) – restless legs in the evening, or repetitive limb movements that disrupt sleep

- head injury (see Chapter 10)

- other medical disorders that interfere with sleep: for example, chronic pain or depression

- drugs – such as longer-acting hypnotic drugs – and side effects of other drugs (e.g. anticonvulsants).

OSA

OSA[10] is a significant cause of EDS. During sleep, relaxation of the upper airway (the throat) leads to reduced airflow and decreased oxygen levels in the blood, which in turn leads to arousal in order to stimulate breathing in response to the primary biological drive to breathe. This pattern of intermittent arousals can continue all night, but the patient is usually unaware because awakenings last a few seconds only, although, classically, the bed partner will report constant noisy cessations of breathing. These arousals, and loss of quality sleep, are what lead to the daytime sleepiness. Collapse of the airway is more pronounced when there is more soft tissue around the neck of an obese patient. It is this that led to the condition being called the Pickwickian syndrome by Burwell *et al.* (1956, p.812), after a character described by Charles Dickens in *The Pickwick Papers*: 'a fat and red-faced boy in a state of somnolency' (Dickens 1993, p.54, first published in 1836–37). Burwell *et al.* (1956) also cite an early-nineteenth-century medical text referring to a 'very fat' tradesman of about 30 whose somnolency was such that 'he could scarce keep awake whilst he described his situation' although 'in all other respects he was well' (p.811). This would plainly have been a problem in those days, but OSA is now a major problem as it is a risk factor for road traffic accidents. For example, Phillips and Kryger (2011) cite estimates that the risk of road traffic accident increases by between two and seven times amongst people with OSA compared with people unaffected by it. OSA also increases the risk of cardiovascular disease and of stroke (Yaggi *et al.* 2005). Prevalences amongst middle-aged people of 2 per cent in females and 4 per cent in men have been estimated (Young *et al.* 1993), although OSA is likely to become more common with increasing rates of obesity.[11]

The main symptom of OSA is EDS, whilst at night there tends to be loud snoring and interruptions in breathing. The individual might wake in the morning with a dry mouth, sore throat and a headache. Other signs that might increase suspicion of the presence of OSA include obesity – having a collar size of more than 17 inches is a simple indicator of increased risk. Suspected sleep apnoea needs full investigation (usually after initial home oximetry screening: see Chapter 8), with overnight monitoring of measures of blood oxygen saturation, respiratory effort and nasal airflow. An index of breathing pauses or reductions (hypopnoeas) per hour is calculated as an apnoea-hypopnoea index (AHI). Over five per hour is the usual cut-off point for diagnosis, although in severe cases the AHI is over 50.

Weight reduction can be very effective in management, but the treatment most widely used is continuous positive airway pressure (CPAP). The patient wears a nasal mask at night through which a machine blows air to keep the airway open. Improvement in the patient's sleep quality, and in quality of life, can be noticed quickly, although many patients find the equipment troublesome or uncomfortable and give up with it. However, the equipment is quite portable and surprisingly quiet, and the resolution of daytime symptoms often convinces the patient to use it.

Narcolepsy

Narcolepsy is a serious and chronic neurological disorder. It is characterized by excessive daytime sleepiness and brief attacks of weakness upon emotional arousal, known as cataplexy. It was first described in France in 1880 by the neurologist Gelineau, and has the reputation in medicine for being the condition with the longest time from onset to diagnosis – maybe as long as 20 years in some cases. This is perhaps due to sufferers being labelled as simply idle (appearing to fall asleep all the time), narcolepsy being misdiagnosed as epilepsy, or the associated hallucinations being misdiagnosed as a psychiatric disorder.

The most common presenting complaint of narcolepsy is excessive sleepiness, with the sudden onset of sleep or 'sleep attacks'. As well as sleepiness there are often attacks of cataplexy, where there is sudden loss of muscle tone without loss of consciousness. This can lead to dropping to the ground but it can be partial, with head nodding, sagging of the jaw or weakening of the knees: patients often describe the feeling that someone has hit the back of their knees. It is particularly associated with the experience of emotions such as laughing or anger. Some people with narcolepsy might therefore attempt to control the onset of cataplexy by avoiding emotional stimuli, thereby withdrawing from everyday life to some extent. Cataplexy is thought to be caused by intrusion of rapid eye movement (REM)* sleep, in which there is a loss of muscle tone (see Chapter 2), into wakefulness.

Other common symptoms of narcolepsy are sleep paralysis (the inability to move for a minute or two at the end of sleep), vivid dream-like experiences at the start or end of sleep (known as hypnogogic and hypnopompic hallucinations respectively), disturbed nocturnal sleep and automatic behaviours (the continued error-prone performance of a task at a time of mounting sleepiness). Sleep paralysis can also occur in narcolepsy. Secondary symptoms related to sleepiness include visual blurring, diplopia and difficulties with memory and concentration. In combination, the symptoms of narcolepsy can have a major impact on relationships, education, employment, driving and quality of life. However, it is possible to pursue a career despite narcolepsy as some well-known people have shown: actor Arthur Lowe (Captain Mainwaring in the UK television series *Dad's Army*) is probably one of the more high profile British people and film actress Nastassja Kinski is another example. French cyclist Franck Bouyer used prescribed medication to stay awake, but for several years was unable to race because the drug was a banned substance in the sport.

The prevalence of narcolepsy with cataplexy has been estimated at about 1 in 2000 – or 47 in 100,000 (Ohayon *et al.* 2002). The disorder most commonly starts in the teens or early twenties but it can present as early as two years old or as late as middle age. Men and women are equally affected. The cause of narcolepsy has only recently been understood, the scientific knowledge having developed in three phases. First, in the 1960s it was shown that many of the features of narcolepsy reflected a dysregulation of REM sleep. This accords with the onset of REM sleep in electroencephalogram (EEG)-recorded daytime naps, as well as the symptoms of cataplexy, sleep paralysis, vivid dreams and hallucinations when waking or going off to sleep. Cataplexy and sleep paralysis, for example, occur when the loss of muscle tone (atonia) associated with REM sleep intrudes or persists into wakefulness. Second, in the 1980s workers in Japan discovered that over 90 per cent of people with narcolepsy have a certain tissue type (known as HLA DR2) that suggested that autoimmunity might have a role in the disorder (Juji *et al.* 1984).

The third step forward came in the late 1990s when two independent groups of researchers identified a hypothalamic neurotransmitter that was named orexin by one group and hypocretin by the other. In 1999 an inherited abnormality in the hypocretin receptor in dogs was shown to cause genetically determined canine narcolepsy. Nishino *et al.* (2000) reported that concentrations of hypocretin were markedly reduced in the cerebrospinal fluid of people having narcolepsy associated with cataplexy. Hypocretin is thought to stabilize the state of wakefulness: a deficiency is thought to weaken the arousal side of a sleep/wake switch in the brain (see Chapter 2). It is believed that the onset of narcolepsy is often related to an infection that may cause an autoimmune attack on hypocretin cells in the hypothalamus. A seasonal increase in onset of symptoms of narcolepsy in the spring suggests that it peaks after winter infections (Han *et al.* 2011).

The diagnosis of narcolepsy involves careful history-taking, HLA tissue typing and sleep laboratory investigations including the multiple sleep latency test (MSLT) which measures how quickly the patient falls asleep and goes into REM sleep during the day (see Chapter 8). The presence of EDS, cataplexy and a positive result in the MSLT allow a definite diagnosis of narcolepsy. However, in many cases there are only two out of three features, and the final diagnosis will be clinical and should be made by a sleep specialist.

There has been less research on the patient experience of narcolepsy than there has on the experience of insomnia, but some surveys involving questionnaires and psychological measures have been carried out. In a study involving 42 children with narcolepsy (under the age of 18), Stores, Montgomery and Wiggs (2006) used measures of aspects of behaviour, emotional state, quality of life, educational progress and impact on families. They found worse scores on these measures for the children with narcolepsy compared with a control group. Daniels *et al.* (2001) found a greater degree of depression and lower scores on a quality of life scale amongst adult members of a narcolepsy support network when compared with the general UK population. The biggest impact was on role limitation: respondents were restricted in the amount and type of work they could do; there was a tendency to avoid social situations; and respondents reported difficulty in some everyday tasks (such as cooking, ironing and childcare).

The management of narcolepsy consists of treating the excessive daytime sleepiness with amphetamines or modafinil whilst cataplexy usually responds to antidepressant drugs. Recently, a new drug, gamma-hydroxybutyrate, has been licensed for the treatment of narcolepsy and it has been shown to be useful in the treatment of EDS and cataplexy in particular. It is, however, very expensive and currently difficult to get on prescription in the UK. Strange as it may seem, some people with narcolepsy require sleeping tablets to improve night-time sleep.

Apart from medication, regular nocturnal sleep habits and attention to sleep hygiene can help to minimize excessive sleepiness; there is also some evidence that planned naps can be used to optimize daytime performance. Schools and employers should be made aware that narcolepsy is a disabling condition and that people who have it are not lazy. Additional information and support for people with narcolepsy can be accessed through Narcolepsy UK.[12]

9.4. Parasomnias

Parasomnias are a group of undesirable, episodic, behaviours that usually occur during sleep or are exaggerated by sleep. They are often precipitated by stress and are usually divided into those occurring in REM sleep and those in slow-wave sleep (SWS). There are also entirely normal phenomena that occur in sleep that might trouble the individual, but are not considered to be parasomnia. The most common of these is probably the hypnic jerk, or 'sleep start', often associated with a sensation of falling; others include sleeptalking (somniloquy), nocturnal groaning (catathrenia) and teeth-grinding (bruxism). A variant of the hypnic jerk is a phenomenon known as exploding head syndrome, which is thought to be an auditory manifestation of the same process, where the person hears a sound of an explosion or has a sense of bursting of the head (Pearce 1989). The main parasomnias are summarized in Table 9.2.

REM sleep parasomnias include REM sleep behaviour disorder (RSBD) and nightmares. In RSBD there is vigorous activity often accompanying (and acting out) vivid dreams; it occurs almost exclusively in men (over 50) and there is a strong association with Parkinson's disease. Essentially, in RSBD there is a failure in the mechanism that normally leads to the atonia that prevents the acting out of dreams. As bad dreams, nightmares[13] naturally occur in REM sleep and the person wakes frightened, with detailed recall, but oriented and alert (in contrast to night terrors – see below). Sleep paralysis is considered to be a normal occurrence (Mahowald 2011) and happens when the atonia of REM sleep persists after wakening. Although it may be a feature of narcolepsy, it can occur commonly in the general population and, whilst it may be very frightening, it is harmless.

Table 9.2. Summary of parasomnias

Parasomnia	Sleep stage	Behaviour	Orientated on waking	Recall	Treatment
Night terrors (First half of the night)	SWS	Scream, often sitting up in bed Fearful Flight/fright behaviour	No	No	Clonazepam, paroxetine Sleep hygiene Manage stress
Sleepwalking (First half of the night)	SWS	Automatic	No	No	As night terrors
Nightmares (Second half of the night)	REM	Frightened after waking	Yes	Yes	Guided imagery training
REM behaviour disorder Men over 50; associated with Parkinson's disease	REM	Violent action, e.g. lashing out at bed partner during sleep; after sleep, memory of a frightening dream	Yes	Yes	Medical treatment difficult Clonazepam sometimes used Make sleeping environments as safe as possible

SWS: Slow-wave sleep
REM: Rapid eye movement sleep

SWS parasomnias, which include night terrors and sleepwalking, are thought to be exacerbated by sleep deprivation, where the amount of SWS may be temporarily increased afterwards. They have also been thought to be caused by alcohol consumption, although this has been questioned recently by Pressman *et al.* (2007) who found no experimental evidence that alcohol predisposes or triggers sleepwalking. Pressman (2011) challenges other misconceptions about parasomnias, including sleepwalking – for example, that it is dangerous for a sleepwalker to be woken during an episode.[14] The most common SWS parasomnias are disorders of arousal; that is, the disorder occurs when the individual is aroused from SWS. There is therefore a strong association with other sleep problems that cause arousal, such as OSA, which means that successful treatment of one disorder (OSA) can lead to improvement of the other.

Night terrors (or sleep terrors) occur when the person wakes abruptly, often screaming, in a very distressed state, unresponsive to comforting (unlike waking from a nightmare). In extreme cases the individual may fear going to bed and remain awake until sleep is irresistible. Night terrors can therefore be very disruptive but they may also be particularly dangerous if there is an attempt to escape – especially from an unfamiliar place such as a hotel bedroom. The same applies in the case of sleepwalking where the individual is similarly unresponsive to others; typically the person walks around, perhaps goes to the toilet, and returns to bed. However, much more complex behaviour is possible in sleepwalking and there are rare cases where crimes are committed.[15] Many sleepwalkers never seek medical advice and the behaviour is tolerated in the family home, but they often present at sleep clinic on starting a first relationship, or moving in with a partner, or perhaps on leaving home to go to university.

SWS parasomnias may be treated with benzodiazepine medication – typically clonazepam – but it is also important for the individual to keep regular hours of sleep so as not to become sleep-deprived. Furthermore, it can be helpful to learn to manage the stress that often precipitates the episodes: this can be particularly effective.

9.5. Circadian rhythm sleep disorders

These are disturbances of the normal sleep rhythm when the person's innate 24-hour rhythm is out of synchrony with the environment (they are considered in more detail in Chapter 3). The most common of these is jet lag. It is usually more difficult to cope with when travelling west to east whereupon difficulty falling asleep is the problem (because the day is shortened); on going east to west early waking can occur. To adjust, the traveller should allow one day per hour of time difference. It also helps to adapt to the new time zone by adjusting quickly to the local time and regime, especially mealtimes. Bright light in the morning for alertness or staying indoors or low light prior to sleeping can help adaptation. Melatonin may help at bedtime for up to four days, or a short-acting hypnotic, such as one of the z-drugs, may be used.

Most people get over jet lag and are unlikely to present in a sleep clinic, but more serious are disorders where the sleep pattern is either advanced or delayed. Partly because it is uncommon anyway, few people complain about advanced sleep phase syndrome: they have an extreme 'lark' tendency and rise early and go to bed early. Having a more extreme 'owl' tendency poses significant difficulties for the individual with delayed sleep phase syndrome (DSPS), where sleep and wake times are delayed by between three and six hours compared to conventional times. It may affect up to 10 per cent of young people to some degree, although the prevalence in the general population is less than 0.2 per cent. Where the individual has to rise early for work or school, they may experience both EDS and initial insomnia, especially if they have used caffeine to stay awake. Actigraphy* can be useful to record the sleep pattern over a couple of weeks (see Chapter 8), but management is less straightforward. It is important that the person rises regularly and sees bright light (perhaps by using a light box) and uses subdued light in a winding down period before bedtime; use of melatonin can also be helpful.

9.6. Conclusion

Without sufficient sleep life can be more difficult, and the despair of some people who present at sleep clinic is testament to the importance of sleep. Whilst this chapter has illustrated the diversity of sleep disorders, it has also shown how sleep problems and sleep disorders can be closely related to other illness. It has been seen that in fact sleep disorders are at the interface between the three states of being (wakefulness, sleep and REM sleep). Management is possible for most sleep disorders and is a combination of medication and cognitive and behavioural strategies, although in the UK non-pharmacological management is not yet widely available and can be difficult to access.

Acknowledgements

The authors are grateful to Dr Sue Wilson of the University of Bristol and to Dr Johanna Herrod, consultant neuropsychiatrist, of the Burden Centre for Neuropsychiatry, Bristol, for their comments on earlier drafts.

Notes

1. Sleeping pills do not themselves cause fractured hips in anyone, but they can cause unsteadiness (see Chapter 11) and this can be a risk for elderly people if they get up in the night whilst still sedated. However, it has been suggested that hypnotic medication use is not a risk factor for hip fracture, but that the underlying insomnia is what causes the association between use of hypnotics and falls (Avidan *et al.* 2005).

2. Although sleep disturbance was observed by James Parkinson in 1817, it is only more recently that it has received attention: see Dhawan *et al.* (2006) who note that it is important to try to improve sleep since it may bring temporary improvement in motor symptoms. It is increasingly recognized that REM sleep behaviour disorder (RSBD) is closely associated with Parkinson's disease.

3. Churchill's sleeping habits were unorthodox and he was prone to work late into the night during the Second World War and he slept in the afternoon. He is recorded as saying the following of his sleep pattern:

    > You must sleep some time between lunch and dinner, and no half-way measures. Take off your clothes and get into bed. That's what I always do. Don't think you will be doing less work because you sleep during the day. That's a foolish notion held by people who have no imagination. You will be able to accomplish more. You get two days in one – well, at least one and a half, I'm sure. When the war started, I had to sleep during the day... (Graebner 1965, p.55)

    Churchill went on to add that this also 'enables you to be at your best in the evening when you join your wife, family and friends for dinner' (p.55).

4. See: http://ezinearticles.com/?Famous-People-Who-Suffered-From-Insomnia &id=669506, accessed on 25 September 2011.

5. International Classification of Diseases (World Health Organization 1992). The latest version of the ICD (ICD–10–CM) is largely consistent with the ICSD-2,

although alongside psychophysiologic insomnia, it retains the term 'primary insomnia'.

6. *Diagnostic and Statistical Manual of Mental Disorders*, Fourth Edition (DSM-IV) (American Psychiatric Association 2000).

7. The International Classification of Sleep Disorders (American Academy of Sleep Medicine 2005).

8. *Psychophysiologic* is the term mostly favoured in the USA whereas *psychophysiological* is commonly used in the UK, and is used here in this chapter.

9. Professor Kevin Morgan of Loughborough University has observed (at the 'Sleep, Well-being and Active Ageing: New Evidence for Policy and Practice' Project Conference held on 28 October 2010, at Church House Conference Centre, London) that long-term problems such as insomnia accumulate with age, so whilst insomnia is a problem of old age, it is not *because* of old age. He cites a survey of 12,560 over-65s, where almost 20 per cent reported chronic insomnia symptoms and just over half of those indicated that sleep became a problem before the age of 65.

10. Obstructive sleep apnoea (OSA) is known by several names including obstructive sleep apnoea syndrome (OSAS) and obstructive sleep apnoea/hyponoea syndrome (OSAHS). In keeping with the other chapters in this book the term OSA is used here. Central sleep apnoea is a separate condition, which is less common than OSA. It is defined as a complete cessation of respiratory drive in that there is no respiratory effort for some period of time. The most important type of central sleep apnoea is Cheyne-Stokes respiration (CSR), that is, a series of waxing and waning respiratory efforts. This can occur with acute high altitude exposure in healthy subjects and sometimes in patients with heart failure or stroke. Treatment is nasal oxygen in patients for whom OSA has been ruled out.

11. One news report refers to a 'tidal wave of sleep disorders related to obesity' (available at www.bbc.co.uk/news/uk-scotland-15184632, accessed on 6 November 2011).

12. See: www.narcolepsy.org.uk.

13. The term 'nightmare' is used here in the modern sense to mean a very distressing dream. The original meaning is discussed in Chapter 15.

14. Pressman (2011) observes that it is actually quite difficult to wake a sleepwalker, and that the risk to others is greater if the sleepwalker reacts defensively.

15. The first successful use of the 'sleepwalking defence' was in 1846 in Massachusetts (see Bornemann and Mahowald 2011). More recently, the tragic case of Brian Thomas who strangled his wife as they slept in their campervan brought the issue of crime committed in sleep to public attention (Morris 2009).

References

American Academy of Sleep Medicine (2005) *International Classification of Sleep Disorders: Diagnostic and Coding Manual*, 2nd edn. Westchester, IL: American Academy of Sleep Medicine.

American Psychiatric Association (2000) *Diagnostic and Statistical Manual of Mental Disorders*, 4th edn. Text Revision (DSM-IV-TR). Washington, DC: American Psychiatric Association.

Avidan, A.Y., Fries, B.E., James, M.L., Szafara, K.L., Wright, G.T. and Chervin, R.D. (2005) 'Insomnia and hypnotic use, recorded in the minimum data set, as predictors of falls and hip fractures in Michigan nursing homes.' *Journal of the American Geriatrics Society 53*, 6, 955–962.

Bell, J.F. and Zimmerman, F.J. (2010) 'Shortened nighttime sleep duration in early life and subsequent childhood obesity.' *Archives of Pediatrics and Adolescent Medicine 164*, 9, 840–845.

Bornemann, M.A.C. and Mahowald, M.W. (2011) 'Sleep Forensics.' In M.H. Kryger, T. Roth and W.C. Dement (eds) *Principles and Practice of Sleep Medicine*, 5th edn. St Louis, MO: Elsevier Saunders.

Bradley, T.D. and Floras, J.S. (2009) 'Obstructive sleep apnoea and its cardiovascular consequences.' *Lancet 373*, 9657, 82–93.

Burwell, C.S., Robin, E.D., Whaley, R.D. and Bickelmann, A.G. (1956) 'Extreme obesity associated with alveolar hypoventilation: a Pickwickian syndrome.' *American Journal of Medicine 21*, 5, 811–818.

Buysse, D.J. (2003) 'Diagnosis and Classification of Insomnia Disorders.' In M.P. Szuba, J.D. Kloss and D.J. Dinges (eds) *Insomnia: Principles and Management*. Cambridge: Cambridge University Press.

Carey, T.J., Moul, D.E., Pilkonis, P., Germain, A. and Buysse, D.J. (2005) 'Focusing on the experience of insomnia.' *Behavioral Sleep Medicine 3*, 2, 73–86.

Chaput, J.P., Lambert, M., Gray-Donald, K., McGrath, J.J. *et al.* (2011) 'Short sleep duration is independently associated with overweight and obesity in Quebec children.' *Canadian Journal of Public Health 102*, 5, 369–374.

Charon, F., Dramaix, M. and Mendlewicz, J. (1989) 'Epidemiological survey of insomniac subjects in a sample of 1,761 outpatients.' *Neuropsychobiology 21*, 3, 109–110.

Chevalier, H., Los, F., Boichut, D., Bianchi, M. *et al.* (1999) 'Evaluation of severe insomnia in the general population: results of a European multinational survey.' *Journal of Psychopharmacology 13*, 4, Suppl. 1, S21–S24.

Chilcott, L.A. and Shapiro, C.M. (1996) 'The socioeconomic impact of insomnia: an overview.' *PharmacoEconomics 10*, Suppl. 1, 1–14.

Daniels, E., King, M.A., Smith, I.E. and Shneerson, J.M. (2001) 'Health-related quality of life in narcolepsy.' *Journal of Sleep Research 10*, 1, 75–81.

Dhawan, V., Healy, D.G., Pal, S. and Chaudhuri, K.R. (2006) 'Sleep-related problems of Parkinson's disease.' *Age and Ageing 35*, 3, 220–228.

Dickens, C. (1993) *The Pickwick Papers*. Ware: Wordsworth Editions Limited. (Original work published in 1836–37.)

Edinger, J.D., Bonnet, M.H., Bootzin, R.R., Doghramji, K. *et al.* (2004) 'Derivation of research diagnostic criteria for insomnia: report of an American Academy of Sleep Medicine work group.' *Sleep 27*, 8, 1567–1596.

Espie, C.A. (2006) *Overcoming Insomnia and Sleep Problems*. London: Robinson.

Espie, C.A. (2009) '"Stepped care": a health technology solution for delivering cognitive behavioural therapy as a first line insomnia treatment.' *Sleep 32*, 12, 1549–1558.

Espie, C.A., Broomfield, N.M., MacMahon, K.M.A., Macphee, L.M. and Taylor, L.M. (2006) 'The attention–intention–effort pathway in the development of psychophysiologic insomnia: a theoretical review.' *Sleep Medicine Reviews 10*, 4, 215–245.

Graebner, W. (1965) *My Dear Mister Churchill*. London: Michael Joseph.

Green, A., Hicks, J. and Wilson, S. (2008) 'The experience of poor sleep and its consequences: a qualitative study involving people referred for cognitive-behavioural management of chronic insomnia.' *British Journal of Occupational Therapy 71*, 5, 196–204.

Han, F., Lin, L., Warby, S.C., Faraco, J. *et al.* (2011) 'Narcolepsy onset is seasonal and increased following the 2009 H1N1 pandemic in China.' *Annals of Neurology 70*, 3, 410–417.

Horne, J. (2010) 'Primary insomnia: a disorder of sleep, or primarily one of wakefulness?' *Sleep Medicine Reviews 14*, 1, 3–7.

Juji, T., Satake, M., Honda, Y. and Doi, Y. (1984) 'HLA antigens in Japanese patients with narcolepsy.' *Tissue Antigens 24*, 5, 316–319.

Kripke, D.F., Simons, R.N., Garfinkel, L. and Hammond, E.C. (1979) 'Short and long sleep and sleeping pills: is increased mortality associated?' *Archives of General Psychiatry 36*, 1, 103–116.

Kryger, M.H., Roth, T. and Dement, W.C. (eds) (2011) *Principles and Practice of Sleep Medicine*, 5th edn. St Louis, MO: Elsevier Saunders.

LeBlanc, M., Mérette, C., Savard, J., Ivers, H., Baillargeon, L. and Morin, C.M. (2009) 'Incidence and risk factors of insomnia in a population-based sample.' *Sleep 32*, 8, 1027–1037.

Maclean, A.W., Davies, D.R. and Thiele, K. (2003) 'The hazards and prevention of driving while sleepy.' *Sleep Medicine Reviews 7*, 6, 507–521.

Mahowald, M.W. (2011) 'Other Parasomnias.' In M.H. Kryger, T. Roth and W.C. Dement (eds) *Principles and Practice of Sleep Medicine*, 5th edn. St Louis, MO: Elsevier Saunders.

Mazza, S., Pépin, J.L., Naëgelé, B., Rauch, E. *et al.* (2006) 'Driving ability in sleep apnoea patients before and after CPAP treatment: evaluation on a road safety platform.' *European Respiratory Journal 28*, 5, 1020–1028.

Morrell, M.J., Jackson, M.L., Twigg, G.L., Ghiassi, R. *et al.* (2010) 'Changes in brain morphology in patients with obstructive sleep apnoea.' *Thorax 65*, 908–914.

Morris, S. (2009) 'Devoted husband who strangled wife in his sleep walks free from court.' *Guardian* 20 November. Available at www.guardian.co.uk/uk/2009/nov/20/brian-thomas-dream-strangler-tragedy, accessed on 3 October 2011.

NICE (National Institute for Clinical Excellence) (2004) *Guidance on the Use of Zaleplon, Zolpidem and Zopiclone for the Short-term Management of Insomnia*. London: NICE.

NIH (National Institutes of Health) (2005) 'NIH State-of-the-Science Conference Statement on Manifestations and Management of Chronic Insomnia in Adults.' *NIH Consensus and State-of-the-Science Statements 22*, 2, 1–30. Available at http://consensus.nih.gov/2005/insomniastatement.pdf, accessed on 12 June 2012.

Nishino, S., Ripley, B., Overeem, S., Lammers, G.J. and Mignot, E. (2000) 'Hypocretin (Orexin) deficiency in human narcolepsy.' *The Lancet 355*, 9197, 39–40.

Ohayon, M.M., Priest, R.G., Zulley, J., Smirne, S. and Paiva, T. (2002) 'Prevalence of narcolepsy symptomatology and diagnosis in the European general population.' *Neurology 58*, 12, 1826–1833.

Pearce, J.M.S. (1989) 'Clinical features of the exploding head syndrome.' *Journal of Neurology, Neurosurgery and Psychiatry 52*, 7, 907–910.

Perlis, M., Shaw, P.J., Cano, G. and Espie, C.A. (2011) 'Models of Insomnia.' In M.H. Kryger, T. Roth and W.C. Dement (eds) *Principles and Practice of Sleep Medicine*, 5th edn. St Louis, MO: Elsevier Saunders.

Phillips, B.A. and Kryger, M.H. (2011) 'Management of Obstructive Sleep Apnea-Hypopnea Syndrome.' In M.H. Kryger, T. Roth and W.C. Dement (eds) *Principles and Practice of Sleep Medicine*, 5th edn. St Louis, MO: Elsevier Saunders.

Pressman, M.R. (2011) 'Common misconceptions about sleepwalking and other parasomnias.' *Sleep Medicine Clinics 6*, 4, xiii–xvii.

Pressman, M.R., Mahowald, M.W., Schenck, C.H. and Bornemann, M.C. (2007) 'Alcohol-induced sleepwalking or confusional arousal as a defense to criminal behavior: a review of scientific evidence, methods and forensic considerations.' *Journal of Sleep Research 16*, 2, 198–212.

Riemann, D. and Perlis, M.L. (2009) 'The treatments of chronic insomnia: a review of benzodiazepine receptor agonists and psychological and behavioral therapies.' *Sleep Medicine Reviews 13*, 3, 205–214.

Roth, T. (2007) 'Insomnia: definition, prevalence, etiology, and consequences.' *Journal of Clinical Sleep Medicine 15*, 3, Suppl. 5, S7–S10.

Sandor, P. and Shapiro, C.M. (1994) 'Sleep patterns in depression and anxiety: theory and pharmacological effects.' *Journal of Psychosomatic Research 38*, Suppl. 1, 125–139.

Siriwardena, S.N., Apekey, T., Tilling, M., Harrison, A. *et al.* (2009) 'Effectiveness and cost-effectiveness of an educational intervention for practice teams to deliver problem focused therapy for insomnia: rationale and design of a pilot cluster randomised trial.' *BMC Family Practice 10*, 9. Available at www.biomedcentral.com/1471-2296/10/9, accessed on 6 October 2011.

Smith, M.T., Perlis, M.L., Park, A., Smith, M.S. *et al.* (2002) 'Comparative meta-analysis of pharmacotherapy and behavior therapy for persistent insomnia.' *American Journal of Psychiatry 159*, 1, 5–11.

Stein, M.D. and Friedmann, P.D. (2005) 'Disturbed sleep and its relationship to alcohol use.' *Substance Abuse 26*, 1, 1–13.

Stores, G., Montgomery, P. and Wiggs, L. (2006) 'The psychosocial problems of children with narcolepsy and those with excessive daytime sleepiness of uncertain origin.' *Paediatrics 118*, 4, e1116–e1123.

Summers-Bremner, E. (2008) *Insomnia: A Cultural History*. London: Reaktion Books Ltd.

Thorpy, M.J. (2011) 'Classification of Sleep Disorders.' In M.H. Kryger, T. Roth and W.C. Dement (eds) *Principles and Practice of Sleep Medicine*, 5th edn. St Louis, MO: Elsevier Saunders.

Vermeeren, A. (2004) 'Residual effects of hypnotics: epidemiology and clinical implications.' *CNS Drugs 18*, 5, 297–328.

Wiedman, J. (1999) *Desperately Seeking Snoozin'*. Memphis, TN: Towering Pines Press.

Wilson, S. and Nutt, D. (2008) *Sleep Disorders*. Oxford: Oxford University Press.

Wilson, S.J., Nutt, D.J., Alford, C., Argyropoulos, S.V. *et al.* (2010) 'British Association for Psychopharmacology consensus statement on evidence-based treatment of insomnia, parasomnias and circadian rhythm disorders.' *Journal of Psychopharmacology 24*, 11, 1577–1601.

World Health Organization (1992) *International Statistical Classification of Diseases and Related Health Problems*, 10th Revision (ICD-10). Geneva: World Health Organization.

Yaggi, H.K., Concato, J., Kernan, W.N., Lichtman, J.H. *et al.* (2005) 'Obstructive sleep apnea as a risk factor for stroke and death.' *New England Journal of Medicine 353*, 19, 2034–2041.

Young, T., Palta, M., Dempsey, J., Skatrud, J., Weber, S. and Badr, S. (1993) 'The occurrence of sleep-disordered breathing among middle-aged adults.' *New England Journal of Medicine 328*, 17, 1230–1235.

10

Sleep and Psychiatry

Dietmar Hank, Jane Hicks and Sue Wilson

10.1. Introduction

Sleep problems are about three times more common in people with psychiatric disorders. They may be a symptom of the disorder, appearing at the same time as other symptoms, or sometimes a little before, as in depression and anxiety disorders. They may also be the result of changes to the brain's sleep mechanisms in organic disorders, such as dementia, or in head injury or neurodevelopmental disorders. As well as such links between psychiatric disorder and sleep problems, there are effects in the other direction. For example, if people suffer from insomnia for a long time, they are twice as likely as people who sleep normally to be diagnosed with depression or anxiety in the future. Another example is that behaviours and attitudes to sleep in psychiatric disorders may impinge on the mechanisms of sleep regulation, and thus give rise to sleep disturbance. These bidirectional associations are explored in this chapter, which considers a selection of conditions that are seen by psychiatrists and neuropsychiatrists.[1]

10.2. Anxiety disorders

Anxiety disorders affect up to 20 per cent of the population, of which a large proportion have generalized anxiety disorder (GAD). GAD is defined by excessive anxiety and worrying on most days, over a period of six months or more. This occurs in association with at least three of the following symptoms: sleep disturbance, restlessness, being easily fatigued, irritability, muscle tension and concentration difficulties. For diagnosis, symptoms must give rise to distress and cause impairment in functioning.

Insomnia is the subjective complaint of poor sleep (described in Chapter 9), and anxiety is an integral element, as worry about sleep is one of the main perpetuating factors influencing the development of chronic insomnia. Many people with insomnia experience mounting anxiety towards bedtime as fears about not sleeping, and the possible consequences next day, become more salient. This increased anxiety leads to high arousal (at a time when arousal levels need to be decreasing) and to a reduced chance of falling asleep – thereby creating a vicious cycle. Anxiety and insomnia are therefore closely related. Accordingly, Bonnet and Arand (1997) found that people with insomnia had an increased metabolic rate, and concluded that insomnia was 'perhaps more of a disorder of arousal than a disorder of sleep' (p.587). It may be a theoretical distinction – and of little obvious relevance to the individual on the ground (or in bed) – but the relationship between the two disorders is still unclear, especially whether insomnia is a precipitating factor in GAD, or *vice versa*, because not all reports have descriptions of the course of the conditions.

Amongst people with GAD, estimates of the incidence of insomnia vary widely according to the instruments used and populations studied. GAD affects approximately 5 per cent of adults, rising to 10 per cent in people between the ages of 55 and 85 (Beekman *et al.* 1998; Wittchen and Jacobi 2005). Most authors agree that there is at least a twofold risk of an insomnia diagnosis in patients with GAD compared to the population as a whole, although this may be much higher. A recent UK population survey found an insomnia diagnosis to be six times more likely in GAD (Stewart *et al.* 2006).

Objective laboratory measures of sleep in patients with GAD and sleep complaints have revealed that they have longer times to initiate sleep, and more waking during the night than controls (Papadimitriou and Linkowski 2005). Since hyperarousal is a key symptom of GAD it is thought that this gives rise to the sleep problems described. However, in a recent study of anxiety symptoms (Argyropoulos *et al.* 2007), the authors point to the independence of the symptoms of hyperarousal and sleep maintenance insomnia, suggesting that not all insomnia in GAD is related to hyperarousal.

Many studies of patients with *insomnia* find that, sleep-focused anxiety aside, the incidence of diagnosed anxiety disorders is higher than it is in good sleepers. For example, in a population survey in France, about a quarter of people with a diagnosis of insomnia also had a diagnosed anxiety disorder (Ohayon 1997). One approach when investigating the association between sleep problems and anxiety in insomnia is to exclude people with symptoms of a psychiatric disorder: whilst this rules out cases of insomnia secondary to psychiatric illness, it risks excluding people whose insomnia leads to the psychiatric symptoms. In a review of studies with and without these exclusions, Riedel and Lichstein (2000) found that when people with evidence of psychiatric disorders were ruled out, nearly half of the studies found significantly higher subclinical anxiety ratings in people with insomnia than normal sleepers.

As well as a risk of concurrent anxiety with insomnia there is a risk of *subsequent* anxiety disorder in insomnia patients. A large American study 20 years ago (Ford and Kamerow 1989) interviewed 7954 adults on two occasions one year apart and was the first to highlight the strong association between sleep disturbance and subsequent anxiety. This association has been reported in further studies: in a survey of 1200 young adults in Michigan, the risk of a new anxiety disorder showed a twofold increase amongst respondents who had insomnia three years earlier compared with those who were previously good sleepers (Breslau *et al.* 1996). In a questionnaire survey of adults over 18 in the UK there was again a twofold increased risk of new anxiety disorder if subjects had reported one sleep problem occurring 'on most nights' a year earlier (Morphy *et al.* 2007). In a longer study in Norway, with two surveys ten years apart (Neckelmann, Mykletun and Dahl 2007), the risk of having an anxiety disorder diagnosis at the second time point increased by about one-and-a-half times if insomnia had been present at the first time point, and about five times if insomnia was present at both time points, indicating the higher risk of long-standing insomnia.

People with panic disorder also have a slightly raised risk of sleep disorder, with at least a third experiencing nocturnal panic attacks.

Most of these attacks occur at the border between light (stage 2) sleep and deep slow-wave sleep (SWS) (Mellman 2006), or at the onset of sleep: they are therefore not associated with dreaming. People in this situation also tend to have a heightened arousal at bedtime, fearing sleep when they might have a panic attack. These panic attacks tend to respond better to antidepressants than to benzodiazepines (Mellman and Uhde 1989). Cognitive behaviour therapy (CBT) can also be effective in management (see Craske and Tsao 2005).

The anxiety disorder with the highest prevalence of sleep disorders is post-traumatic stress disorder (PTSD). The most distressing sleep symptom is nightmares, with the content often containing images of real experiences, and 50–70 per cent of people with PTSD suffer from these (Spoormaker and Montgomery 2008). Insomnia is also prevalent, with 40–50 per cent reporting significant insomnia. Treating these symptoms is a key target in overall amelioration of the disorder.

10.3. Depression

Major depressive disorder is characterized by overwhelming low mood with anhedonia (loss of interest or enjoyment in usually pleasurable activities) as well as other symptoms. There is such a strong association between major depression and sleep disturbance that some researchers have suggested that a diagnosis of depression in the absence of sleep complaints should be made with caution (Jindal and Thase 2004). Sleep disturbance may be the reason that depressed patients first seek help, and is one of the few proven risk factors for suicide (Agargun, Kara and Solmaz 1997). If sleep problems remain after other symptoms are ameliorated, there is a significantly increased risk of relapse and recurrence.

In clinical samples, difficulty in initiating or maintaining sleep (including early morning wakening), or both, have been reported in about three-quarters of all depressed patients (Hamilton 1989; Yates et al. 2007). In epidemiological studies examining insomnia and depression, sleep symptoms occurred in 50–60 per cent of a sample of young adults aged 21–30 (Breslau et al. 1996). In a UK population sample (n = 8580) (Stewart et al. 2006), the incidence of insomnia symptoms in a wide age range of patients with depression increased with age. Overall, 83 per cent of depressed patients had at least one insomnia symptom compared with 36 per cent who did not have depression. This ranged from 77 per cent in the 16–24 age group, to 90 per cent in the 55–64 age group.

Hypersomnia is less common and tends to be a feature of atypical depression.[2] It is more prevalent in the young, with about 40 per cent of patients under 30, compared with 10 per cent of those in their fifties, experiencing the symptom (Posternak and Zimmerman 2001), and a higher incidence in females of all ages. Some people experience both insomnia and hypersomnia during the same depressive episode.

Disturbed sleep is a very distressing symptom which has a huge impact on quality of life in depressed patients (Katz and McHorney 2002). Investigating this association, Paterson, Nutt and Wilson (2009) surveyed the views of patients with depression and asked about their symptoms and associated sleep difficulties. Members of Depression Alliance, a UK-based charity for people with depression, were sent a postal questionnaire which asked respondents if they suffered from sleep difficulties when they were depressed. A total of 97 per cent of respondents reported sleep difficulties during depression, and 59 per cent of these indicated that poor sleep significantly affected their quality of life. The majority believed their sleep difficulties started at the same time as their depression. About two-thirds had sought extra treatment for their sleep problems, including prescribed sleeping pills, over-the-counter sleeping aids and extra visits to their doctor.

As well as the distressing symptoms of sleep disturbance experienced by patients, changes in objective sleep architecture* are well documented in depression (Benca *et al.* 1992). Compared with normal controls, sleep continuity of depressed subjects is often impaired, with increased wakefulness (more frequent and longer periods of wakefulness during the night), and reduced sleep efficiency.* Sleep onset latency* is significantly increased and total sleep time reduced. The time taken to commence rapid eye movement (REM) sleep (REM latency) is often shortened and the duration of the first period of REM sleep is increased. The number of eye movements in REM sleep (REM density) is also increased. The total amount of deep SWS is often decreased in depression, compared with normal controls. This reduction may be related to decreased regional cerebral blood flow seen in some frontal areas of the brain during SWS in imaging studies

(Maquet *et al.* 1997), and it may be a consequence of the abnormalities in this area described in depression (Drevets 2007).

Sleep abnormalities in depression, both subjective and objective, point to a disruption in both homeostatic and circadian drives to sleep. The alteration in timing or evolution of slow-wave activity may be thought of as a disruption in normal sleep homeostasis, resulting in a decreased pressure to sleep. Alterations in REM timing, increases in wake and stage 1 (S1) sleep and early morning waking point to the circadian process being affected; these symptoms in depression patients suggest an earlier onset of key sleep rhythms, or phase advance. Whether the circadian rhythm disruption is a cause, a consequence or a co-morbid condition of depression is the subject of much research at present, as the underlying genetic control of the mammalian clock is becoming clearer, and investigation of clock genes in depression more common (see also Chapter 3).

10.4. Schizophrenia

The diagnostic symptoms of schizophrenia include hallucinations (mostly auditory)[3] and delusions, often with a persecutory nature. The disorder affects up to 1 per cent of the population, typically starts in late teenage or early adult years, and tends to take a lifelong course. It is thought to result from a combination of genetic factors and environmental factors or stress. Noting the complex neuropathology of schizophrenia, with widespread alteration in brain mechanisms, Wulff and colleagues observe that it is 'hardly surprising that abnormal sleep has been described in patients with schizophrenia since the 1920s' (Wulff *et al.* 2010, p.593).

People with schizophrenia frequently complain of insomnia (delayed sleep, fragmented sleep and reduction in total sleep time) and more severely, during periods of psychotic agitation, there may be total sleep loss. Sleep quality is reduced, with restlessness and nightmares. Sleep/wake reversal is more common in people with schizophrenia. The subjective complaints are largely corroborated in studies using objective measures such as polysomnography (PSG) which show reduced sleep time, poor sleep efficiency and some reduction in deep SWS (Benson and Feinberg 2011).

A meta-analysis has also shown that unmedicated patients with schizophrenia tend to show increased sleep latency, reduced total sleep time and reduced sleep efficiency (Chouinard *et al.* 2004). Patients never treated with antipsychotic medication, compared with patients who had come off medication, also showed increased total wake time and a reduced proportion of S2 sleep. REM sleep does not appear to be significantly different, either in quality or quantity, between patients with schizophrenia and healthy controls, although there is a tendency for REM latency to be shorter in individuals with schizophrenia. This might be explained by a relative lack of SWS in this population (Benson 2006, 2008). People with schizophrenia have also been found to have reduced asymmetry of delta wave count – a marker of SWS – in the frontal cortex of the brain when compared to healthy controls, who showed a right-sided dominance (Sekimoto *et al.* 2007). These factors – reduced SWS and the different symmetry patterns in patients with schizophrenia – are thought to contribute to the pathophysiology of the disorder, especially to negative symptoms[4] such as apathy, lack of spontaneity, flat affect and impoverished speech. Sekimoto *et al.* (2007) found that delta wave activity during SWS was inversely related to the magnitude of the negative symptoms – the worse the negative symptoms, the lower the delta count.

Since the 1950s the main treatment for schizophrenia has been antipsychotic medication, which can have an effect on sleep and sleep architecture. Some of these medications, both older ones such as chlorpromazine, and newer ones such as olanzapine, have sedative properties that improve sleep, but sometimes tend to make people sleepy in the daytime. Increased SWS has been found with a number of antipsychotic medications, including olanzapine (Sharpley, Vassallo and Cowen 2000). Some antipsychotic medication can, however, cause further sleep problems, including sleepwalking, restless leg syndrome, periodic limb movement in sleep and, where there is a gain in weight, obstructive sleep apnoea (OSA). After antipsychotic medication has been discontinued, severe insomnia can herald the relapse of a psychotic illness (Benson 2006).

Recent research looking at sleep/wake rhythms in people with schizophrenia has shown that a proportion of patients have delayed sleep periods, and some seem to lack a proper 24-hour sleep/wake rhythm altogether (Wulff *et al.* 2012). It may be that disruption of the biological clock is a symptom of schizophrenia itself, since it seems to be independent of the type or dose of medication being taken. Reviewing this evidence, and evidence of the importance of a normal rest/activity cycle with a well-marked difference between day and night-time activity (Bromundt *et al.* 2011), Wilson and Argyropoulos (2012) suggest that it may be justified to use specific chronotherapeutic treatments (light therapy and enhancing sleep and daily activity) in rehabilitation after an acute episode of the illness.

10.5. Neurodegenerative conditions

Alzheimer's disease

Alzheimer's disease (AD) is a 'neurodegenerative disorder characterized by progressive decline in memory and other cognitive domains' (Petit, Montplaisir and Boeve 2011, p.1038). Sleep problems result from degenerative changes to the nervous system and it is estimated that sleep disturbance is present in 25 per cent of people with mild to moderate AD and in about 50 per cent of more severe cases (Petit *et al.* 2011). People with AD may experience sleep difficulties such as excessive daytime sleep, or napping, initial insomnia, fragmentation of night-time sleep, a reduction of SWS and confusional episodes during the night. Another problem is 'sundowning' – an increase of problem behaviours in the afternoon or evening as well as nocturnal wandering which is partly explained by changes in the biological clock (the suprachiasmatic nucleus of the hypothalamus – see Chapter 3). Disturbance of sleep in patients with AD is associated with agitation, and aggressive behaviours, which have a considerable impact on the patient's quality of life and greatly increase the burden for caregivers. Sleep disturbance is a significant factor contributing to the breakdown of home-based care and subsequent institutionalization.[5]

As well as deterioration in neurons instrumental for the circadian rhythm, natural with age and advanced in people with AD, pathways important for the initiation and maintenance of sleep also appear to be affected (see Wulff *et al.* 2010). Furthermore, medical disorders (such as airway diseases, heart disease and diabetes) and psychiatric disorders (such as anxiety and depression) commonly found in older people and sufferers of AD, can also contribute to sleep disorders. Sleep-disordered breathing is not uncommon in patients and, apart from disrupting sleep, it may further negatively impact on daytime behaviours and cognitive functioning. Housebound and institutionalized patients frequently lack adequate exposure to daylight, spend more time in bed, are less physically active and enjoy fewer social activities, all of which can contribute to insomnia (Dauvilliers 2007). A number of medications prescribed in dementia can give rise to sleep problems, insomnia in particular: acetylcholinesterase inhibitors, used to treat symptoms of mild and moderate Alzheimer's, can induce sleep onset insomnia, whereas antipsychotic medication used for behavioural problems can induce hypersomnia (Iranzo 2010).

The management of sleep problems in AD, as in other cases, can be pharmacological or behavioural. McCurry *et al.* (2004) show in case studies how a detailed assessment and individualized management can bring about improvements in sleep, including simple measures such as excluding a pet cat from the bedroom and minimizing access to more distracting or stimulating aspects of their environment during the night. In a subsequent larger trial involving daily walks, light therapy and sleep hygiene* education (such as regular bedtime and rising times, and limited opportunities to nap in the daytime), McCurry *et al.* (2005) achieved a 32 per cent reduction in night-time wakening compared with controls – an improvement maintained at six-month follow-up. For more on non-pharmacological management see Deschenes and McCurry (2009).

Treating sleep problems in AD with medication also needs an individual approach according to circumstances (Iranzo 2010). A particular difficulty is side effects: for example, benzodiazepines may cause sedation and confusion whereas antidepressants, which might also decrease sleep latency, may cause somnolence, dizziness and weight gain (Deschenes and McCurry 2009). A further difficulty is that there is a lack of evidence for some medication helping insomnia in patients with AD: for example, Deschenes and McCurry (2009) note that there are no data for the use of z-drugs (see Chapter 11) with this population, or for melatonin. However, melatonin, in combination with light therapy, may be helpful for regulating circadian rhythms (Iranzo 2010).

Parkinson's disease

Parkinson's disease (PD) is a progressive neurological disorder characterized by rigidity, resting tremor and slowness of movement, amongst other symptoms. Arnulf, Reading and Vidialhet (2010) observe that 'the whole gamut of sleep disorders may be seen in [PD], occasionally in the same patient' (p.100). Wulff *et al.* (2010) cite estimates of 80–90 per cent of PD patients having a sleep disorder. Dhawan *et al.* (2006) suggest that disturbance of sleep might precede motor symptoms. A particular problem is maintaining sleep; there is also an association with REM sleep behaviour disorder (RSBD) (see Chapter 9) and daytime sleepiness may result from both poor night-time sleep and the neurodegenerative process. Trenkwalder and Arnulf (2011) suggest that the sleep/wake problems in parkinsonism may be caused by a combination of three factors: degenerative damage in the areas of the brain that regulate sleep and arousal, problems caused by the disease (such as difficulty moving in bed during awakenings) and side-effects of medication for PD that could cause nocturnal movements, insomnia or sleepiness. Given the complexity of the problems involved, treatment needs to be tailored to the individual (see Arnulf *et al.* 2010; Trenkwalder and Arnulf 2011).

10.6. Intellectual disability

Intellectual disability (ID)[6] can be defined as a disability 'characterized by significant limitations both in intellectual functioning and in adaptive behaviour, which covers many everyday social and practical skills'.[7] The disability originates before the age of 18. Sleep disorders are highly prevalent amongst people with ID, but often are not recognized and remain untreated. Doran, Harvey and Horner (2006) state that 'people with developmental disorders experience more fragmented sleep and a higher incidence of sleep disorders than do individuals in the general population' (p.14). They go on to suggest that a person with ID will not have the ability to compensate for sleep problems – hence behavioural and/or health problems are exacerbated. Brylewski and Wiggs (1999) provide evidence for this is in their community study of adults with ID in Oxfordshire. It was found that individuals with sleep problems (taking over an hour to settle, or waking in the night) were more likely to display irritability, stereotypy or hyperactivity than good sleepers, although it could not be stated that one caused the other, nor whether both related to something else.

Estimates of sleep disturbance amongst people with ID in one review ranged from 13 to 86 per cent across the spectrum – including all degrees of ID, all age groups and the presence of other health problems (Didden and Sigafoos 2001). Doran *et al.* (2006) cite an estimate that perhaps 39 per cent of adults with severe ID meet diagnostic criteria for insomnia (whereas in the general population it is about a tenth of people: see Chapter 9). Parasomnias (14%) and sleep-related breathing problems (15%) were common in a community-based group of adults with ID (Brylewski and Wiggs 1998). Sleep problems are common in children with ID too (Didden *et al.* 2002).

Although not everyone with an autistic spectrum disorder (ASD) has an ID, it is one area where there has been recent interest. In their review, Richdale and Schreck (2009) found that most studies 'confirm that insomnia and in particular sleep onset difficulties are a hallmark of sleep in ASD, though...circadian sleep disturbances and parasomnias also occur' (p.406). A relative lack of deep sleep (SWS) in favour of lighter sleep has been found in some PSG studies. Furthermore, increasing severity of sleep disturbance appears to be associated with more autism symptoms. Richdale and Schreck (2009) propose that a biopsychosocial viewpoint implies that sleep problems could result from one, or a combination of, biological or genetic factors, psychological or behavioural characteristics, and family and environmental factors. For example, altered melatonin production (linked to a particular pattern of melatonin genes common in autism) and timing might give rise to insomnia and change in the circadian sleep rhythm in this population. Behavioural issues, such as the need for routines and rituals, can give rise to settling difficulties and there may be family or home factors that are not conducive to good sleep.

With such a wide range of sleep difficulties, in the context of a wide range of ability, treatment of sleep problems in people with ID will depend on careful assessment. Didden and Sigafoos (2001) outline the behavioural procedures that are available, including chronotherapy (systematically delaying bedtime until the desired times are achieved), sleep/wake scheduling and light therapy. Small-scale studies suggest that brief and relatively simple interventions such as sleep hygiene, stimulus control and sleep restriction therapy (see Chapter 9) as well as relaxation techniques can be effective (Gunning and Espie 2003; Hylkema and Vlaskamp 2009). Amongst pharmacological measures, melatonin can be effective as a treatment for people with ID and chronic sleep disturbance in helping to get off to sleep. Adverse reactions are few and in the short term melatonin appears to be free of rebound insomnia, withdrawal symptoms and tolerance. However, some questions remain over the longer-term effects of melatonin, particularly during puberty and regarding the reproductive system (Braam *et al.* 2008; Sajith and Clarke 2007).

10.7. Traumatic brain injury
In people under the age of 40, traumatic brain injury (TBI) is the leading cause of disability. In the USA it is estimated that, annually, between 180 and 250 people per 100,000 are admitted to hospital with TBI: 20 to 30 per 100,000 die (Bruns and Hauser 2003). Following TBI psychiatric disorders such as depression, anxiety and substance use are common, as are persistent changes in personality. According to Ouellet, Savard and Morin (2004), between 30 and 70 per cent of TBI patients experience sleep problems, with a likely negative impact on other symptoms and rehabilitation. The reasons are several and Verma, Anand and Verma (2007) list possible mechanisms for TBI causing sleep disorders including: direct and indirect brain injury, damage to neck and back causing pain, weight gain and pre-existing abnormality exacerbated by head trauma.

Insomnia is the most common subjective complaint, both in the acute stages and months, or even years after brain injury – although, as noted by Orff, Ayalon and Drummond (2009), it is 'inherently defined by self-report' (p.156). In an Australian study involving 63 people with TBI (between 20 days and over three years post-injury), 80 per cent of respondents reported long sleep onset latency or increased night-time wakening, compared with 23 per cent of matched controls (Parcell *et al.* 2006); it was also found that more frequent night-time awakenings were more commonly associated with milder injury. A consequence of poor sleep at night can be excessive daytime sleepiness, and in a survey by Cohen *et al.* (1992), subjectively reported sleepiness was found in 14 per cent of hospitalized TBI patients but in 38 per cent of discharged patients after two to three years. Sleep initiation and maintenance problems were more frequently reported in hospitalized patients, but excessive daytime somnolence was more common amongst discharged patients. Watson *et al.* (2007) found sleepiness to be present in about half of TBI patients after one month in a prospective study involving 514 brain-injured people. More severe head injury appeared to result in greater sleepiness and after a year, approximately a quarter of brain-injured respondents continued to experience sleepiness.

PSG studies are inconclusive probably because the site, severity and degree of persistence of the damage varies in the samples that have been investigated; their findings range from altered sleep architecture, lower sleep efficiency and prolonged nocturnal awakenings, to a lack of evidence for objective sleep impairment. However, objectively diagnosed sleep disorders are common: in one PSG study (Castriotta *et al.* 2007), of 87 adults with at least three months history of TBI, across the severity spectrum, 46 per cent were found to have a sleep disorder. The most common diagnosis was obstructive sleep apnoea (OSA) (23%), followed by post-traumatic hypersomnia (11%), periodic limb movements in sleep (7%) and narcolepsy (6%). Excessive daytime sleepiness (i.e. MSLT* score of less than ten minutes – see Chapter 8) was found in 26 per cent of participants. Cause or severity of head injury was not related to sleep measures in PSG studies. As the researchers observed (Castriotta *et al.* 2007), it is possible that conditions like narcolepsy and OSA might have been undiagnosed before the TBI but may have contributed to the cause of the accidental injury. Therefore, whilst there may be an association between TBI and sleep disorder, as is the case with anxiety and other psychiatric disorders, the direction of causality may be unclear.

Daytime sleepiness is one of the most commonly reported sleep symptoms following TBI, and is important because it may make behavioural therapies and rehabilitation much more difficult. One cause of daytime sleepiness is circadian rhythm sleep disorders (CRSD), and case reports, small studies and clinical experience suggest TBI might be associated with CRSD. In one study (Ayalon *et al.* 2007) this was the case for 36 per cent of participants with insomnia complaints following mild TBI. Delayed sleep phase syndrome (DSPS) (see Chapter 9) was slightly more frequent than irregular sleep/wake pattern (ISWP), but both conditions were much more frequent than the expected prevalence amongst sleep clinic insomnia patients, where DSPS was found in 7 to 16 per cent of cases and where ISWP was rare (Reid and Zee 2011). Although this has not been a consistent finding – for example, Steele *et al.* (2005) found no shift in their sample of ten patients – Baumann (2010) suggests that post-traumatic insomnia might be overestimated and actually be a function of disruption of circadian rhythms. Ayalon *et al.* (2007) speculate that in the presence of normal brain scans (CT and MRI) a possible cause might be microscopic damage to the circadian system or that factors that often accompany mild TBI (depression, anxiety, trauma, pain and change in daily routines) might also contribute to the change in rhythm.

Although there is good evidence for the effectiveness of psychological and behavioural therapies for insomnia (Morin *et al.* 2006), there is a lack of published evidence on their use for insomnia following TBI. Given the likely increased susceptibility of the traumatized brain to hypnotic medications that may cause additional, adverse daytime symptoms, other treatment should be the priority. Bright light therapy and melatonin are effective in the treatment of CRSD and would also seem to be options in the treatment of these problems in TBI (Bjorvatn and Pallesen 2009; Orff *et al.* 2009).

In summary, sleep disorders are common in TBI and appear to be associated with poorer performance on aspects of cognitive testing, psychosocial adjustment, quality of life and recovery. A number of studies raise the question whether pre-existing sleep disorders, in particular excessive daytime tiredness, may be a contributing aetiological factor to TBI. Subjective insomnia complaints in TBI are likely over-reported, as is true for insomnia in general, whereas hypersomnia symptoms are possibly under-reported. High vigilance for sleep problems and low threshold for PSG studies is required in this population. As Agrawal, Cincu and Joharapurkar (2008) state, a more refined understanding is needed of sleep disorders and their management in patients with TBI in order to offer best possible care and optimize rehabilitation.

10.8. Conclusion

Sleep symptoms are a major concern in many conditions in psychiatry, and if there is a common theme in this chapter it is interdependence, or close relationships. The chapter has shown the delicate balance necessary for a good sleep/wake pattern. Figure 3.3 in Chapter 3 illustrates just a part of that complexity, but it is sufficient for us to appreciate at a simple level, that matches clinical experience, how it does not take much to upset the equilibrium.

In the case of GAD the relationship with sleep disturbance is so close that insomnia and anxiety are commonly found together – whichever may come first – and the same kinds of treatment – whether medication or psychological (CBT) – can be effective in both. A similar close relationship with disrupted sleep has been observed in depression, but in this case there might be objective changes in sleep architecture and possible disruption of circadian cycles. Circadian rhythm disruption also appears to be a factor in the case of schizophrenia and is a promising area of research. It has been suggested that as well as medication and light therapy, enhancement of daily activity could be of significant help. The same applies in relation to AD where sleep problems result from degenerative changes: there is still scope to improve sleep.

Given the range of problems that may occur in the context of ID, negative consequences for sleep are not surprising. The relative lack or research into sleep problems in ID perhaps relates to societal attitudes, or perhaps to an assumption that little can be done. It is notable that in a substantial textbook on sleep medicine (Kryger, Roth and Dement 2011) there is no section devoted to sleep in ID. However, given the close relationship between sleep and learning, discussed elsewhere in this book (Chapter 7), it seems all the more important to address sleep difficulties, because improved sleep might facilitate learning, maximize potential and enhance quality of life. Similarly, changes in sleep as a result of TBI might be expected, given the far-reaching consequences of head trauma. Whilst studies show many objective changes in sleep after brain injury, it has been suggested that sleep disturbance can also be a causal factor: that is, sleep disorders can make accidents more likely if they cause sleep deprivation. It may also be that subsequent disability is exacerbated by sleep disorder in addition to sequelae of the injury.

Sleep is important for both general and mental health. In the case of mental health, as seen in this chapter, it is inextricably linked. Research is increasingly showing how close this relationship is and offers prospects for improved management both of disrupted sleep and of psychiatric disorders, where changes to sleep/wake cycles are part of the condition. There is considerable scope for real improvement of quality of life by improving the sleep quality of people with the whole range of conditions seen in psychiatry.

Acknowledgement

The authors acknowledge the editorial contribution of Andrew Green.

Notes

1. This indeterminate expression is deliberately chosen since a discussion of the categorization and naming of the diverse range of disorders considered in this chapter is beyond the scope of this book. It is not possible to cover all disorders, and it is not intended to imply that sleep disturbance is not an issue in any that are not mentioned here.

2. Atypical depression is actually common. Parker *et al.* (2002) cite these two essential criteria: 'mood reactivity (criterion A) and two or more of the following features (criterion B): increased appetite or weight gain, hypersomnia, leaden paralysis, and long-standing interpersonal rejection sensitivity' (p.1472).

3. Visual hallucinations are also possible in schizophrenia. Dement *et al.* (1970) discuss the relationship, and differences, between hallucinations and dreaming and why we cannot dream whilst we are awake.

4. 'Negative symptoms' is the term used to differentiate the type of symptoms listed here which are different from 'positive' symptoms such as delusions, hallucinations and disordered thought.

5. The continuing importance of sleep for older people, in their own homes and in care homes, has been recognized in a four-year collaborative research project between several universities – SomnIA: Sleep in Ageing – which concluded in 2010. See www.somnia.surrey.ac.uk/index.html, accessed on 17 December 2011.

6. Various terms are used in the literature and some that are quoted here are not terms of our choice. As noted above, a discussion on terminology is beyond our scope here.

7. American Association on Intellectual and Developmental Disabilities, available at www.aamr.org/content_100.cfm?navID=21, accessed on 11 December 2011.

References

Agargun, M.Y., Kara, H. and Solmaz, M. (1997) 'Sleep disturbances and suicidal behavior in patients with major depression.' *Journal of Clinical Psychiatry 58*, 6, 249–251.

Agrawal, A., Cincu, R. and Joharapurkar, S.R. (2008) 'Traumatic brain injury and sleep disturbances.' *Journal of Clinical Sleep Medicine 4*, 2, 177.

Argyropoulos, S.P., Ploubidis, G.B., Wright, T.S., Palm, M.E. *et al.* (2007) 'Development and validation of the Generalized Anxiety Disorder Inventory (GADI).' *Journal of Psychopharmacology 21*, 2, 145–152.

Arnulf, I., Reading, P. and Vidialhet, M. (2010) 'Sleep Disorders in Idiopathic Parkinson's Disease.' In S. Overeem and P. Reading (eds) *Sleep Disorders in Neurology: A Practical Approach.* Chichester: Wiley-Blackwell.

Ayalon, L., Borodkin, K., Dishon, L., Kanety, H. and Dagan, Y. (2007) 'Circadian rhythm sleep disorder following mild traumatic brain injury.' *Neurology 68*, 14, 1136–1140.

Baumann, C.R. (2010) 'Sleep-Wake Disorders Following Traumatic Brain Injury.' In S. Overeem and P. Reading (eds) *Sleep Disorders in Neurology: A Practical Approach.* Chichester: Wiley-Blackwell.

Beekman, A.T.F., Bremmer, M.A., Deeg, D.J.H., van Balkom, A.J.L.M. *et al.* (1998) 'Anxiety disorders in later life: a report from the longitudinal aging study Amsterdam.' *International Journal of Geriatric Psychiatry 13*, 10, 717–726.

Benca, R.M., Obermeyer, W.H., Thisted, R.A. and Gillin, J.C. (1992) 'Sleep and psychiatric disorders: a meta-analysis.' *Archives of General Psychiatry 49*, 8, 651–668.

Benson, K.L. (2006) 'Sleep in schizophrenia: impairments, correlates, and treatment.' *Psychiatric Clinics of North America 29*, 4, 1033–1045.

Benson, K.L. (2008) 'Sleep in schizophrenia.' *Sleep Medicine Clinics 3*, 2, 251–260.

Benson, K.L. and Feinberg, I. (2011) 'Schizophrenia.' In M.H. Kryger, T. Roth and W.C. Dement (eds) *Principles and Practice of Sleep Medicine*, 5th edn. St Louis, MO: Saunders.

Bjorvatn, B. and Pallesen, S. (2009) 'A practical approach to circadian rhythm sleep disorders.' *Sleep Medicine Reviews 13*, 1, 47–60.

Bonnet, M.H. and Arand, D.L. (1997) 'Hyperarousal and insomnia.' *Sleep Medicine Reviews 1*, 2, 97–108.

Braam, W., Didden, R., Smits, M. and Curfs, L. (2008) 'Melatonin treatment in individuals with intellectual disability and chronic insomnia: a randomized placebo-controlled study.' *Journal of Intellectual Disability Research 52*, 3, 256–264.

Breslau, N., Roth, T., Rosenthal, L. and Andreski, P. (1996) 'Sleep disturbance and psychiatric disorders: a longitudinal epidemiological study of young adults.' *Biological Psychiatry 39*, 6, 411–418.

Bromundt, V., Köster, M., Georgiev-Kill, A., Opwis, K. *et al.* (2011) 'Sleep-wake cycles and cognitive functioning in schizophrenia.' *British Journal of Psychiatry 198*, 269–276.

Bruns, J. Jr and Hauser, W.A. (2003) 'The epidemiology of traumatic brain injury: a review.' *Epilepsia 44*, Suppl. 10, 2–10.

Brylewski, J. and Wiggs, L. (1998) 'A questionnaire survey of sleep and night-time behaviour in a community-based sample of adults with intellectual disability.' *Journal of Intellectual Disability Research 42*, 2, 154–162.

Brylewski, J. and Wiggs, L. (1999) 'Sleep problems and daytime challenging behaviour in a community-based sample of adults with intellectual disability.' *Journal of Intellectual Disability Research 43*, 6, 504–512.

Castriotta, R., Wilde, M.C., Lai, J.M., Atanasov, S., Masel, B.E. and Kuna, S.T. (2007) 'Prevalence and consequences of sleep disorders in traumatic brain injury.' *Journal of Clinical Sleep Medicine 3*, 4, 349–356.

Chouinard, S., Poulin, J., Stip, E. and Godbout, R. (2004) 'Sleep in untreated patients with schizophrenia: a meta-analysis.' *Schizophrenia Bulletin 30*, 4, 957–967.

Cohen, M., Oksenberg, A., Snir, D., Stern, M.J. and Groswasser, Z. (1992) 'Temporally related changes of sleep complaints in traumatic brain injured patients.' *Journal of Neurology, Neurosurgery, and Psychiatry 55*, 4, 313–315.

Craske, M.G. and Tsao, J.C.I. (2005) 'Assessment and treatment of nocturnal panic attacks.' *Sleep Medicine Reviews 9*, 3, 173–184.

Dauvilliers, Y. (2007) 'Insomnia in patients with neurodegenerative conditions.' *Sleep Medicine 8*, Suppl. 4, 27–34.

Dement, W., Halper, C., Pivik, T., Ferguson, J. *et al.* (1970) 'Hallucinations and Dreaming.' In D.A. Hamburg, K.A. Pribaum and A.J. Stunkard (eds) *Perception and its Disorders*. Baltimore, MD: The Williams & Wilkins Company.

Deschenes, C.L. and McCurry, S.M. (2009) 'Current treatments for sleep disturbances in individuals with dementia.' *Current Psychiatry Reports 11*, 1, 20–26.

Dhawan, V., Healy, D.G., Pal, S. and Chaudhuri, K.R. (2006) 'Sleep-related problems of Parkinson's disease.' *Age and Ageing 35*, 3, 220–228.

Didden, R. and Sigafoos, J. (2001) 'A review of the nature and treatment of sleep disorders in individuals with developmental disabilities.' *Research in Developmental Disabilities 22*, 4, 255–272.

Didden, R., Korzilius, H., van Aperlo, B., van Overloop, C. and de Vries, M. (2002) 'Sleep problems and daytime problem behaviours in children with intellectual disability.' *Journal of Intellectual Disability Research 46*, 7, 537–547.

Doran, S.M., Harvey, M.T. and Horner, R.H. (2006) 'Sleep and developmental disabilities: assessment, treatment, and outcome measures.' *Mental Retardation 44*, 1, 13–27.

Drevets, W.C. (2007) 'Orbitofrontal cortex function and structure in depression.' *Annals of the New York Academy of Sciences 1121*, 499–527.

Ford, D.E. and Kamerow, D.B. (1989) 'Epidemiologic study of sleep disturbances and psychiatric disorders: an opportunity for prevention?' *Journal of the American Medical Association 262*, 1479–1484.

Gunning, M.J. and Espie, C.A. (2003) 'Psychological treatment of reported sleep disorder in adults with intellectual disability using a multiple baseline design.' *Journal of Intellectual Disability Research 47*, 3, 191–202.

Hamilton, M. (1989) 'Frequency of symptoms in melancholia (depressive illness).' *British Journal of Psychiatry 154*, 2, 201–206.

Hylkema, T. and Vlaskamp, C. (2009) 'Significant improvement in sleep in people with intellectual disabilities living in residential settings by non-pharmaceutical interventions.' *Journal of Intellectual Disability Research 53*, 8, 695–703.

Iranzo, A. (2010) 'Sleep in Other Neurodegenerative Diseases.' In S. Overeem and P. Reading (eds) *Sleep Disorders in Neurology: A Practical Approach*. Chichester: Wiley-Blackwell.

Katz, D.A. and, McHorney, C.A. (2002) 'The relationship between insomnia and health-related quality of life in patients with chronic illness.' *Journal of Family Practice 51*, 3, 229–235.

Kryger, M.H., Roth, T. and Dement, W.C. (eds) (2011) *Principles and Practice of Sleep Medicine*, 5th edn. St Louis, MO: Saunders.

Jindal, R.D. and Thase, M.E. (2004) 'Treatment of insomnia associated with clinical depression.' *Sleep Medicine Reviews 8*, 1, 19–30.

Maquet, P., Degueldre, C., Delfiore, G., Aerts, J. *et al.* (1997) 'Functional neuroanatomy of human slow-wave sleep.' *Journal of Neuroscience 17*, 8, 2807–2812.

McCurry, S.M., Logsdon, R.G., Vitiello, M.V. and Teri, L. (2004) 'Treatment of sleep and nighttime disturbances in Alzheimer's disease: a behaviour management approach.' *Sleep Medicine 5*, 4, 373–377.

McCurry, S.M., Gibbons, L.E., Logsdon, R.G., Vitiello, M.V. and Teri, L. (2005) 'Nighttime insomnia treatment and education for Alzheimer's disease: a randomized, controlled trial.' *Journal of the American Geriatrics Society 53*, 5, 793–802.

Mellman, T.A. (2006) 'Sleep and anxiety disorders.' *Psychiatric Clinics of North America 29*, 4, 1047–1058.

Mellman, T.A. and Uhde, T.W. (1989) 'Sleep panic attacks: new clinical findings and theoretical implications.' *American Journal of Psychiatry 146*, 9, 1204–1207.

Morin, C.M., Bootzin, R.R., Buysse, D.J., Edinger, J.D., Espie, C.A., Lichstein, K.L. (2006) 'Psychological and behavioural treatment of insomnia: update of the recent evidence (1998–2004).' *Sleep 29*, 11, 1398–1414.

Morphy, H., Dunn, K.M., Lewis, M., Boardman, H.F. and Croft, P.R. (2007) 'Epidemiology of insomnia: a longitudinal study in a UK population.' *Sleep 30*, 3, 274–280.

Neckelmann, D., Mykletun, A. and Dahl, A.A. (2007) 'Chronic insomnia as a risk factor for developing anxiety and depression.' *Sleep 30*, 7, 873–880.

Ohayon, M.M. (1997) 'Prevalence of DSM–IV diagnostic criteria of insomnia: distinguishing insomnia related to mental disorders from sleep disorders.' *Journal of Psychiatric Research 31*, 3, 333–346.

Orff, H.J., Ayalon, L. and Drummond, S.P.A. (2009) 'Traumatic brain injury and sleep disturbance: a review of current research.' *Journal of Head Trauma Rehabilitation 24*, 3, 155–165.

Ouellet, M-C., Savard, J. and Morin, C.M. (2004) 'Insomnia following brain injury: a review.' *Neurorehabilitation and Neural Repair 18*, 4, 187–198.

Papadimitriou, G.N. and Linkowski, P. (2005) 'Sleep disturbance in anxiety disorders.' *International Review of Psychiatry 17*, 4, 229–236.

Parcell, D.L., Ponsford, J.L., Rajaratnam, S.M. and Redman, R. (2006) 'Self-reported changes to nighttime sleep after traumatic brain injury.' *Archives of Physical Medicine and Rehabilitation 87*, 2, 278–285.

Parker, G., Roy, K., Mitchell, P., Wilhelm, K., Malhi, G. and Hadzi-Pavlovic, D. (2002) 'Atypical depression: a reappraisal.' *American Journal of Psychiatry 159*, 9, 1470–1479.

Paterson, L.M., Nutt, D.J. and Wilson, S.J. (2009) 'NAPSAQ-1: National Patient Sleep Assessment Questionnaire in depression.' *International Journal of Psychiatry in Clinical Practice 13*, 1, 48–58.

Petit, D., Montplaisir, J. and Boeve, B.F. (2011) 'Alzheimer's Disease and Other Dementias.' In M.H. Kryger, T. Roth and W.C. Dement (eds) *Principles and Practice of Sleep Medicine*, 5th edn. St Louis, MO: Saunders.

Posternak, M.A. and Zimmerman, M. (2001) 'Symptoms of atypical depression.' *Psychiatry Research 104*, 2, 175–181.

Reid, K.J. and Zee, P.C. (2011) 'Circadian Disorders of the Sleep-Wake Cycle.' In M.H. Kryger, T. Roth and W.C. Dement (eds) *Principles and Practice of Sleep Medicine*, 5th edn. St Louis, MO: Saunders.

Richdale, A.L. and Schreck, K.A. (2009) 'Sleep problems in autism spectrum disorders: prevalence, nature, and possible biopsychosocial aetiologies.' *Sleep Medicine Reviews 13*, 6, 403–411.

Riedel, B.W. and Lichstein, K.L. (2000) 'Insomnia and daytime functioning.' *Sleep Medicine Reviews 4*, 3, 277–298.

Sajith, S.G. and Clarke, D. (2007) 'Melatonin and sleep disorders associated with intellectual disability: a clinical review.' *Journal of Intellectual Disability Research 51*, 1, 2–13.

Sekimoto, M., Kato, M., Watanabe, T., Kajimura, N. and Takahashi, K. (2007) 'Reduced frontal asymmetry of delta waves during all-night sleep in schizophrenia.' *Schizophrenia Bulletin 33*, 6, 1307–1311.

Sharpley, A.L., Vassallo, C.M. and Cowen, P.J. (2000) 'Olanzapine increases slow-wave sleep: evidence for blockade of central 5-HT2C receptors in vivo.' *Biological Psychiatry 47*, 5, 468–470.

Spoormaker, V.I. and Montgomery, P. (2008) 'Disturbed sleep in post-traumatic stress disorder: secondary symptom or core feature?' *Sleep Medicine Reviews 12*, 3, 169–184.

Steele, D.L., Rajaratnam, S.M., Redman, J.R. and Ponsford, J.L. (2005) 'The effect of traumatic brain injury on the timing of sleep.' *Chronobiology International 22*, 1, 89–105.

Stewart, R., Besset, A., Bebbington, P., Brugha, T. *et al.* (2006) 'Insomnia comorbidity and impact and hypnotic use by age group in a national survey population aged 16 to 74 years.' *Sleep 29*, 11, 1391–1397.

Trenkwalder, C. and Arnulf, I. (2011) 'Parkinsonism.' In M.H. Kryger, T. Roth and W.C. Dement (eds) *Principles and Practice of Sleep Medicine*, 5th edn. St Louis, MO: Saunders.

Verma, A., Anand, V. and Verma, N.P. (2007) 'Sleep disorders in chronic traumatic brain injury.' *Journal of Clinical Sleep Medicine 3*, 4, 357–362.

Watson, N.F., Dikmen, S., Machamer, J., Doherty, M. and Temkin, N. (2007) 'Hypersomnia following traumatic brain injury.' *Journal of Clinical Sleep Medicine 3*, 4, 363–368.

Wilson, S. and Argyropoulos, S. (2012) 'Sleep in schizophrenia: time for closer attention.' *British Journal of Psychiatry 200*, 4, 273–274..

Wittchen, H.-U. and Jacobi, F. (2005) 'Size and burden of mental disorders in Europe.' *European Neuropsychopharmacology 15*, 4, 357–376.

Wulff, K.L., Dijk, D.-J., Middleton, B., Foster, R.G., Joyce, E.M. (2012) 'Sleep and circadian rhythm disruption in schizophrenia.' *British Journal of Psychiatry 200*, 4, 308–316.

Wulff, K.L., Gatti, S., Wettstein, J.G. and Foster, R.G. (2010) 'Sleep and circadian rhythm disruption in psychiatric and neurodegenerative disease.' *Nature Reviews Neuroscience 11*, 8, 589–599.

Yates, W.R., Mitchell, J., Rush, A.J., Trivedi, M. *et al.* (2007) 'Clinical features of depression in outpatients with and without co-occurring general medical conditions in STAR*D: confirmatory analysis.' *Primary Care Companion to the Journal of Clinical Psychiatry 9*, 1, 7–15.

11

Medication and Sleep

Sue Wilson

11.1. Introduction

This chapter provides an overview of drugs and substances that can promote or prevent sleep, or have been connected with sleep in the past. It mostly covers drugs prescribed by doctors, but also looks at drugs that can be bought over the counter, including those found in health shops, as well as recreational and street drugs. However, before considering the effects of drugs in the brain, it is helpful to understand some of the mechanisms of the brain through which these drugs can act. (See also Chapters 2 and 3.)

11.2. The brain and neurotransmitters

The human brain is an incredibly complex organ made up of about 100 billion nerve cells, or neurones, which have a huge number of potential interconnections. Nerve cells pass messages to each other by producing a very brief impulse of electrical activity – a process known as firing. The impulse travels down the nerve at about 200mph and is passed on to the next nerve cell (or sometimes to many nerve cells) at a place where the two nerves are very close to each other, called a synapse (see Figure 11.1). This is done by a chemical process in which the firing nerve releases a chemical called a neurotransmitter into the space between the nerves (synaptic cleft). On reaching the next nerve the neurotransmitter affects its electrical excitability, making it more or less likely to fire in its turn — although whether a nerve cell fires or not also depends on the inputs it receives from perhaps several other neurones. The messages passed at synapses can make the nerve more likely to fire (excitatory transmission) or less likely (inhibitory transmission), and the net effect depends on how many excitatory and inhibitory messages there are.

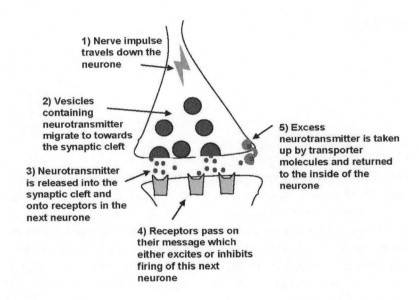

1) Nerve impulse travels down the neurone

2) Vesicles containing neurotransmitter migrate to towards the synaptic cleft

3) Neurotransmitter is released into the synaptic cleft and onto receptors in the next neurone

4) Receptors pass on their message which either excites or inhibits firing of this next neurone

5) Excess neurotransmitter is taken up by transporter molecules and returned to the inside of the neurone

Figure 11.1. A synapse, the connection between one nerve and the next

The main excitatory neurotransmitter in the brain is glutamate, a salt of glutamic acid, an amino acid found in many foods (the sodium salt of glutamic acid is also known as monosodium glutamate). The main inhibitory neurotransmitter is another amino acid, known as gamma-aminobutyic acid, or GABA. Amongst other neurotransmitters are noradrenaline, dopamine, serotonin, acetylcholine, histamine and adenosine. Neurotransmitters are made in neurones, using precursor chemicals ('ingredients' from the bloodstream) already present in the brain. Eating food containing molecules of one of the precursors is unlikely to affect nerve transmission, because of a sophisticated mechanism called the blood-brain barrier. This is a highly evolved protective system of membrane barriers and specialized pumps in the walls of small blood vessels which allow only certain substances to cross from the bloodstream into the brain – usually smaller molecules recognized as safe. A major consideration for the development of a new drug is therefore its formulation into a molecule which will cross the blood-brain barrier either because of its similarity to other molecules which can cross, or its 'disguise', enabling it to use existing pumps.

When the neurotransmitter crosses the synaptic cleft onto the membrane of the next nerve (postsynaptic membrane) it reaches proteins called receptors embedded in the cell membrane, each type of which responds only to a particular neurotransmitter. Once there, the receptor then causes downstream changes in the chemistry of the nerve cell to make it in its turn more or less likely to fire. After the neurotransmitter has acted on the postsynaptic receptor it is cleared from the synaptic space by specialized proteins called reuptake transporters (i.e. taking the neurotransmitter back into the nerve cell) on the neurones or the surrounding supporting cells, either to be broken down and disposed of, or to be recycled inside the cell for rerelease in the future (see Figure 11.1).

An example of nerve transmission would be what occurs on hearing a simple noise such as a click. The hair cells in the ear cause the acoustic nerve to fire, transmitting an electrical impulse into the brain to a synapse with a neurone in a relay station (interneurone) in the brainstem, the part of the base of the brain where it joins to the spinal cord. This releases the neurotransmitter glutamate onto a glutamate receptor on the interneurone causing it to fire. Glutamate transporters remove the excess transmitter. Two more such synapses in relay stations in upper brainstem and midbrain are passed in the same way before the impulse reaches the 'thinking' part of the brain, the cortex or outer layer (see Figure 11.2). The sound is perceived there, about a tenth of a second after the soundwave reached the ear, and a message sent to other parts of the brain for interpretation and understanding. At each of these relay points, particularly the last, the interneurones can be affected not only by the excitatory incoming information from the ear, but by many influences from other parts of the brain; for instance, listening for the click might cause other neurones from the conscious parts of the brain to release excitatory transmitters onto the interneurones which would enhance the effect of the incoming nerve impulse. Being asleep might mean that GABA synapses on to that same connecting neurone dampen the effect and make it less likely to pass on the auditory message to the cortex. At the cortex, a balance of inputs from many neurones all over the brain could mean that heightened attention on something else, such as a riveting television programme, might influence whether the sound of the click is passed on to the interpretation process and therefore 'registered' by the person.

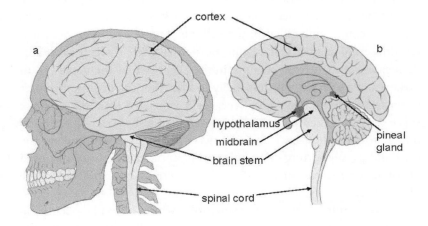

Figure 11.2. Diagram of the human brain: side view (a) and as seen from the midline (b)

As well as glutamate and GABA, there are many other neurotransmitters that are used to pass messages from one nerve to another, each with its own set of receptors that are not responsive to other neurotransmitters. Most drugs that affect the brain do so by affecting receptors, and they can do this by:

- simulating the action of a brain neurotransmitter on the postsynaptic receptor (these are called agonists)

- blocking its action on postsynaptic receptors (antagonists)

- changing the receptor's sensitivity.[1]

Other drugs work by increasing the amount of neurotransmitter present in the synapse, either by increasing its release into the synaptic cleft, blocking its transportation out of the cleft or preventing the action of enzymes that break it down.

11.3. Drugs that promote sleep

All drugs that can be prescribed by doctors have undergone rigorous and extensive testing to establish that they are safe and that they work. A comprehensive overview of their use in insomnia has been carried out by the British Association for Psychopharmacology (Wilson *et al.* 2010). There has been little rigorous testing of the effectiveness of the drugs bought over the counter for insomnia (although their safety and use as anti-allergy drugs have usually been investigated), so a reference for further reading is given at the end of this chapter.

Prescription medication
HYPNOTIC DRUGS

Sleeping pills that are prescribed to people with insomnia are known as hypnotics and have nothing to do with hypnotizing anyone (Hypnos was the Greek god of sleep). Nearly all of these drugs affect the action of just one brain neurotransmitter, GABA, which is the most widely distributed inhibitory neurotransmitter in the brain, and 'damps down' the excitability of neurones in all areas of the brain. Increasing GABA function causes sedation and sleep but also causes muscle relaxation, memory impairment and unsteadiness; it can therefore impair performance of skills such as driving. Reduction of GABA's effects results in arousal, anxiety, restlessness, insomnia and exaggerated reactivity.

There is a robust system of nerve cells and pathways using different neurotransmitters which form a pathway that leads up from the brainstem to the relay stations and to the cortex in order to maintain arousal. This is known as the ascending arousal system and involves neurones using the neurotransmitters noradrenaline, acetylcholine, dopamine, serotonin and histamine (see Chapter 2). This network of neurones is very active whilst we are awake, sending messages up to various parts of the brain to make them more attentive and receptive to incoming signals from the senses. During sleep the network's activity is damped down by inhibitory nerve pathways such as those involving

GABA, so that incoming information from outside is not perceived, therefore the brain does not react to it.

The main type of GABA receptor in the brain, the GABA-A receptor, is a fast-acting receptor that acts directly on the nerve cell membrane to make the cell less likely to fire. The majority of sleeping pills, the benzodiazepines and 'z-drugs' (see below), enhance the effects of GABA by lowering the level of GABA that is needed to activate the GABA-A receptor. They do not act directly on the receptor but only modulate the ability of GABA to do so – 'helping' its calming effects. Because they are indirect modulators of GABA and require its presence for their effect, the brain can in principle compensate for an overdose of these drugs by reducing GABA production; if there is no GABA then they will not work. It is believed that this explains the very high safety margin of hypnotic drugs – taking an overdose is not lethal, unless combined with other more dangerous substances. This contrasts with the older drugs like barbiturates that did not rely on the brain's own GABA for their action. However, sleeping pills remain likely to cause sedation when the person wants to be awake, as well as unsteadiness, loss of balance and memory problems, because of the fact that GABA receptors all over the brain are being affected – not only those regulating arousal state but also those in areas controlling movement and memory. Whilst the drug is in the body, if there is a situation where a person needs to be up and about, rather than in bed asleep, it can increase the likelihood of falls, which is why they are prescribed with caution in the elderly. These GABA drugs all interact with alcohol, so that together they produce more and longer-lasting sleep-inducing effects, and alcohol itself has other dangerous sedative effects through different receptor systems; all pack inserts for these drugs have a warning not to take them with alcohol.

Benzodiazepines such as diazepam (Valium[2]) have a long duration of action and are used to treat short-term anxiety. Benzodiazepines with a shorter action such as temazepam are used to treat sleeplessness, but nowadays the most commonly used sleep-improving drugs which modulate GABA-A receptors are the z-drugs: zopiclone, zolpidem and zaleplon. This is because they have the shortest duration of action (see Figure 11.3) and so are less likely to cause hangover or drowsiness in the morning when people want to be alert and drive safely. However, there is still likely to be a significant level of zopiclone in the bloodstream at

8 a.m. after taking it at 11 p.m., particularly if the person has had any alcohol during the previous evening; this is why doctors advise caution about driving when taking these tablets.

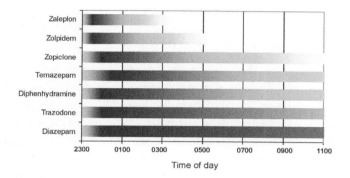

Figure 11.3. Duration of action of various drugs taken at 23:00
Darker shading represents more effect. For example, zaleplon and zolpidem reach their maximum effect quickly and 'wear off' quickly whereas temazepam takes longer to work and is still producing sleepiness by mid-morning. Diazepam is included for comparison, but is usually only used in the daytime for anxiety.

At present there is a recommendation that doctors do not prescribe these drugs continuously for more than four weeks. That is because in the 1970s and 1980s some people became dependent on benzodiazepines, usually when they were prescribed for daytime use in anxiety, and it was decided that taking them for a shorter period would prevent this. Because the newer z-drugs act at the same receptor, they were also subjected to the same restrictions. In fact, many people have been taking either benzodiazepines or z-drugs for longer periods than this, and research into long-term effects is still being carried out. Other people are reluctant to take sleeping pills because they do not want to become addicted. Whilst such concern is understandable, it is worth considering the definition of addiction used by most of the medical profession. Addiction includes three or more, together, of the following:

- a strong desire or sense of compulsion to take the substance

- difficulties in controlling substance-taking behaviour in terms of its onset, termination or levels of use

- increasing the dose of the drug, sometimes to levels that would be dangerous to a first-time user (tolerance)

- constantly thinking about and looking forward to taking the drug
- drug-seeking behaviour that replaces alternative pleasures or interests
- increased amount of time necessary to obtain or take the substance or to recover from its effects.

Most people, given the choice, would prefer not to take sleeping pills if they could sleep without them. They do not experience a compulsive desire to take them, or spend time in drug-seeking behaviour. Unprescribed dose increases above recommended doses in patients with insomnia are uncommon, and tolerance to hypnotic drug effects is not a frequent problem in clinical experience; many patients use the same dose of hypnotic for months or years and still feel it works. However, dependence on sleeping pills does happen to some people; commonly there is a kind of psychological dependence based on the fact that the treatment works to reduce people's sleep disturbance, and therefore they are unwilling to stop. If they do stop, there can be relapse, where original symptoms return. A temporary worsening of sleep, usually with increased time to get off to sleep, is reported during the withdrawal period for most sleeping pills, even in studies where normal sleepers take them for research purposes. If this temporary change of sleep after stopping is so great as to make sleep worse than before taking the medication, it is called rebound insomnia. Research has shown that brain GABA-A receptors do change in function during long-term treatment with benzodiazepine receptor modulators; the brain is constantly trying to return to the status quo when being affected by drugs, and so the receptors change in their sensitivity to the drug. Once the drug is taken away, the receptors take time to return to pre-medication status. If people are warned about this and can plan their tailing off the drug at a convenient time, the problem need not be significant.

Of course, sleep without sleeping pills is an aim of most people with insomnia, and psychological treatments like cognitive behaviour therapy (CBT – see Chapter 9) are very effective in helping them to do this. Learning the strategies involved in such therapy can improve the experience of coming off sleeping pills and subsequent episodes of poor sleep can be better managed without pills.

ANTIDEPRESSANTS

Sometimes antidepressants are prescribed for sleep problems, especially if there are some depressive symptoms (see Chapter 10), but they do not work on the GABA system like the hypnotic drugs. The antidepressants most commonly prescribed for sleep are trazodone and mirtazapine and they work by blocking types of serotonin receptors (called 5HT2) and types of histamine receptors (called H1). Both serotonin and histamine contribute to the ongoing arousal system and so blocking these receptors reduces arousal. There is no time restriction on prescribing these but no one has studied whether they continue to help people sleep after prolonged use. They usually have a long duration of action and so they are likely to cause morning drowsiness or clumsiness. Other antidepressants such as amitriptyline or doxepin (called tricyclics because of their chemical structure) affect these serotonin receptors and many other brain receptors, as well as some in the body, and therefore they can produce unwanted side effects such as dry mouth, dizziness, nausea and changes in heart rate. These tricyclic antidepressants are dangerous in overdose because of their effects on the heart and circulation, unlike drugs such as trazodone or mirtazapine or specific serotonin reuptake inhibitors (SSRIs) that are much safer.

MELATONIN

Another drug that is sometimes prescribed for sleeplessness is melatonin. Melatonin is a hormone that occurs naturally in the body and the brain and is often called the 'darkness' hormone because it is only secreted during the hours of darkness. It is produced by the pineal gland that is located in the centre of the brain and is about the size of a pea (see Figure 11.2). The melatonin signal forms part of the system that regulates the sleep/wake cycle on a roughly 24-hour rhythm (see Chapter 3). Taking melatonin, in a carefully timed regime, has proved useful in helping people with jet lag to resynchronize themselves to the desired schedule (Sack et al. 2007), and has recently been shown to have a modest effect on improving sleep quality in people over the age of 55 who have insomnia (Wade et al. 2007), probably compensating for the diminished melatonin rhythm that occurs with age. In the UK, melatonin is only available on prescription, but many people obtain it in overseas airports or from countries where it is classed as a food supplement.

Drugs available over the counter

Over-the-counter painkillers such as aspirin and paracetamol have never been shown to affect sleep itself, although there is no doubt that when sleep is disturbed by pain, adequate pain relief will ameliorate this. It is important for people on these or other painkillers to take them at the optimum time for pain relief to occur at the time for sleep.

ANTIHISTAMINES

Histamine neurones in the hypothalamus, a part of the brain concerned with sleep regulation, send their messages up to the cortex to maintain arousal and attention. An antihistamine is a drug that is usually taken to alleviate allergic reactions such as rashes or hay fever; the older antihistamines are able to pass the blood-brain barrier and therefore cause sedation when taken during the day. These older antihistamines, such as promethazine and diphenhydramine, are the main ingredients of over-the-counter sleep remedies, and doctors can prescribe them for insomnia, although this is not common. There has been little research into their use in insomnia, but it seems from the limited available evidence that they may have a modest sleep-promoting effect in milder insomnia, which may not be maintained beyond a few days. They also have a longer duration of action than the z-drugs, and so may cause more morning drowsiness, and like antidepressants, have unwanted actions at other receptors which give rise to side effects.

HERBAL SLEEP AIDS

The ingestion of various herbs such as valerian, hops, chamomile and many others is a popular strategy for poor sleepers. It is unknown how these remedies might work on brain receptors as the active chemicals in them have yet to be identified. There are some reports of a modest sleep-improving effect of valerian, but one that seems not to last more than one or two nights in many people, and reports are often contradictory. Generally, evidence for the effectiveness of herbal remedies is sparse and often not reported in a scientific way. St John's wort is worthy of a special mention, not because it is effective for insomnia (there is very little research, and it can sometimes make it worse), but because it has potentially dangerous interactions with many other medications, including those that are taken for depression, heart problems, blood pressure and many other disorders. It is therefore not a good choice for those with sleep problems.

The substance 5-hydroxytryptophan (5HTP) is a naturally occurring amino acid found in some foods such as turkey, milk, potatoes, pumpkin and various green vegetables, and can be seen in health shops with a recommendation for use in insomnia. It is a precursor for serotonin, a neurotransmitter in the brain with some involvement in sleep (see above), although, as mentioned, it is not clear how much effect increases in dietary 5HTP would influence levels in the brain. However, there is some low-level evidence of improved sleep in a few people and it is safe in small doses. The American Academy of Sleep Medicine (AASM) produced a statement in 2005 based on extensive research. This provides a good overview of the issues with non-prescription remedies for insomnia (Meoli *et al.* 2005).

Recreational and 'street' drugs

ALCOHOL

Alcohol is one of the most common ways worldwide to self-medicate for sleep problems, but although it may accelerate sleep onset, its overall effect is sleep-disturbing. In healthy good sleepers who are light social drinkers, the effects on the night's sleep of going to bed with a blood alcohol concentration (BAC) of about 0.03 per cent, or after about two units of alcohol, are small.[3] Deep sleep is increased slightly in the first half of the night and decreased in the latter half. If the BAC is 0.1 per cent (i.e. after five or six units) there is a larger effect, with sleep starting more quickly, and more deep sleep early in the night, but more awakenings in the latter half of the night – in these research studies the overall effect is to lessen sleep. This is probably because alcohol has effects at the GABA receptor, but not in the same way as hypnotic drugs mentioned above. It causes a less controlled increase in inhibitory activity of GABA neurones, not dependent on GABA itself, and has some effects to decrease the main excitatory neurotransmitter, glutamate; this can result in depression of respiration, and in large doses, death (about 200 people per year die of accidental alcohol poisoning in the UK). However, alcohol remains the most popular self-administered treatment for insomnia, and this has often been reported as a pathway to alcohol dependence. In people who become dependent on alcohol, the deep sleep is actually reduced in amount every night, and once drinking ceases it takes some weeks or months to return to normal levels.

OPIATES

Opiates comprise recreational drugs such as opium (which is usually eaten or smoked) and heroin (which is injected or smoked) as well as medically prescribed drugs. The latter include diamorphine (pure heroin, injected for pain relief), morphine (usually as an oral syrup for pain relief), tablets such as codeine and oxycodone, and methadone (an oral syrup, used as a substitute for heroin in addicts).

Opium has been used for many centuries to relieve pain and used to be thought to induce sleep; all opiates are controlled drugs.[4] They have a marked pain-reducing effect but their effects on sleep (now we can measure them scientifically) are controversial, because acute doses of morphine actually disrupt sleep in addicts and in healthy volunteers, and prevent people with post-operative pain from sleeping properly. We have no idea why this should be. What is clear is that opiates induce euphoria and alteration of dreaming, with more frequent and more vivid dreams in sleep, and dreamy 'visions' in the awake state. Laudanum, a mixture of morphine and fortified wine, was used widely in the nineteenth century to reduce pain and help sleep, although it is unclear which of its components was contributing to the effects. Many people became addicted to this potent mix of alcohol and opium. What is known, however, is that all opiates used for pleasure are addictive and require larger and larger doses to induce the pleasant effects. They should never be considered by people just needing a good night's sleep because of the strong likelihood of addiction, and also because opiates all work as agonists at specific opiate receptors in the brain which are involved in pain and respiration and therefore may compromise breathing during sleep. Overdose often results in respiratory arrest and this is how heroin addicts die when they take an unexpectedly pure shot of heroin. These opiate receptors respond to the body's own opiates, known as endorphins, and also to externally administered opiate drugs. The involvement of these receptors in sleep is the subject of current research and is still not worked out, but they may be important for sleep regulation, because addicts withdrawing from opiates suffer prolonged insomnia. Opiate withdrawal triggers an increase in function of some of the other neurotransmitters involved in arousal such as noradrenaline and dopamine, so this may result in a hyperaroused state.

CANNABIS

Many people say they use cannabis in the evening to help them sleep. This effect may be mediated through enhanced relaxation at bedtime, as there are few objective effects on sleep. Cannabis contains many chemical compounds, but the main two psychoactive ones are tetrahydrocannabinol (THC) and cannabidiol (CBD). THC appears to have no objectively measured effects on sleep in healthy volunteers, but increases sleepiness on awakening in the morning after high doses. On the other hand, CBD produces more wakefulness during sleep after high doses, and less morning sleepiness. These effects may counteract each other, but relative THC/CBD proportions in cannabis preparations vary as do individuals' reaction to the drug. There is some evidence that cannabis receptors are involved in pain perception, and a medically prescribed nasal spray containing THC and CBD is in clinical trials for the relief of chronic pain in various long-term illnesses including multiple sclerosis; in those studies there is a preliminary improvement in sleep reported in the patients (Russo, Guy and Robson 2007).

Whereas there are numerous cannabinoid receptors in the brain, their function is only just beginning to be established, and is a subject of much research. They appear to respond to the body's own cannabinoid neurochemicals by affecting nerve cell signalling through a complex interaction with other neurotransmitters; this leads to effects on stress mechanisms and pain, but revelations about cannabis receptor function are likely in the next few years.

11.4. Wake-promoting drugs

Although this chapter has concentrated mainly on drugs that promote sleep, or are thought at some time to promote it, it is important to consider sleep as part of a 24-hour cycle. Therefore those drugs and compounds that promote wakefulness and prevent sleep are also of interest.

Caffeine

Caffeine is present in coffee, cola and 'energy' drinks and, to a lesser extent, tea. It is known to be wake-promoting, probably because it antagonises receptors of adenosine, a sleep-promoting neurotransmitter in the brain. In experimental studies caffeine produced an increase in time to fall asleep of about 60 per cent, and modestly increased wakening at night when taken in doses of about 150mg (1–2 cups of brewed coffee) at bedtime (Paterson *et al.* 2009). The effects on waking of caffeine are very variable from person to person and can change as we get older. Many people describe how they were able to drink lots of coffee late at night whilst a student, and yet in their forties and fifties they find that coffee after 6 p.m. keeps them awake at night. Of course, it may be that instant coffee with a low caffeine content is what was widely available then (in the 1970s), but there is basic evidence that the effects of caffeine are longer-lasting with increasing age. The increase in duration of action could be due to a slower metabolism in the liver with age, or to an increased sensitivity to caffeine's activating effects.

Stimulant drugs

Amphetamine-like stimulants are all controlled drugs and can be prescribed, but are often sold as street drugs. They increase wakefulness by increasing the amount of neurotransmission in dopamine and noradrenaline neurones at synapses. They do this by mimicking the action of the transmitter and to some extent by blocking its reuptake. These drugs are detrimental to sleep, and patients who take them for medical purposes such as control of excessive sleepiness in narcolepsy take care to time the dosing so that the stimulant effects do not impinge on desired sleep. The main prescribed drugs are dexamfetamine (Dexedrine) and methylphenidate (Ritalin). Cocaine is a stimulant which also prevents synaptic reuptake of the arousing neurotransmitters dopamine and noradrenaline, without the transmitter-mimicking action of amphetamines; it is a drug of abuse which is snorted or smoked (crack) and can disrupt sleep for a few hours after ingestion. Modafinil is a non-amphetamine wake-promoting drug used to treat disorders of daytime sleepiness. Its mode of action is unclear but does not involve dopamine release or reuptake. Its action is of fairly slow onset and, probably because it does not cause a 'rush', it is not abused.

Ecstasy (3,4-methylenedioxy-N-methylamphetamine, MDMA)
This drug increases serotonin release and people take it because it gives a feeling of euphoria, a sense of intimacy with others, reduces anxiety and elevates mood. It also promotes wakefulness as serotonin is part of the arousal system, and people who use it tend to do so at parties and stay up all night to dance and socialize. Surveys have shown that sleep is fragmented for two nights after weekend use and two studies of long-term users have been reported to have subjectively unsatisfactory sleep (Carhart-Harris *et al.* 2009; Dughiero, Schifano and Forza 2001). This might be because prolonged ecstasy use has long-lasting effects on the brain's serotonin system, or could be related to a lifestyle that includes weekend sleep deprivation and irregular sleep/wake pattern.

11.5. Conclusion
We now know a great deal about how drugs work in the brain, mostly derived from laboratory-based and preclinical experiments, but there is still a huge amount to learn. Despite the effectiveness of psychological treatments for insomnia, we are always likely to need hypnotic medication for short-term use and perhaps in the longer term too, if psychological treatments remain difficult to access. However, we do not yet know the relative roles of drugs and these behavioural therapies, and whether combining them has any advantage; meanwhile, the search for the 'perfect' drug for insomnia continues. The following list of ideal properties suggests that it may be an unattainable goal as no single drug is likely to tick all the boxes:

- rapid absorption
- rapid sleep induction
- works through the night
- induces 'normal' sleep pattern
- no residual effects in the morning
- specific mechanism of action
- low risk of mortality in overdose
- no rebound insomnia
- no dependence

- no tolerance
- no effects on balance or movement
- no interaction with other drugs or alcohol
- no effects on breathing during sleep.

There are two main problems with drugs that are currently available for insomnia. The first problem is with offset of action: at present if we want a drug to work throughout the night, the downside is that there will be residual sleepiness in the morning. The second problem is the focus of action: we do not yet have an effective insomnia drug which only targets the sleep centres in the brain, so there are unwanted effects from other parts of the brain influenced by the same neurotransmitters. Research on new drugs that takes account of these issues is continuing. It is also important to investigate individual responses to drugs that may be largely genetically determined and research into personalized, tailored treatments according to a person's genetic make-up is likely to be very fruitful in the future.

As for keeping awake, it has been seen that various possibilities currently exist: these range from the widely used caffeine to the more dangerous and illegal substances. There is a safe wake-promoting drug in modafinil which is used for narcolepsy and already used unprescribed by people who wish to stay awake. However, whereas people usually take hypnotics in the hope of getting a 'normal' amount of sleep in order to cope during the day, they use stimulants (in absence of a sleep disorder) to push the boundaries and to achieve more. This is a lifestyle choice and a matter for discussion elsewhere.

This chapter was completed in November 2010.

Notes

1. These drugs are known as allosteric modulators.
2. Prescription drugs have a generic or official name, for example, diazepam and zopiclone (which is always in lowercase) and one or several other brand names which drug companies give it – a proprietary name, usually with a capital letter, for example, Valium and Zimovane.
3. Two units to alcohol are roughly a 120–150ml glass of wine, or ¾ pint of beer (5%), or two 25ml measures of spirits.
4. Some drugs are controlled under the Misuse of Drugs legislation. Stricter legal controls apply to controlled drugs to prevent them being obtained illegally,

misused or causing harm. These legal controls govern how controlled medicines may be stored, produced, supplied and prescribed.

References

Carhart-Harris, R.L., Nutt, D.J., Munafò, M. and Wilson, S.J. (2009) 'Current and former ecstasy users report different sleep to matched controls: a web-based questionnaire study.' *Journal of Psychopharmacology 23*, 3, 249–257.

Dughiero, G., Schifano, F. and Forza, G. (2001) 'Personality dimensions and psychopathological profiles of ecstasy users.' *Human Psychopharmacology: Clinical and Experimental 16*, 8, 635–639.

Meoli, A.L., Rosen, C., Kristo, D., Kohrman, M. *et al.* (2005) 'Oral nonprescription treatment for insomnia: an evaluation of products with limited evidence.' *Journal of Clinical Sleep Medicine 1*, 2, 173–187.

Paterson, L.M., Nutt, D.J., Ivarsson, M., Hutson, P.H. and Wilson, S.J. (2009) 'Effects on sleep stages and microarchitecture of caffeine and its combination with zolpidem or trazodone in healthy volunteers.' *Journal of Psychopharmacology 23*, 5, 487–494.

Russo, E.B., Guy, G.W. and Robson, P.J. (2007) 'Cannabis, pain, and sleep: lessons from therapeutic clinical trials of *Sativex®*, a cannabis-based medicine.' *Chemistry and Biodiversity 4*, 8, 1729–1743.

Sack, R.L., Auckley, D., Auger, R.R., Carskadon, M.A. *et al.* (2007) 'Circadian rhythm sleep disorders: part I, basic principles, shift work and jet lag disorders. An American Academy of Sleep Medicine review.' *Sleep 30*, 11, 1460–1483.

Wade, A.G., Ford, I., Crawford, G., McMahon, A.D. *et al.* (2007) 'Efficacy of prolonged release melatonin in insomnia patients aged 55–80 years: quality of sleep and next-day alertness outcomes.' *Current Medical Research and Opinion 23*, 10, 2597–2605.

Wilson, S.J., Nutt, D.J., Alford, C., Argyropoulos, S.V. *et al.* (2010) 'British Association for Psychopharmacology consensus statement on evidence-based treatment of insomnia, parasomnias and circadian rhythm disorders.' *Journal of Psychopharmacology 24*, 11, 1577–1601.

Further reading

Porter, R. and Teich, M. (eds) (1995) *Drugs and Narcotics in History*. Cambridge: Cambridge University Press.

12

Too Tired to Sleep

Alex Westcombe and Hazel O'Dowd

12.1. Introduction

If a random selection of people were asked to define the links between sleep and tiredness, they would probably come up with a fairly simple formula: increasing tiredness precedes going to bed, which is followed by falling asleep, and the tiredness is resolved in the morning. However, they would probably mention some exceptions to this too, including feeling completely exhausted yet being unable to get to sleep, or not feeling refreshed on waking despite apparently sleeping well. Such exceptions imply that tiredness does not have a direct relationship with sleep. In other words, it is not always the case that the more tired someone gets, the closer they are to sleep – nor that the more they sleep, the less tired they become.

This chapter aims to explore the nature of sleep and tiredness, their components and interactions. Chronic fatigue syndrome/myalgic encephalomyelitis (CFS/ME)[1] is considered in detail as an example of how tiredness and sleep-related difficulties are often seen together. It might appear strange to emphasize tiredness in a book about sleep, but a person's experience of sleep can only be understood by their perceptions when awake.

12.2. Exploring the concepts of tiredness, sleepiness and fatigue

Tiredness

Although 'tiredness' is, at least in British English, a commonly used term, it is not necessarily an exact one. It can be used to cover a range of experiences, as demonstrated by Olympic rower Annabel Vernon:

> ...I could probably think of a hundred different ways of being tired. Training for 30 hours a week or thereabouts is essentially a constant process of getting tired and recovering, getting tired and recovering, and so on. There's walking-up-stairs tired, falling-asleep-everywhere tired, generally-a-bit-grumpy tired, counting-strokes-on-an-ergo tired, losing-your-sense-of-humour tired...
> (Vernon 2011)

There seem to be three key elements here: a need for sleep, physical fatigue and mood. Concentrating on the first two, an Oxford English Dictionary definition for 'tired' is 'in need of sleep or rest; weary'. Dement, Hall and Walsh (2003) defined tiredness as suboptimal *sleepiness*, whereas Olson (2007) placed it at the lowest level of a hierarchy – below *fatigue* and exhaustion. It appears appropriate, therefore, to divide 'tiredness' into sleepiness and fatigue, and then to explore both in more detail. The issues of mood and motivation are returned to later.

Sleepiness

Interpreting the definitions of Mathis and Hess (2009) in a slightly different way, sleepiness could be defined in terms of the experience (a craving for sleep, reduced concentration, wandering thoughts, heavy eyelids), how it is observed (yawning, eye-rubbing, heavy head, lowering eyes, objective measures of time taken to fall asleep), and the consequences (diminished alertness and cognitive performance).

Johns (2010) also makes a distinction between feeling sleepy (which he specifically terms 'drowsiness') and the likelihood of actually falling asleep (which he calls 'sleep propensity'). He also emphasizes the variations in sleepiness – between and within individuals – and what might affect them. First, it is possible to measure an 'average' sleepiness rating for an individual: the Epworth Sleepiness Scale (ESS)

(Johns 1991) comprises a list of different situations and asks people to rate how likely they would be to fall asleep in each of them. An average can be taken of these scores, which gives an idea of someone's general likelihood, across a variety of situations, to fall asleep. It is also the case that particular settings have their own sleep potential: for example, someone is more likely to fall asleep when resting horizontally in a quiet, dark room compared to when they are walking outside. Johns contends that these factors are quite reliable and consistent across many people. There is also the combination of the two factors: how the individual interacts with the setting. Johns stresses the neurological impact of light perception (the importance of which is discussed in Chapter 3) and postural muscle tension on the sensory nervous system. He also alludes to more psychological factors, giving the example of how someone might fill out the ESS if they were being assessed for their capacity to drive; two of the specific questions ask people how likely they are to fall asleep whilst sat in a car (Johns 2010).

Another example could be the meaning attached to sleepiness in a particular setting. For example, the levels of sleepiness might be more important to someone who is worried about their sleep quality, which might make them more aware of sensations of sleepiness/drowsiness than someone who is not so concerned. Similarly, feeling sleepy whilst driving on a busy motorway at night might be more significant for someone than it would be when they are trying to finish watching a film in the middle of a lazy afternoon. Vernet et al. (2010) suggest that motivation could play a part: people in their study with idiopathic hypersomnia[2] who had a significant problem with sleepiness during the day said they felt more awake when doing more pleasurable activities, activities which were of more value to them.

If sleepiness is seen to be made up of many elements, this can help explain why different measures do not always correlate well with each other. There is ample evidence, for example, of a lack of a close relationship between the multiple sleep latency test (MSLT)* and the ESS (although there are some factors which influence the strength of the relationship – see Short, Lack and Wright 2010). Instead of deciding that the ESS is just inferior to the MSLT, it is more helpful to consider that both techniques are measuring different elements of sleepiness (Shen, Barbera and Shapiro 2006).

Fatigue

Fatigue also has many facets, and attempts to distinguish them, for example:

- primary: where no other disease process is thought to be responsible

- secondary: the result of another disease (such as cancer or lupus)

- central: diffuse, possibly mediated in the central nervous system

- peripheral: associated with the periphery of the body: usually expressed by reductions in function of specific muscles.

Olson and Morse (2005) suggest six elements: muscular, cognitive, emotional, body sensation, sleep disruption and social disruption. Of these, cognitive fatigue is described in terms of diminished cognitive function, particularly regarding attention and decision-making. Montana *et al.* (2010) have reported some tentative links between physical and cognitive elements of fatigue, but they are generally considered separate elements. A final element is psychological fatigue, which can be defined in terms of 'weariness' and reduced motivation (Shen *et al.* 2006).

There are many different self-report measures of fatigue, some of which are unidimensional, whilst others are multidimensional (see Whitehead 2009 for a review of fatigue in chronic illness). They have different emphases too. For example, the frequently used Fatigue Severity Scale (FSS) (Krupp *et al.* 1989) emphasizes the consequences of the fatigue on general life more than it focuses on the experience of fatigue itself. Fatigue, in all its forms, is also influenced by many factors, via numerous biological, pathological and social processes (DeLuca 2005).

Sleep and sleep quality

'Sleep' is defined in fairly straightforward, biological ways using objective criteria, as covered in Chapters 2 and 8. This entire book attests to the many other influences on sleep – behavioural, cultural, psychological and social – and they need not all be addressed here. However, the nature of 'intent' and habit regarding sleep are considered alongside some of the influences on how people perceive their sleep and think about it.

Except where there is pathological sleepiness or narcolepsy, if a situation requires wakefulness, people are usually able to prevent themselves falling asleep. This could be whilst operating dangerous machinery or where it would be socially inconvenient (e.g. during a conversation with one's spouse). Other people might actively try to avoid sleep for as long as they can, when, for example, fearing distressing dreams or other negative experiences. This is exemplified by one of James Lee Burke's traumatized characters in the novel *Rain Gods*: 'Paradoxically, for Pete, sleeplessness was not the problem, it was the solution' (Burke 2008, p.314).

Looking at sleep rather than wakefulness, it has been suggested that humans are capable of sleeping when they do not *need* to – likened to being able to eat in the absence of hunger (Horne 2010). More accurately, however, people can only make efforts to increase the likelihood of going to sleep; they cannot bring about the state of sleep themselves. This decision to try to sleep might be in harmony with biological processes (at night, or mid-afternoon), and therefore more likely to succeed, or it might not. Increasing sleepiness is not the only driver to sleep; it could be due to wanting to avoid boredom or other aversive feelings.[3] It could also be in the anticipation of a forthcoming deficit, in line with the military exhortation to eat, sleep and excrete whenever possible (as it is never certain when the next opportunity might arise). Finally, 'habit' can have a role; as a colleague reported: 'My client said he doesn't sleep because he is tired, or because he is sleepy, or because he necessarily wants or needs to. It is just what he does at 2 o'clock in the afternoon.'

With regard to what people think about their own sleep, sleep 'quality' ratings are influenced by a variety of dimensions (Harvey *et al.* 2008). These include the duration of time awake during the intended sleep period, waking frequency, difficulties getting (or returning) to sleep and daytime consequences attributed to the sleep episode. What element of sleep is relevant to an individual will also be important: for one person, the most significant quality criterion is the time to fall asleep initially; for another person it is the difficulty in falling back to sleep, or frequency of waking (Krystal and Edinger 2008).

The time spent asleep (sleep duration) is likely to be an important criterion for many people, but not everyone is accurate in estimating it. There is a lot of individual variation in this, but, particularly in people with insomnia, there is a tendency for individuals to underestimate their own sleep duration compared with normal sleepers (Means *et al.* 2003). There is also evidence that other people have a tendency to think they have been asleep for longer than they actually were (Trajanovic *et al.* 2007).

Beyond estimates of sleep duration, ratings of sleep quality are influenced by how people feel on waking, and during the day (Green, Hicks and Wilson 2008; Harvey *et al.* 2008). One concept relating to daytime experience is how 'refreshed' people feel when they wake up. Indeed, 'unrefreshing' or 'non-restorative' sleep are often mentioned both in the sleep *and* fatigue literature. Just as there are suggestions that people's rating of sleep duration can be inaccurate, there is plenty of evidence that some sleep can be considered to have been unrefreshing even in the absence of objective evidence of disrupted sleep (Stone *et al.* 2008). The key point here is the presence of an implicit link between feeling unrefreshed and sleep quality: it is the sleep that is considered to be at fault.

12.3. The relationships between sleep, sleepiness and fatigue

Sleep and sleepiness

Given the different elements of sleepiness, it is perhaps to be expected that the association between sleep and sleepiness is not straightforward. A patient recently said to one of us, 'I am not sleepy, but if I sit down I can fall asleep at any point.' Someone might therefore be unaware of any feeling of sleepiness, but as soon as they close their eyes, or their head 'hits the pillow', they rapidly fall asleep. There are two possibilities here: there was no preceding episode of sleepiness and the transition to sleep was a learned response (where the pillow rapidly evokes a cascade of sleep-inducing hormones and neurotransmitters) or there *was* a biological sleep need, but this was not in conscious awareness.

Alongside these links between sleep and sleepiness in normal sleep/wake cycles, excessive daytime sleepiness can be a diagnostic indicator of a formal sleep disorder. Excessive daytime sleepiness (EDS) is associated with hypersomnia, narcolepsy and disorders characterized by repeated disruptions of sleep such as periodic limb movement disorder and obstructive sleep apnoea (OSA). These are discussed in more detail in other chapters, but it is worth noting that not all sleep disorders are linked to sleepiness. For example, and perhaps counterintuitively, daytime sleepiness is not necessarily more pronounced in people with insomnia (Singareddy, Bixler and Vgontzas 2010). One argument put forward for this is that the physiological and psychological hyperarousal, which is considered to be associated with people with insomnia, overrides any sleepiness linked to insufficient sleep (Shekleton, Rogers and Rajaratnam 2010).

Sleepiness and fatigue

Sleepiness and fatigue are frequently experienced alongside each other in everyday life: most people feel sleepy and fatigued at similar times during a 24-hour cycle and these reduce after an episode of sleep. Yet, they are different.[4] Statistical correlations between self-report measures tend to be low to moderate (Hossain *et al.* 2005); in other words, sleepiness and fatigue are related, but not strongly. There is also some evidence that if sleep is deliberately reduced under experimental conditions in people with insomnia, the effects on sleepiness and fatigue vary; namely, sleepiness stays the same and fatigue increases (Bonnet and Arand 1998).

Before continuing, however, it is worth noting that particularly high correlations have been found between some individual items on the ESS and some on the FSS – the scales used by Hossain *et al.* (2005) and others – which might lead to an overestimation of the statistical relationship between them (Merkelbac, Schulz and Fatigue Collaborative Study Group 2006). In investigating this further, Bailes *et al.* (2006) examined items from both the ESS and the FSS and also reported that the measures were confounded – elements within each were measuring the same as the other. However, using statistical techniques they were able to create two new distinct sets of items: one representing fatigue and one representing sleepiness. Put differently, when they put all the items from both questionnaires into one 'pot' they were able to draw them out differently, to create two, new, clearer dimensions.

It has already been stated that both fatigue and sleepiness are multidimensional, therefore any relationships between them should ideally be viewed similarly. One element that is part of both fatigue and sleepiness is cognitive function. For example, 'alert' and 'drowsy' can be equally used to describe sleepiness or cognitive fatigue. Returning to the term 'tiredness', Vernet *et al.* (2010) appear to define it in terms of cognitive fatigue, and signs on UK motorways tell drivers 'Tiredness can kill. Take a break.' This is not referring to drivers' inability to depress the pedals because their legs are too fatigued, but to their diminished cognitive capacity to drive safely – presumably because of sleepiness. More specifically, the driver accident literature tends to use the words 'driver fatigue' rather than 'driver sleepiness' as a correlate of reduced driving skill (e.g. Dawson and McCulloch 2005). (For further discussion of sleepiness and vigilance in terms of fitness to drive see, for example, Mathis and Hess 2009.)

Sleep and fatigue

Within sleep-related research, there is evidence that fatigue can be experienced by people with OSA (Chotinaiwattarakul *et al.* 2009) and insomnia (Shekleton *et al.* 2010). Indeed, Singareddy *et al.* (2010) emphasize that if their patients with insomnia report significant daytime sleepiness (rather than them being 'tired or fatigued'), that raises the suspicion that another underlying sleep disorder is present.

Within fatigue-related research, the largest body of evidence involving assessment of sleep is in CFS/ME. Most simply, CFS/ME is defined as the presence of long-term fatigue that has an impact on someone's life. It is a diagnosis of exclusion: that is, other reasons for the fatigue need to be ruled out before a diagnosis of CFS/ME can be made.[5] In the absence of irrefutable biological markers, several different sets of diagnostic criteria exist, all of which are based on self-report. Symptoms include post-exertional malaise, cognitive difficulties, headaches, sore throats and pain. Sleep disruption has long been considered to be important in CFS/ME, and self-reported poor sleep is also included, with varying emphasis, in most of the diagnostic criteria.

Many studies exist which have looked at the role of sleep and sleep disorders in CFS/ME. They have demonstrated that a proportion of people with CFS/ME do have previously undiagnosed formal sleep disorders, although, crucially, this is not at a higher rate than in healthy populations (Reeves *et al.* 2006). There are also many studies that have demonstrated a difference between people with CFS/ME and healthy controls in a specific aspect of sleep. There are also others that found contradictory results. One particular example of this is Fischler *et al.* (1997) who reported less slow-wave sleep (SWS)* in their clinical CFS/ME group, whereas Le Bon *et al.* (2007) and Neu *et al.* (2009) reported more. This outcome is particularly notable as the authors are from the same research group. Studies continue to find greater problems in people with CFS/ME than without, including in homeostatic drive – how people recover from disrupted sleep in the next significant sleep episode (Armitage *et al.* 2007; Decker *et al.* 2009). One final point worth considering is whether, when studies have found a small but statistically significant difference between groups, or changes in a variable, these differences or changes are *clinically* important. In other words, whether they are enough to actually account for noticeable day-to-day variations in broader symptoms or experiences within an individual or between groups of people. Overall, the evidence of sleep disruption is not consistent enough to conclude that CFS/ME is primarily a disorder of sleep: there is too much fatigue, and too little consistent sleep disturbance for the sleep to be the key. That said, sleep is still disrupted for many people in this population, to a greater or lesser extent.

Irrespective of the degree of objectively measured sleep difficulties, the overwhelming majority of people with CFS/ME would consider their own sleep quality to be poor. This can be in terms of high levels of unrefreshing sleep (Majer *et al.* 2007),[6] symptoms of insomnia (Fossey *et al.* 2004) and restlessness (Unger *et al.* 2004). Increased daytime sleepiness is not, however, consistently reported. For example, Watson *et al.* (2004) found a difference but Unger *et al.* (2004) did not.

12.4. Mediating and moderating factors

It is clear that tiredness, sleep, sleepiness and fatigue are all complex concepts themselves, each with different facets and elements. Their measurement is also not as precise as may be hoped. At this point it is tempting to give up trying to explain any of it – especially any of the associations – and to go back to bed. An alternative is to acknowledge the challenges and to look further into some of the factors that might have roles to play in mediating or moderating the connections between them. Methodological issues are addressed first, followed by perceptions, the influence of time, and then diagnosis. CFS/ME is used as an example throughout. This is partly due to the body of CFS/ME literature which mentions sleep and its consequences, and partly because it is our clinical area of interest: sleep is mentioned frequently, and is a matter of concern, for most of our patients.

Methodology: techniques and populations

Although the sleep laboratory is considered the best location for objective measurement of sleep, it is far from a normal sleep environment. Participants are asked to sleep in an unfamiliar bed, with various electrodes and wires attached to them, possibly under the gaze of a video camera. There may also be an additional structure imposed including set times for lights out and waking, and stopping any sleep-affecting medication two weeks beforehand. All or any of these could jeopardize the chance of readings reflecting the individual's normal night-to-night sleep.[7] The risk of a 'first-night effect' (where sleep is worse on the first night – akin to the experience of people without sleep problems when staying for the first night in a hotel) has long been recognized (see Le Bon et al. 2003). Reeves et al. (2006) suggest that three nights of polysomnography (PSG)* could be required to get accurate results, especially given the indications that recovery sleep might be an issue on the second night for people with CFS/ME (Armitage et al. 2007). Some studies carry out home-based measurement, using PSG or actigraphy,* which improve the chances of measuring something approaching the usual sleep pattern, although such methods also have some shortcomings (Creti et al. 2010).

The second complication is that CFS/ME is a heterogeneous illness (e.g. Vollmer-Conna, Aslakson and White 2006). Put differently, a group of people with CFS/ME will all share an experience of major fatigue, but there will be variations in the number and severity of the other symptoms they have such as sore throats, joint pain or headaches. There will also be a range of differences in sleep problems. Our clinical experience is that some people sleep excessively and, conversely, others have insufficient sleep.[8] This does have an implication for investigating sleep's role in CFS/ME. Taking a simplistic example, if one subgroup have excessive sleep, but another have insufficient sleep, it is possible that these will 'balance each other out' so the average amount of sleep for the entire population is not actually different from a healthy comparison group.

Another potential complication is the nature of the people who actually take part in research, who might not be representative of the wider CFS/ME population. Research volunteers could have a greater interest in sleep than others, either because they hope that sleep will have a curative role for them or they are particularly focused on, and worried about, their sleep. Perhaps more significantly, volunteers are likely to be generally 'higher functioning' (i.e. they are able to do more than others with more severe symptoms) and therefore are more able to complete long investigations and questionnaire batteries. The possibility remains that there is a group of people with CFS/ME who are more severely affected by symptoms but who cannot take part in demanding research studies. They might, however, actually have more consistently serious disturbed sleep than the people who have already been investigated.

Perceptions, expectations and beliefs

Basic psychological research would support a role for individual perceptions and patterns of thinking on sleep. For example, perceptual styles have been identified in people with CFS/ME that involve greater levels of focus on symptoms, with more negative meanings being attached to these symptoms (Moss-Morris and Petrie 2003). Additionally, self-defined poor sleepers appear more able to distinguish levels of fatigue than better sleepers (Neu et al. 2010), and people with CFS/ME-like fatigue rate their sleep as more unrefreshing than people with non-CFS/ME fatigue (Nisenbaum et al. 2004). Hossain et al. (2005) speculate on the effects of beliefs about fatigue and sleepiness; sleepiness might be under-reported as it is considered a sign of weakness, whereas fatigue is a consequence of real work and effort.

According to Harvey et al. (2008), people with insomnia appear to require more elements on which to base decisions on their sleep quality than people without the diagnosis. It is impossible from these data to determine causality: did the cognitive factors and beliefs about sleep make it more likely that someone would develop insomnia, or are they a result of an increased focus on sleep, given its central role in the experiences of people with insomnia? Harvey et al. (2008) speculate on the existence of a specific bias where otherwise ambiguous cues on how someone is feeling (aches, sore eyes) are attributed to the most salient reason for them: if someone has insomnia, this is more likely to be their lack of sleep.[9] They also mention that anxiety and depression might play a part in this whole process of perception and belief. These factors could be independent of the insomnia itself.

A more reductionist view is that psychological factors also have a measurable biological base, or at least that biology has a role. Jones (2008) suggests that 'the sense of the physiology of the body' (p.123) – or 'interoception' – is actually biologically mediated. Rahman *et al.* (2011) provide some evidence that nocturnal heart rate influences self-perceptions of sleep in people with CFS/ME. Whilst Neu *et al.* (2007) reported more microarousals in sleep patterns in people with CFS/ME than in controls, they did not find a link to sleep being self-rated as poorer. Despite this, the authors speculated that there was still a biological process that was influencing sleep beliefs, but that this had not yet been measurable.

Alongside a possible role of perceptual biases (biologically mediated or not), simple expectations also have a role. As noted earlier, many people find that sleep reduces feelings of fatigue, and, similarly, Bhui, Dinos and Morelli (2011) reported that people talk about fatigue levels in the context of their sleep quality. In CFS/ME, however, the high degree of reported unrefreshing sleep suggests that there is an expectation that sleep should reduce fatigue, but in fact it does not.

A much larger section – or in fact a chapter – could have been written on the psychology of sleep. These brief, and rather varied examples are included to demonstrate the potential roles psychological factors can have. This is not, of course, to say that people's symptoms are somehow 'fabricated' or in 'people's heads', just that amongst the many influences on sleep, sleepiness and fatigue, beliefs and perceptions have a part to play.

Time course, behaviour and dynamics

Very nearly all research into sleep, sleepiness and fatigue is cross-sectional: it looks at relationships that are measured at one point in time. In the case of CFS/ME in particular, the position on the time course of the symptoms might be important. For example, systemic infection is known to be one of the 'triggers' for CFS/ME and it is also recognized that infection can lead to increased sleep drive (Imeri and Opp 2009). One possible subsequent sequence is: the sleep drive persists beyond the infection, leading to sleep/wake patterns remaining unbalanced, and then longer sleep (or time in bed, seeking sleep) leads to reduced daytime activity levels, which in turn decrease nocturnal sleep quality (both actual and perceived), perpetuating the sleep disruption.

There are risks for increased fatigue and sleepiness here, which themselves might then drive behaviours to reduce them (by someone trying to sleep more) and so on. Imeri and Opp (2009) also note that sleep disruption itself can affect immune function, which would of course increase the likelihood of more infections.

The presence of sleep disruption in some people with CFS/ME could therefore be a consequence of how they have reacted to their CFS/ME symptoms, rather than it being a primary cause. (Vernet *et al.* 2010 made a similar suggestion: that people with a diagnosis of idiopathic insomnia might spend so much energy trying to stay *awake*, they become more 'fatigued'.) Considering CFS/ME to be a 'dynamic' disorder where symptoms, beliefs, biology and behaviour constantly interact provides a structure with greater potential for interpreting some of the complexities of the relationships to sleep. This parallels the idea of the sleep/wake *cycle* where the tensions between sleep and wakefulness are constantly changing.

Diagnosing and labelling

Because CFS/ME is a diagnosis of exclusion, and there are several different criteria in existence, formally diagnosing CFS/ME is not always straightforward. This is also the case with sleep disorders. One of the shared difficulties is diagnostic overlap between disorders of sleep, fatigue, pain and mood. For example, a lot of people with CFS/ME report insomnia and many people with insomnia report daytime fatigue: the dividing line is not entirely clear. CFS/ME is an illness of many parts and Vernet *et al.* (2010) commented that their sample with idiopathic hypersomnia reported fatigue as well as other multiple symptoms. Depression has a clear relationship to sleep disruption (Baldwin and Papakostas 2006) and fatigue (Ferentinos *et al.* 2009). Experiences of, for example, apathy and a lack of motivation or drive could be seen in people with CFS/ME or depression. Pain is similarly associated with poor sleep (Tang 2008) and depression (Ohayon and Schatzberg 2010). Pain is also one of the diagnostic criteria for CFS/ME: the differential diagnosis between CFS/ME and fibromyalgia/chronic widespread pain can be difficult to make at times (Friedberg 2010).

One way of looking at this overlapping pattern of diagnoses is that they have some link to an underlying biological process, mediated by the central nervous system. For example, hyperarousal is implicated in insomnia (Bonnet and Arand 2010) and centrally mediated neurochemical changes are thought to underpin fibromyalgia and some of the associated sleep disruption (Clauw 2010).[10] CFS/ME has been linked with altered levels of a group of protein regulators called cytokines (Nakamura *et al.* 2010), as has sleep (Kapsimalis *et al.* 2008). Above the neurochemical level, body weight and size might also have a shared role. A high body mass index (BMI) is associated with poor sleep (Watson *et al.* 2010), sleep disorder OSA (Schwab, Remmers and Kuna 2011) and fatigue, where it is hypothesized that the high weight increases 'metabolic strain', thereby depleting energy reserves (Aslakson *et al.* 2009, p.17). Indeed, a BMI of greater than 40 or 45 (depending on the criteria) is actually an exclusion criterion for CFS/ME.

There are obviously, therefore, challenges in diagnosing these various disorders and difficulties, and separating them out meaningfully. There are some guidelines: for example, Moss-Morris and Petrie (2001) suggest that depression and CFS/ME can be differentiated in terms of particular thinking styles, particularly regarding self-esteem and what the symptoms are attributed to, and more recent research implies that there might be differences in brain physiology between CFS/ME and depression (Duffy *et al.* 2011). Another relevant factor could, however, be the nature of the diagnostic setting. Mariman (2009)[11] suggests that the diagnosis that is eventually applied to an individual depends on which specialist the person sees first. If the individual is referred to a fatigue clinic, their symptoms could be seen as fatigue-related. If they are referred to a sleep clinic, those same symptoms might be attributed to sleep disruption, making a diagnosis of sleep disorder more likely. The individual patient is also important: if they present to their specialist with fatigue as their greatest concern, that may influence the diagnosis. If they report tiredness all the time to their doctor, that could be attributed to depression. If they talk specifically about heightened sleepiness, they might be referred for a sleep investigation.

Perhaps the diagnostic conundrums could be left to the theorists, and the actual clinical reality be reflected by accepting the fact that people can have more than one 'disorder' at a time. It is possible to have long-term fatigue and be of high weight, and be depressed, and have pain. Libman *et al.* (2009) make this point particularly about a diagnosis of sleep apnoea and a diagnosis of CFS/ME, arguing that they can conceptually and pragmatically co-exist in a patient.

12.5. Clinical implications

Reflecting on the complexity of the picture so far, the default response would be to return to the usual refrain: we need more and better research. Plainly, that is required, and high quality research – crucially that defines its terms carefully – will increase our understanding further. There are some pointers for clinical practice already.

Whichever the most 'obvious' disorder or difficulty someone presents with, be that fatigue, sleep or mood-related, other difficulties should not be ignored. Irrespective of their independent effect on quality of life, sleep disruptions (whether objective or subjective) are likely to have a role in the maintenance of CFS/ME (White *et al.* 2007) or make recovery more difficult. Interventions that target them remain warranted in CFS/ME.

Although medication has a role in the management of sleep disorders (see Chapter 11), the evidence for effective pharmacological interventions in CFS/ME is unclear. For example, studies using stimulants such as modafinil have yielded inconsistent results (Randall *et al.* 2005). It could be that there is a subset of people for whom some medication might help: van Heukelom *et al.* (2006) reported that melatonin had a greater effect for patients with a certain type of natural melatonin secretion.

Cognitive and behavioural interventions can be effective in reducing levels of insomnia (Harvey 2009) and depression (Kuyken, Dalgleish and Holden 2007). There is also evidence that insomnia-related interventions can affect pain levels (Vitiello *et al.* 2009). For fatigue, a cognitive behavioural approach has led to the remission of CFS/ME symptoms for a subset of people (White *et al.* 2011). The same study demonstrated a similar result for graded exercise, and exercise has a role in improving sleep (Buman *et al.* 2011), depression (Carek, Laibstain and Care 2011) and fibromyalgia type pain (Häuser, Thieme and Turk 2010). In other words, despite long-term sleep and fatigue disorders being complex and multidimensional, and influenced by many different factors, similar cognitive and behavioural interventions can be effective in reducing the load of symptoms. One interpretation of this is that seeking a single categorical diagnosis might prove to be a little less important (at least for people on the borderline between different diagnoses) when the treatment may be similar anyway.

Looking at certain beliefs about sleep in particular, there is a case for helping patients – especially those with CFS/ME – to distinguish sleepiness from fatigue, and both of the terms from 'tiredness'. At the end of an intervention, a patient recently remarked: 'When I am sleepy now, I go to sleep; when I am fatigued, I rest.' That distinction proved to be very useful for her. In CFS/ME, people will not be able to 'sleep themselves better', as a colleague put it, yet that is an implicit belief amongst many people. Challenging that belief could reduce people's tendency to 'chase' sleep in order to reduce the long-term fatigue. This, in turn, helps to reduce the risk of them falling into the trap of trying harder and harder to sleep, which worsens the sleep and fatigue. The best message to put across to patients in terms of sleep management is for someone to do what they can to improve their sleep (see Chapter 9), but then be phlegmatic about the outcome.

It is not just patients who could benefit from having an open mind about their sleep interventions. A patient explained to one of us that she had cut down her daytime sleeping but that it had had no effect on her nocturnal sleep, or on her fatigue levels. She was, however, able to take her tablets and food more regularly and, most importantly, was seeing her friends more: her life had improved. If a clinician had focused only on sleep and fatigue, this outcome would have been seen as treatment failure, when in fact, it was not.

12.6. Conclusion

For most of us, the relationship between sleepiness and fatigue is relatively straightforward, and 'tiredness' just about sums it up. When sleepiness or fatigue become troublesome, the interactions between them become more subtle and also more significant in terms of potential treatment. Even if terms, methodologies and research samples are improved in future research, the dynamic and complex nature of fatigue and sleep, and the fact that both are influenced by so many factors, means that no single theory (be it psychological, biological, physiological, psycho-physiological or diagnostic) is likely to account for the interrelationships in an over-arching, all-encompassing way.

Combined theories that incorporate the dynamic nature of sleep, sleepiness and fatigue might prove more successful and accurate.

Looking at CFS/ME in particular, research into the role of sleep is continuing, as even though sleep disruption is not a fundamental cause of CFS/ME, it does have a role, at least in contributing to the maintenance of the illness. More importantly, it can also be a distressing part of patients' experiences. Sleep-focused interventions are valuable for many aspects of fatigue, pain and mood.

Overall, whilst everyone accepts that sleep is unavoidable, fatigue and sleepiness are too – even if twenty-first-century lifestyles try to make them appear optional. For most people they are part of a normal cycle, but when they become problematic and persistent, they are demonstrably disabling for those who experience them. It is important that we continue to ask the right questions about tiredness, sleep, sleepiness and fatigue, and to listen carefully to the answers, both as researchers and as clinicians.

Notes

1. Some researchers and patient groups distinguish chronic fatigue syndrome (CFS) from myalgic encephalomyelitis/myalgia (ME). Others consider the terms interchangeable. Here, the initialism CFS/ME is used throughout where a diagnosis has been applied or implied.

2. Idiopathic hypersomnia can be defined as 'chronic, daily, excessive daytime sleepiness despite normal sleep' (Vernet *et al.* 2010, p.525), where the sleepiness is not caused by other known factors. Hypersomnia itself also can be defined in terms of time asleep, or time in bed (Kaplan and Harvey 2009).

3. It is also possible that excessive sleeping might itself increase low mood (Kaplan and Harvey 2009).

4. This is not, of course. a novel idea. See, for example, Duntley (2005), Neu *et al.* (2010), Shahid, Shen and Shapiro (2010), and Pigeon, Sateia and Ferguson (2003) for further discussions of this.

5. Sleep disorders are generally considered to be a reason why a diagnosis of CFS/ME should not be given, but the examples provided in the criteria are inconsistent: Fukuda *et al.* (1994) mention sleep apnoea and narcolepsy as exclusion criteria, as do Carruthers *et al.* (2003), who also include restless legs syndrome. Sharpe *et al.* (1991) actually do not mention sleep disorders. Insomnia is not specifically mentioned as an exclusion criterion in any of the criteria.

6. It would, however, be expected that unrefreshing sleep is higher in this group as it is one of the criteria used for a diagnosis of CFS/ME.

7. The direction of the effect might also be difficult to predict, as an imposition of structure for someone whose sleep is disorganized might actually improve their

sleep. Similarly, some psychoactive drugs have complex interactions with sleep and the removal of these might, again, improve sleep. Conversely, sleep could also be worse, given the change in habit and routine.

8. A straw poll in our department revealed large differences in clinicians' beliefs about the level of sleep disorder in their CFS/ME patients. This might be a reflection of insufficient research, or personal or professional interest (do individual clinicians ask different questions?), but it could be another reflection of the heterogeneity of the CFS/ME population.

9. An alternative possibility is that actually having a condition for a long time might mean less attention is paid to it as there is habituation to its effects, where familiarity with symptoms make it more difficult to distinguish levels of them (Hossain *et al.* 2005).

10. Clauw, D. (2010) Presentation at the British Association of CFS/ME Conference. Milton Keynes, UK. 13–14 October.

11. Mariman, A. (2009) Speaking at the International Sleep Medicine Course, Cambridge, England. September.

References

Armitage, R., Landis, C., Hoffmann, R., Lentz, M. *et al.* (2007) 'The impact of a 4-hour sleep delay on slow wave activity in twins discordant for chronic fatigue syndrome.' *Sleep 30*, 5, 657–662.

Aslakson, E., Vollmer-Conna, U., Reeves, W.C. and White, P.D. (2009) 'Replication of an empirical approach to delineate the heterogeneity of chronic unexplained fatigue.' *Population Health Metrics 7*, 17.

Bailes, S., Libman, E., Baltzan, M., Amsel, R., Schondorf, R. and Fichten, C.S. (2006) 'Brief and distinct empirical sleepiness and fatigue scales.' *Journal of Psychosomatic Research 60*, 6, 605–613.

Baldwin, D.S. and Papakostas, G.I. (2006) 'Symptoms of fatigue and sleepiness in major depressive disorder.' *Journal of Clinical Psychiatry 67*, Suppl. 6, 9–15.

Bhui, K.S., Dinos, S. and Morelli, M.L. (2011) 'Ethnicity and fatigue: expressions of distress, causal attributions and coping.' *Sociology Mind Open Access 1*, 4, 156–163.

Bonnet, M.H. and Arand, D.L. (1998) 'The consequences of a week of insomnia. II: patients with insomnia.' *Sleep 21*, 4, 359–368.

Bonnet, M.H. and Arand, D.L. (2010) 'Hyperarousal and insomnia: state of the science.' *Sleep Medicine Reviews 14*, 1, 9–15.

Buman, P., Hekler, B., Bliwise, L. and King, C. (2011) 'Moderators and mediators of exercise-induced objective sleep improvements in midlife and older adults with sleep complaints.' *Health Psychology 30*, 5, 579–587.

Burke, J.L. (2008) *Rain Gods.* London: Phoenix.

Carek, J., Laibstain, E. and Care, M. (2011) 'Exercise for the treatment of depression and anxiety.' *International Journal of Psychiatry in Medicine 41*, 1, 15–28.

Carruthers, B.M., Jain, A.K., De Meirleir, K.L., Peterson, D.L. *et al.* (2003) 'Myalgic encephalomyelitis/ chronic fatigue syndrome: clinical working case definition, diagnostic and treatment protocols.' *Journal of Chronic Fatigue Syndrome 11*, 1, 7–36.

Chotinaiwattarakul, W., O'Brien, L.M., Fan, L. and Chervin, R.D. (2009) 'Fatigue, tiredness, and lack of energy improve with treatment for OSA.' *Journal of Clinical Sleep Medicine 5*, 3, 222–227.

Creti, L., Libman, E., Baltzan, M., Rizzo, D., Bailes, S. and Fichten, C.S. (2010) 'Impaired sleep in chronic fatigue syndrome: how is it best measured?' *Journal of Health Psychology 15*, 4, 596–607.

Dawson, D. and McCulloch, K. (2005) 'Managing fatigue: it's about sleep.' *Sleep Medicine Reviews 9*, 5, 365–380.

Decker, M.J., Tabassum, H., Lin, J.M. and Reeves, W.C. (2009) 'Electroencephalographic correlates of Chronic Fatigue Syndrome.' *Behavioral and Brain Functions 5*, 43.

DeLuca, J. (ed.) (2005) *Fatigue as a Window to the Brain*. London: MIT Press.

Dement, W.C., Hall, J. and Walsh, J.K. (2003) 'Tiredness versus sleepiness: semantics or a target for public education?' *Sleep 26*, 4, 485–486.

Duffy, F.H., McAnulty, G.B., McCreary, M.C., Cuchural, G.J. and Komaroff, A.L. (2011) 'EEG spectral coherence data distinguish chronic fatigue syndrome patients from healthy controls and depressed patients: a case control study.' *BMC Neurology 11*, 82. Available at www.biomedcentral.com/1471-2377/11/82, accessed on 28 April 2012.

Duntley, P. (2005) 'Fatigue and Sleep.' In J. DeLuca (ed.) *Fatigue as a Window to the Brain*. London: MIT Press.

Ferentinos, P., Kontaxakis, V., Havaki-Kontaxaki, B., Paparrigopoulos, T. *et al.* (2009) 'Sleep disturbances in relation to fatigue in major depression.' *Journal of Psychosomatic Research 66*, 1, 37–42.

Fischler, B., Le Bon, O., Hoffmann, G., Cluydts, R., Kaufman, L. and De Meirleir, K. (1997) 'Sleep anomalies in the chronic fatigue syndrome. A comorbidity study.' *Neuropsychobiology 35*, 3, 115–122.

Fossey, M., Libman, E., Bailes, S., Baltzan, M. *et al.* (2004) 'Sleep quality and psychological adjustment in chronic fatigue syndrome.' *Journal of Behavioral Medicine 27*, 6, 581–605.

Friedberg, F. (2010) 'Chronic fatigue syndrome, fibromyalgia, and related illnesses: a clinical model of assessment and intervention.' *Journal of Clinical Psychology 66*, 6, 641–665.

Fukuda, K., Straus, S. E., Hickie, I., Sharpe, M. C., Dobbins, J. G. and Komaroff, A. (1994) 'The chronic fatigue syndrome: a comprehensive approach to its definition and study. International Chronic Fatigue Syndrome Study Group.' *Annals of Internal Medicine 121*, 1, 953–959.

Green, A., Hicks, J., and Wilson, S. (2008) 'The experience of poor sleep and its consequences: a qualitative study involving people referred for cognitive-behavioural management of chronic insomnia.' *British Journal of Occupational Therapy 71*, 5, 196–205.

Harvey, A.G. (2009) 'Insomnia.' In D. McKay, J.S. Abramowitz and S. Taylor (eds) *Cognitive-behavioral Therapy for Refractory Cases: Turning Failure into Success*. Washington, DC: American Psychological Association.

Harvey, A.G., Stinson, K., Whitaker, K.L., Moskovitz, D. and Virk, H. (2008) 'The subjective meaning of sleep quality: a comparison of individuals with and without insomnia.' *Sleep: Journal of Sleep and Sleep Disorders Research 31*, 3, 383–393.

Häuser, W., Thieme, K. and Turk, D.C. (2010) 'Guidelines on the management of fibromyalgia syndrome: a systematic review.' *European Journal of Pain 14*, 1, 5–10.

Horne, J. (2010) 'Primary insomnia: a disorder of sleep, or primarily one of wakefulness? *Sleep Medicine Reviews 14*, 1, 3–7.

Hossain, J.L., Ahmad, P., Reinish, L.W., Kayumov, L., Hossain, N.K. and Shapiro, C.M. (2005) 'Subjective fatigue and subjective sleepiness: two independent consequences of sleep disorders?' *Journal of Sleep Research 14*, 3, 245–253.

Imeri, L. and Opp, M.R. (2009) 'How (and why) the immune system makes us sleep.' *Nature Reviews Neuroscience 10*, 3, 199–210.

Johns, M.W. (1991) 'A new method for measuring daytime sleepiness: the Epworth sleepiness scale.' *Sleep 14*, 6, 540–545.

Johns, M.W. (2010) 'A new perspective on sleepiness.' *Sleep and Biological Rhythms 8*, 3, 170–179.

Jones, J.F. (2008) 'An extended concept of altered self: chronic fatigue and post-infection syndromes.' *Psychoneuroendocrinology 33*, 2, 119–129.

Kaplan, K.A. and Harvey, A.G. (2009) 'Hypersomnia across mood disorders: a review and synthesis.' *Sleep Medicine Reviews 13*, 4, 275–285.

Kapsimalis, F., Basta, M., Varouchakis, G., Gourgoulianis, K., Vgontzas, A. and Kryger, M. (2008) 'Cytokines and pathological sleep.' *Sleep Medicine 9*, 6, 603–614.

Krupp, L.B., LaRocca, N.G., Muir-Nash, J. and Steinberg, A.D. (1989) 'The fatigue severity scale. Application to patients with multiple sclerosis and systemic lupus erythematosus.' *Archives of Neurology 46*, 10, 1121–1123.

Krystal, A.D. and Edinger, J.D. (2008) 'Measuring sleep quality.' *Sleep Medicine 9*, Suppl. 1, S10–S17.

Kuyken, W., Dalgleish, T., and Holden, E.R. (2007) 'Advances in cognitive-behavioural therapy for unipolar depression.' *Canadian Journal of Psychiatry 52*, 1, 5–13.

Le Bon, O., Minner, P., van Moorsel, C., Hoffmann, G. *et al.* (2003) 'First-night effect in the chronic fatigue syndrome.' *Psychiatry Research 120*, 2, 191–199.

Le Bon, O., Neu, D., Valente, F. and Linkowski, P. (2007) 'Paradoxical NREMS distribution in "pure" chronic fatigue patients: a comparison with sleep apnea-hypopnea patients and healthy control subjects.' *Journal of Chronic Fatigue Syndrome 14*, 2, 45–60.

Libman, E., Creti, L., Baltzan, M., Rizzo, D., Fichten, C.S., and Bailes, S. (2009) 'Sleep apnea and psychological functioning in chronic fatigue syndrome.' *Journal of Health Psychology 14*, 8, 1251–1267.

Majer, M., Jones, J.F., Unger, E.R., Youngblood, L.S. *et al.* (2007) 'Perception versus polysomnographic assessment of sleep in CFS and non-fatigued control subjects: results from a population-based study.' *BMC Neurology 7*, 40.

Mathis, J. and Hess, C.W. (2009) 'Sleepiness and vigilance tests.' *Swiss Medical Weekly 139*, 15–16, 214–219.

Means, M.K., Edinger, J.D., Glenn, D.M. and Fins, A.I. (2003) 'Accuracy of sleep perceptions among insomnia sufferers and normal sleepers.' *Sleep Medicine 4*, 4, 285–296.

Merkelbach, S., Schulz, H. and Fatigue Collaborative Study Group (2006) 'What have fatigue and sleepiness in common?' *Journal of Sleep Research 15*, 1, 105–106.

Montana, X., Neu, D., Hoffmann, G., Gilson, M. *et al.* (2010) 'Are physical and mental fatigue related or not?' *Journal of Sleep Research 19*, Suppl. 2, 180.

Moss-Morris, R. and Petrie, J. (2001) 'Discriminating between chronic fatigue syndrome and depression: a cognitive analysis.' *Psychological Medicine 31*, 3, 469–479.

Moss-Morris, R. and Petrie, J. (2003) 'Experimental evidence for interpretive but not attention biases toward somatic information in patients with chronic fatigue syndrome.' *British Journal of Health Psychology 8*, 2, 195–208.

Nakamura, T., Schwander, S.K., Donnelly, R., Ortega, F. *et al.* (2010) 'Cytokines across the night in chronic fatigue syndrome with and without fibromyalgia.' *Clinical and Vaccine Immunology 17*, 4, 582–587.

Neu, D., Cappeliez, B., Hoffmann, G., Verbanck, P., Linkowski, P. and Le Bon, O. (2009) 'High slow-wave sleep and low-light sleep: chronic fatigue syndrome is not likely to be a primary sleep disorder.' *Journal of Clinical Neurophysiology 26*, 3, 207–213.

Neu, D., Mairesse, O., Hoffmann, G., Dris, A. *et al.* (2007) 'Sleep quality perception in the chronic fatigue syndrome: correlations with sleep efficiency, affective symptoms and intensity of fatigue.' *Neuropsychobiology 56*, 1, 40–46.

Neu, D., Mairesse, O., Hoffmann, G., Valsamis, J.B. *et al.* (2010) 'Do "sleepy" and "tired" go together? Rasch analysis of the relationships between sleepiness, fatigue and nonrestorative sleep complaints in a nonclinical population sample.' *Neuroepidemiology 35*, 1, 1–11.

Nisenbaum, R., Reyes, M., Unger, E.R. and Reeves, W.C. (2004) 'Factor analysis of symptoms among subjects with unexplained chronic fatigue: what can we learn about chronic fatigue syndrome?' *Journal of Psychosomatic Research 56*, 2, 171–178.

Ohayon, M.M. and Schatzberg, A.F. (2010) 'Chronic pain and major depressive disorder in the general population.' *Journal of Psychiatric Research 44*, 7, 454–461.

Olson, K. (2007) 'A new way of thinking about fatigue: a reconceptualization.' *Oncology Nursing Forum 34*, 1, 93–99.

Olson, K. and Morse, J. (2005) 'Delineating the Concept of Fatigue Using a Pragmatic Utility Approach.' In J. Cutliffe and H. McKenna (eds) *The Essential Concepts of Nursing.* Oxford: Elsevier Science.

Pigeon, W.R., Sateia, M.J. and Ferguson, R.J. (2003) 'Distinguishing between excessive daytime sleepiness and fatigue. Toward improved detection and treatment.' *Journal of Psychosomatic Research 54*, 61–69.

Rahman, K., Burton, A.R., Galbraith, S., Lloyd, A. and Vollmer-Conna, U. (2011) 'Sleep-wake behavior in chronic fatigue syndrome.' *Sleep 34*, 5, 671–678.

Randall, D.C., Cafferty, F.H., Shneerson, J.M., Smith, I.E., Llewelyn, M.B. and File, S.E. (2005) Chronic treatment with modafinil may not be beneficial in patients with chronic fatigue syndrome. *Journal of Psychopharmacology 19*, 6, 647–660.

Reeves, W.C., Heim, C., Maloney, E.M., Youngblood, L.S. *et al.* (2006) 'Sleep characteristics of persons with chronic fatigue syndrome and non-fatigued controls: results from a population-based study.' *BMC Neurology 6*, 41.

Schwab, R.J., Remmers, J.E. and Kuna, S.T. (2011) 'Anatomy and Physiology of Upper Airway Obstruction.' In M.H. Kryger, T. Roth and W.C. Dement (eds) *Principles and Practice of Sleep Medicine*, 5th edn. St Louis, MO: Elsevier Saunders.

Shahid, A., Shen, J. and Shapiro, C.M. (2010) 'Measurements of sleepiness and fatigue.' *Journal of Psychosomatic Research 69*, 1, 81–89.

Sharpe, M.C., Archard, A.C., Banatvala, J.E., Borysiewicz, L.K. *et al.* (1991) 'A report: Chronic fatigue syndrome: guidelines for research.' *Journal of the Royal Society of Medicine 84*, 2, 118–121.

Shekleton, J.A., Rogers, N.L. and Rajaratnam, S.M. (2010) 'Searching for the daytime impairments of primary insomnia.' *Sleep Medicine Reviews 14*, 1, 47–60.

Shen, J., Barbera, J. and Shapiro, C.M. (2006) 'Distinguishing sleepiness and fatigue: focus on definition and measurement.' *Sleep Medicine Reviews 10*, 1, 63–76.

Short, M., Lack, L. and Wright, L. (2010) 'Does subjective sleepiness predict objective sleep propensity?' *Sleep 33*,1, 123–129.

Singareddy, R., Bixler, E.O. and Vgontzas, A.N. (2010) 'Fatigue or daytime sleepiness?' *Journal of Clinical Sleep Medicine 6*, 4, 405.

Stone, K.C., Taylor, D.J., McCrae, C.S., Kalsekar, A. and Lichstein, K.L. (2008) 'Nonrestorative sleep.' *Sleep Medicine Reviews 12*, 4, 275–288.

Tang, N.K. (2008) 'Insomnia co-occurring with chronic pain: clinical features, interaction, assessments and possible interventions.' *Reviews in Pain 2*, 1, 2–7.

Trajanovic, N.N., Radivojevic, V., Kaushansky, Y. and Shapiro, C.M. (2007) 'Positive sleep state misperception – a new concept of sleep misperception.' *Sleep Medicine 8*, 2, 111–118.

Unger, E.R., Nisenbaum, R., Moldofsky, H., Cesta, A. *et al.* (2004) 'Sleep assessment in a population-based study of chronic fatigue syndrome.' *BMC Neurology 4*, 6.

van Heukelom, R.O., Prins, J.B., Smits, M.G. and Bleijenberg, G. (2006) 'Influence of melatonin on fatigue severity in patients with chronic fatigue syndrome and late melatonin secretion.' *European Journal of Neurology 13*, 1, 55–60.

Vernet, C., Leu-Semenescu, S., Buzare, M.A. and Arnulf, I. (2010) 'Subjective symptoms in idiopathic hypersomnia: beyond excessive sleepiness.' *Journal of Sleep Research 19*, 4, 525–534.

Vernon, A. (2011) 'International rowing to the letter.' Available at www.bbc.co.uk/blogs/annabelvernon/2011/08/international_rowing_to_the_le.html, accessed on 11 January 2012.

Vitiello, M.V., Rybarczyk, B., Von Korff, M. and Stepanski, E.J. (2009) 'Cognitive behavioral therapy for insomnia improves sleep and decreases pain in older adults with co-morbid insomnia and osteoarthritis.' *Journal of Clinical Sleep Medicine 5*, 4, 355–362.

Vollmer-Conna, U., Aslakson, E. and White, P.D. (2006) 'An empirical delineation of the heterogeneity of chronic unexplained fatigue in women.' *Pharmacogenomics 7*, 3, 355–364.

Watson, N.F., Buchwald, D., Vitiello, V., Noonan, C. and Goldberg, J. (2010) 'A twin study of sleep duration and body mass index.' *Journal of Clinical Sleep Medicine 6*, 1, 11–17.

Watson, N.F., Jacobsen, C., Goldberg, J., Kapur, V. and Buchwald, D. (2004) 'Subjective and objective sleepiness in monozygotic twins discordant for chronic fatigue syndrome.' *Sleep 27*, 5, 973–977.

White, P.D., Goldsmith, K.A., Johnson, A.L., Potts, L. *et al.* (2011) 'Comparison of adaptive pacing therapy, cognitive behaviour therapy, graded exercise therapy, and specialist medical care for chronic fatigue syndrome (PACE): a randomised trial.' *Lancet 377*, 9768, 823–836.

White, P.D., Sharpe, M.C., Chalder, T., DeCesare, J.C. *et al.* (2007) 'Protocol for the PACE trial: a randomised controlled trial of adaptive pacing, cognitive behaviour therapy, and graded exercise, as supplements to standardised specialist medical care versus standardised specialist medical care alone for patients with the chronic fatigue syndrome/myalgic encephalomyelitis or encephalopathy.' *BMC Neurology 7*, 6.

Whitehead, L. (2009) 'The measurement of fatigue in chronic illness: a systematic review of unidimensional and multidimensional fatigue measures.' *Journal of Pain and Symptom Management 37*, 1, 107–128.

13

Ambivalent Attitudes Towards Sleep in World Religions

Stephen Jacobs

13.1. Introduction

Although we spend approximately one-third of our lives asleep, in world religions sleep usually only merits passing comments, or is discussed in order to elucidate metaphysical or theological concepts. Ancoli-Israel (2001, p.778) suggests that 'rarely is sleep itself a subject of discussion'. However, as her article on the Hebrew tradition demonstrates, a great deal can be gleaned about religious attitudes towards sleep from these passing comments and tangential discussions. These gleanings indicate that although sleep is regarded as part of the created order, religions tend to hold rather ambivalent attitudes towards it. This ambivalence is particularly pronounced in observations about when it is appropriate to sleep and when to be awake. There are, for example, references in both Christianity and Islam which suggest that sleeping can indicate a lack of vigilance, a failure to overcome physical weakness and the inability to align oneself with the sacred.[1] Conversely, there are also references that suggest that insomnia indicates a lack of faith.

Religious ideas about the nature of sleep are contingent upon metaphysical presuppositions. In this chapter I explore two broad metaphysical models, which I term the linear model and the cyclical model. The linear model, which pertains to the monotheistic traditions of Judaism, Christianity and Islam, suggests a definite beginning to creation and the gradual progression through time to an absolute end. In these traditions sleep is regarded as gift from God, and therefore a mystery. In contrast, the Indian traditions, Hinduism, Buddhism,[2] Jainism and Sikhism, tend to postulate a cyclical model, which suggests never-ending cycles of creation and destruction. In these traditions the cycle of sleep and waking is regarded as analogous to both the cycle of transmigration and the cosmological cycles of creation and dissolution of the manifest universe.

13.2. When is sleep appropriate?

All religions accept sleep as a natural aspect of life, and it tends therefore to be evaluated positively in most traditions. For example, in the monotheistic religions, sleep is regarded as an aspect of the divine created order and is associated with healing and restoration. In the *Pirque D'Rabbi Eliezer – The Chapters of Rabbi Eliezer* (ca. eighth century CE[3]) this association is explicitly stated: 'What did the Holy One, blessed be He, do? He created the sleep of life, so that man lies down and sleeps while He sustains him and [gives] him life and repose' (cited in Ancoli-Israel 2001, p.780).

As part of the created order, sleep is often associated with the cycle of night and day, with night generally regarded as the more appropriate time for sleep. In Islam, for example, it is indicated that Allah created the night for rest and the day for activity. The Qur'an suggests, 'And He it is Who makes the Night as a Robe for you, and makes the Day (as it were) a Resurrection' (*Sūrah* 25 – *Al Furqān* 47).[4] This verse also alludes to the idea that night and sleep are associated with death and the day with life.

Most religious traditions suggest that, just as one has to eat when one is hungry, one should sleep when one is tired, although there are significant exceptions. Most traditions advocate particular times when it is important to overcome the natural inclination to sleep by specifying the most beneficial times for prayer and ritual performance, and by indicating appropriate amounts of, and times for, sleep. Adherence to these exceptions is associated with concepts of the good religious life. Taking too much sleep, being unable to sleep, or sleeping at inappropriate times are regarded as indications of not being in harmony with the sacred. Excessive sleep, like too much food, is regarded as an indulgence. Proverbs (20:13), for example, suggests: 'Do not love sleep or you will grow poor; stay awake and you will have food to spare.'[5] Sleep is equated with indolence which is incompatible with the religious life, an idea that is especially important in Calvinist theology.

Max Weber in his seminal work on the Protestant ethic observed that Calvin, and other Reformation theologians, posited the idea of predestination. That is, God has *chosen* those for salvation and it is not possible to *earn* salvation. The fundamental question is therefore not whether one can be saved, but 'am I one of the elect?' (Weber 2001, p.65, first published in 1930). Calvin's theology postulated that there was no absolute means of determining whether one was one of the elect, but it was nonetheless 'an absolute duty to consider oneself chosen' (Weber 2001, p.66). The Protestant ethic suggested that good works could not earn the believer salvation, but were regarded as an 'indispensible sign of election'. The diligence necessary to convince Protestants that they were amongst the elect entailed 'a systematic self-control' (Weber 2001, p.69) which produced an ascetic disposition that did not necessitate withdrawing from the world. This ascetic disposition condemns idleness as the primary sin, and, in particular, suggests that too much sleep is sinful (Weber 2001, p.104). Every waking hour engaged in work is regarded as spiritually valuable. The implication of this view is that sleep, whilst necessary, is inherently spiritually worthless.

Sleeping during the day is often regarded as slothful, and it is considered as religiously or spiritually beneficial to rise early and to minimize sleep. In the Qur'an (*Sūrah* 3 – *Al Imran*: 17), for example, it is suggested that true Muslims should 'pray for forgiveness in the early hours of the morning'. In most monastic communities the ritual day is structured in a way that curtails sleep. Being awake and being ritually active signify both devotion and the subordination of the physical to the spiritual.

However, there is one important exception to the general consensus that oversleeping signifies slothfulness and is spiritually harmful. The narrative of the sleepers of Ephesus, which according to Smith (1993) was first recorded in a western language in the sixth century CE, relates that seven Christian youths from Ephesus took refuge in a cave to escape persecution from the Romans. They fell asleep, but did not wake for over three hundred years. The story can also be found in the Qur'an (*Sūrah* 18 – *Al Kahf*: 9–26) which emphasizes that sleep was a refuge, not primarily from persecution, but from the idolatrous milieu of the Roman religion. So sleep is represented not only in terms of indolence, but also as a potential haven in times of great adversity.

In Hindu traditions, especially those associated with yoga and meditation, the very early morning is regarded as the best time to meditate. The day is divided into thirty 48-minute periods known as *muhūrtas*, and the time immediately prior to sunrise is referred to as *Brahmā Muhūrta* – 'the time of Brahma'. According to the Hindu teacher Swami[6] Sivananda (2000), *Brahmā Muhūrta* is the time of the day when the mind is least agitated and most clear and therefore the time when meditation is most effective. The concept of *Brahmā Muhūrta* clearly determines the pattern of sleep and waking. It is also thought that the practice of yoga and meditation reduces the amount of time required for sleep. Sivananda, drawing on traditional yogic spiritual psychology, makes a distinction between the brain and mind: the brain is part of the material world, and therefore requires rest, but the mind is a manifestation of the true self (*ātman*[7]): 'Mind is nothing but Atma-Sakti.[8] It is brain that wants rest (sleep), but not the mind. A Yogi who has controlled the mind never sleeps. He gets pure rest from meditation itself' (Sivananda 1998). In other words, once the yogi has fully mastered the techniques of yoga and meditation, he no longer requires any sleep.

In the Sikh code of conduct – the *Sikh Rehat Maryada* – it is suggested that a devout Sikh should also rise early to pray, in what is called the 'ambrosial hours'[9] (Shiromani Gurdwara Parbandhak Committee 1994). There is no absolute consensus on the exact timing of the ambrosial hours, but they are commonly understood to be three hours before dawn. This is regarded as the optimum time for prayer and meditation precisely because most others are asleep. 'The atmosphere is sacred because the vibrations of the mind involved in world matters are not emitted from the masses since they are in deep sleep' (Sikh Information, n.d.).

Both waking and sleeping can be regarded as obstacles to developing a consciousness of the sacred, which is achieved through prayer and meditation. In waking consciousness the mind is distracted by worldly affairs, and the 'vibrations' caused by the worldly preoccupations of others can potentially disrupt the consciousness of the sacred. Conversely, in sleep the mind is at rest and therefore unable to access the sacred. However, because the masses are sleeping, and their minds at rest, the potential disruptions caused by their thoughts are minimized. Presumably, also in the ambrosial hours, those who are not asleep are mostly engaged in prayer and meditation, which also contributes to the sacredness of the atmosphere.

In most religious traditions there are also times when the normal patterns of sleep and waking may be altered by ritual requirements. For example, during the important festival the Night of Shiva (*Śivarātri*), some Hindus go without either sleep or food for 24 hours. In Hindu metaphysics, creation is said to have three qualities known as the three *guṇas*. These are: *sattva* – balance and harmony; its opposite *rajas* – activity, dynamism and agitation; and the negative aspect *tamas* – inertia and stagnation. Yoga and meditation aim to develop one's *sattvic* nature and minimize one's *rajasic* and *tamasic* natures. Sleep is regarded as *tamasic*, and is therefore a very different state of being from meditation. During the Night of Shiva, to go without sleep is regarded as a strategy for overcoming one's *tamasic* nature. Fasting is considered as a way of subjugating one's *rajasic* nature. Once *tamas* and *rajas* are diminished, this enables one's *sattvic* nature to prevail. According to Mircea Eliade (1969) 'when *sattva* predominates, consciousness is calm, clear, comprehensible; dominated by *rajas*, it is agitated, uncertain, unstable; overwhelmed by *tamas*, it is dark, confused, bestial' (p.23). Predomination of *sattva* facilitates an understanding of the true nature of reality, which is a necessary precursor for liberation from the cycle of transmigration. There is clearly an ambivalent attitude underlying the rationale for forgoing sleep. Sleep is regarded as being an inherent aspect of the created order but, conversely, conquering the desire to sleep signifies the ability to transcend the created order.

In Christianity there are also circumstances when sleep is regarded as inappropriate. In Matthew's Gospel Jesus admonished the disciples for sleeping whilst he prayed alone in the garden at Gethsemane just prior to his arrest. Jesus asked Peter and the other disciples after waking them, 'Could you men not keep watch with me for one hour?' Jesus continued that the disciples should 'Watch and pray so that you will not fall into temptation. The spirit is willing, but the body is weak' (Matthew 26:40–41). The implication is that sleep is purely a physical and bodily phenomenon, but that at specific and significant times, the spirit needs to overcome the natural proclivity of the body to sleep.

Religions therefore tend to represent sleep as an inherent aspect of the created order. However, the sacred transcends the created order and at certain times most religions advocate the necessity for overcoming nature, including the desire to sleep, in order to facilitate access to the sacred. Too much sleep tends to be characterized as indolent, and therefore incompatible with the religious life.

13.3. Sleep, vigilance and vulnerability

The ambivalence of religious attitudes towards sleep is nowhere more obvious than in narratives that pertain to the intertwining themes of vigilance and vulnerability. Matthew clearly equates wakefulness with vigilance, and sleep with weakness and temptation. These notions are emphasized when Jesus indicates to the disciples that they should keep watch because 'you do not know on what day your Lord will come' (Matthew 24:42–43). Jesus stresses this point by recounting that the owner of a house would have kept watch if he had known what time of the night the thief would have broken into his house. In other words, if you are asleep, you are not vigilant and can expect to lose something of value. Of course what is of ultimate value is salvation. Paul expresses a similar point in Romans when he admonishes his readers:

> The hour has come for you to wake up from your slumber, because our salvation is nearer now than we first believed. The night is nearly over; the day is almost here. So let us put aside the deeds of darkness and put on the armour of light. (Romans 13:11–12)

Paul uses sleep as a metaphor for ignorance, and in particular ignorance of the salvific teachings of Jesus, which are equated with light and, by extension, with the day and wakefulness.

The corollary of the idea that wakefulness is associated with vigilance is the concept that night and sleep are associated with being particularly vulnerable. This vulnerability is not only because we are inherently less aware of our surroundings whilst asleep, but also because many religious traditions equate night with darkness and peril. Darkness is also associated with malevolent forces (see Ekirch 2006). This is of particular significance in Christianity, where God is associated with light and the devil with darkness. This idea was reinforced in medieval Christianity, which represented the devil as an insomniac – a being who can find no rest (Summers-Bremner 2008).

The concept of vulnerability whilst sleeping suggests that it is crucial to have divine protection at night. Consequently, many religious traditions indicate that it is especially important to remember God and/or to pray immediately prior to retiring. Devout Sikhs, for example, should recite a prayer known as *Sohila* before sleeping. This not only brings protection, but also, it is sometimes claimed that it can cure insomnia because it focuses the mind on the 'Infinite One' and therefore nullifies anxiety.

The Anglican evening prayer traditionally recited on retiring requests that God 'Lighten our darkness... And by thy great mercy defend us from all perils and dangers of this night' (Church of England 1771). Although the night is perilous, and sleep leaves us vulnerable, as the evening prayer suggests, God who never sleeps will guard the believer from peril. Psalm 3:5–6 suggests 'I lie down and sleep; I wake again, because the Lord sustains me. I will not fear the tens of thousands drawn up against me on every side.' This Psalm is attributed to David and is said to have been composed whilst he fled from Absalom's uprising. David can relax his vigilance and sleep well, despite the danger of attack, because he has faith that God is eternally vigilant and will protect the faithful whilst they sleep. A similar sentiment is expressed in the Sikh sacred text, the Guru Granth Sahib (GGS): 'The Infinite One is pervading among all. So sleep in peace, and do not worry' (GGS 176:7).[10]

13.4. Oh God, why can't I sleep?
Insomnia is sometimes represented as indicating that believers lack faith and the trust that God will protect them in their hours of greatest

vulnerability. Mark's Gospel (4:35–38) tells how Jesus and the disciples were in a boat when a storm arose. Mark suggests that whilst the disciples were scared, Jesus slept. The disciples woke Jesus and enquired if he was not concerned whether or not they would drown. Having calmed the storm, Jesus asked them why they were fearful, and suggested that it was a lack of faith in the love, omnipotence and omnipresence of God that made them afraid and therefore unable to sleep. This appears to contradict the narrative of Jesus admonishing the disciples when they fell asleep in the Garden of Gethsemane: in that case, a demonstration of faith demands perpetual vigilance (to be awake) to the sacred, whereas the account of the stormy sea suggests that faith in the sacred requires the adherent to relax their vigilance (sleep), no matter what the profane circumstances might be, and failure to sleep signifies faithlessness.

In Islam there is some indication that an ability to sleep is indicative of true commitment to Allah. In the battle of Uhud, the second major encounter between the fledgling Muslim community and the Meccans opposed to Muhammad, the Muslims suffered a defeat.[11] The Qur'an suggests:

> After (the excitement)
> Of the distress, He sent down
> Calm on a band of you
> Overcome with slumber
> While another band
> Was stirred to anxiety
> By their own feelings
> Moved by wrong suspicions
> Of Allah.
>
> (*Sūrah* 3 – *Āl 'Imrān*: 154)

This verse refers to two types of Muslims: those truly embracing the new faith, and those embracing it in name only, who are referred to as hypocrites (*munafiqun*). Only the truly faithful could sleep, whilst those inwardly doubting Allah were anxious and unable to sleep.

In Indian, and Indian-derived, traditions – especially those connected with yoga and meditation – an agitated mind is believed to be an obstacle to an understanding of the sacred ground of being. Most forms of meditation involve techniques for stilling the mind which are regarded both as therapeutic and as having religious and spiritual benefits. In Tibetan dream yoga it is believed that it is not only possible to control the mind whilst awake, but also whilst we are dreaming. Going to sleep with an agitated mind will necessarily lead to a disturbed night's sleep, which will therefore not be refreshing for the sleeper. Tenzin Rinpoche, a teacher in the Tibetan Bön tradition, observes: 'It is beneficial to prepare for sleep, to take it seriously. Purifying the mind as much as possible before sleep, just as before meditating, generates more presence and positive qualities' (Rinpoche 1998, p.97).

Rinpoche (1998) suggests that restful sleep is spiritually as well as physically beneficial. He recommends various breathing and visualization techniques, which create 'a protective, sacred environment' that is 'calming and relaxing and promotes restful sleep' (p.103). These techniques have the potential to ensure that the restorative benefits of sleep are optimized. However, Rinpoche (1998) intimates that there are three types of sleep: the sleep of ignorance, which is 'a great darkness'; samsaric sleep, which is a 'great delusion'; and clear light sleep that 'occurs when the body is sleeping but the practitioner is neither lost in darkness or dreams, but instead abides in pure awareness' (pp.145–146). The techniques of yogic sleep can, therefore, bring the practitioner into a state of awareness, similar to that produced in meditation, and this awareness has the potential to liberate the individual from the cycle of transmigration.

The complex and sometimes contradictory evaluations of waking and sleeping have been explored in this and the previous section. For example, the monotheistic religions tend to see relaxed sleep as a sign of faith in God, although in Christianity there is also a suggestion that the faithful should be vigilant and eternally awake to the possibility of salvation. All religious traditions indicate that it is important to calm the mind before sleep, and therefore advise prayer or meditation immediately prior to sleep. However, the rationale for this suggestion is informed by very different metaphysical presuppositions about the nature of the sacred, and this is explored in the following section.

13.5. Understanding sleep – understanding the sacred

Religious traditions often speculate about the nature of sleep as a means of considering the nature of the sacred. For example, in Christianity the viewing of sleep as integral to the created order is a way of emphasizing the distinction between the creator and the created. Psalm 121:3 suggests that God 'neither slumbers nor sleeps'. Similarly, in the Qur'an (*Sūrah* 2 – *Al Baqarah*: 255) Allah is 'The Self-Subsisting, Eternal [and] no slumber can seize Him, nor sleep'. The belief that neither God nor Allah sleeps not only highlights the radical otherness of the sacred, but also relates to the idea that both God and Allah are eternally vigilant and watch over the faithful.

Sleep is also often regarded as a mystery, and consequently as a sign of the reality of the sacred. In the Qur'an it is suggested that within creation there are various 'Signs' that indicate the existence of Allah. In his commentary on *Sūrah* 30 (*Al Rūm*), Ali (1999) suggests that 'Allah's Signs are many, and so are His mysteries: yet each does point to His Unity, Goodness, Power and Mercy' (Ali 1999, p.1012). The Qur'an (30:23) unequivocally states 'And among His Signs is the sleep that ye take'.

Whereas the monotheistic traditions indicate that God does not sleep, in Hinduism an important narrative and an icon represent the god Vishnu as sleeping. The cyclical nature of sleep and waking is used to illustrate the cyclical nature of the Hindu worldview according to which the world is not created *ex nihilo*, as in Christian doctrine – nor is time regarded as linear with a definite beginning and end. The cosmos is not so much created and destroyed, but alternates between states of being manifest and unmanifest. The analogy often used is that of a spider that both spins and reabsorbs its web. The idea is expanded in the mythic narratives and iconography that represent the god Vishnu reclining on the serpent Śeṣa afloat on the cosmic ocean. When Vishnu is asleep in this form, the universe is perceived to be in a latent and unmanifest state. When Vishnu awakes, a lotus containing the creator deity Brahma emerges from his navel, and the phenomenal universe is manifest.

The period that Vishnu is awake is referred to as a day of Brahma, and according to Hindu cosmology lasts 4320 million solar years. The night of Brahma, when the manifest world – symbolically represented by Brahma in the lotus – is reabsorbed back into the sleeping deity, is equally long (see Zimmer 1974, pp.13–17 and pp.35–36). In this mythic narrative, Brahma is associated with the manifestation of the phenomenal cosmos, and is regarded as analogous to the waking state. Vishnu is clearly associated with the dream state. However, there is a third important deity in the Hindu pantheon, namely Shiva, who is often associated with the dissolution of the phenomenal cosmos. The corollary of this is that Shiva is associated with the state of deep sleep. The name Shiva might well derive from the root *śin*, meaning 'to sleep'. Hence, according to Danielou:

> Śiva is described as he in whom 'all go to sleep', 'he who puts things to sleep', etc. His power is represented by the eternal night in which all goes to sleep. (Danielou 1991, p.269)

A narrative associated with the representation of the sleeping Vishnu relates how the sage Marandeya, whilst wandering from one place of pilgrimage to another, slips from the mouth of the slumbering deity. Much to his surprise, all the familiar things of the world have disappeared and he finds himself afloat on an endless ocean, next to the sleeping deity resting on the coils of a serpent. Marandeya questions whether he is himself dreaming. He then falls back into the mouth of the sleeping Vishnu, and he is once again in a familiar landscape. He wonders if his experience of the infinite ocean and the sleeping deity was itself a dream (see O'Flaherty 1984, p.111).

The story of Marandeya explores an important theme in Hindu philosophy, namely, an enquiry into the nature of reality. A consideration of dreams and dreaming is an important aspect of this philosophical speculation according to which Marandeya's experience of Vishnu asleep in the cosmic ocean is in fact more real than his experience of wandering in the familiar landscape. The phenomenal world of sensory experience is ultimately not real. The world that we experience in our waking state is produced by the power of what Hindu philosophers call *māyā* – a term that is often poorly translated as 'illusion', but better interpreted as 'misperception'.[12] Just as we might misperceive the dream world as real whilst we are actually dreaming, we also misperceive the waking state to be ultimately real. However, whilst we are convinced by the reality of this world, we will continue to endure an endless cycle of birth, death and re-birth analogous to the cycle of waking and sleeping.

Whilst different in numerous respects from Hinduism, many forms of Buddhism share this cyclical view of life. In Buddhism, enlightenment is regarded as being completely awake – or being fully aware that all aspects of the phenomenal world are impermanent and therefore fundamentally unsatisfactory. As an enlightened being the Buddha is considered to be fully awake; in comparison, we, even in our apparently waking state, are in fact asleep. In other words, the relationship between the sleeping state and being awake is analogous to the relationship between the waking state and enlightenment.

In Indian traditions in general, sleep is regarded as a state of consciousness. Reflection on the nature of sleep can lead to an understanding of the nature of being. Nowhere is the ontology of sleep more fully examined than in the texts known as the *Upaniṣads*.[13] In a fairly typical exchange recounted in the *Bṛhadaranyaka Upaniṣad* the Emperor Janaka asks the sage Yajnavalkya 'what serves as light for man?' (4:3:2). Yajnavalkya lists such things as the sun, the moon, fire, and so on. However, all these are external sources, and Janaka is not satisfied with any of these answers. Ultimately Yajnavalkya replies that it is the self (*ātman*) that is the light of man (4:3:6). In his commentary on this verse Swami Nikhilananda observes:

> One cannot see dream objects without light. While dreaming too, one meets friends, parts with them, and goes to different places – all without the help of some sort of [external] light. From deep sleep, again, one awakes with the remembrance that one slept happily and knew nothing; this shows that some sort of light functions in deep sleep too. (Nikhilananda 1990, p.263)

Nikhilananda's point is that whilst it is obvious that there is consciousness (light) in the dream state, there is also consciousness in the deep-sleep state. This light is considered as the true self (*ātman*), which is equated with *turīya*, the primordial consciousness, and which underlies waking, dream and deep-sleep states. Nikhilananda's commentary indicates that an analysis of the dream state and the deep-sleep state leads to the conclusion that perception and awareness are ultimately not contingent on anything external. Consequently this suggests that there is a level of consciousness that is self-illuminating as well as being the fundamental ground of all consciousness. The deep-sleep, dreaming and waking states might be considered levels of consciousness that increasingly occlude the consciousness of one's true self (*ātman*).

In the *Māndukya Upaniṣad*, this idea is linked to the mystical syllable 'OM' (\). This syllable is actually the conflation of three phonemes – 'A', 'U' and 'M'.[14] 'A' is said to be the first sound produced at the back of the throat; 'M' is the last sound produced at the front of the lips; and 'U' occurs in the middle. OM, therefore, is regarded as the primordial sound that not only encompasses all possible sound but is everything, according to the *Māndukya Upaniṣad*, whose opening verse states: 'OM – this whole world is that syllable' (*Māndukya Upaniṣad*: 1, in Olivelle 1998, p.289). 'A' is equated with the waking state in which there is a consciousness of external objects. 'U' is equated with the dream state when consciousness is turned inwards. 'M' is associated with the deep-sleep state in which there are no desires or dreams (*Māndukya Upaniṣad*: 5). Finally, the conflation of the three phonemes is identified as the fourth state (*turīya*), in which consciousness rests in itself. The *Māndukya Upaniṣad* (12) indicates that 'the Self (*ātman*) is OM'. This awareness leads to the liberation from the wheel of transmigration. In other words, a contemplation of the three states of consciousness leads to the conclusion that there must be a fourth state of being which transcends not only the cycle of waking, dreaming and sleep, but also the cycle of life, death and re-birth.

The corresponding patterns between the cycles of sleep, transmigration and creation can be illustrated as in Figure 13.1. This suggests that a contemplation of the daily pattern of sleeping, dreaming and waking can lead to deeper existential and metaphysical knowledge. This knowledge can in turn lead to liberation from all of these cycles.

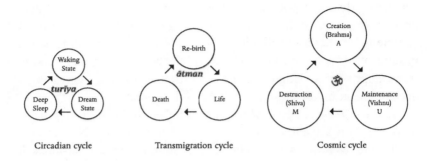

Figure 13.1. Analogous cycles in Hindu thought

It has been argued in this section that a contemplation of the patterns of sleep and waking can lead to a deeper understanding of the nature of the sacred. Conversely, the different metaphysical ideas about the nature of creation also inform different religions' understanding about the nature of sleep. However, as other chapters show, sleep includes two distinct states: non-rapid eye movement (NREM) sleep, which includes deep sleep, and REM sleep – the dream state. All religious traditions have a great deal to say about dreams and dreaming (see Bulkeley 2008), and many religions consider dreams as a form of sacred communication.

13.6. Dreaming as sacred communication

There are traditions of dream interpretation in most religions, or a general belief that certain images within dreams can be portents of things to come in the physical world; for example, in hagiographical accounts of the Buddha's life, it is suggested that, before his birth, his mother had a dream which was interpreted by a Brahmin as indicating that she would have a son who would either rule the world or renounce it. Whilst the interpretation of dreams suggests that there is some intrinsic connection between the dream world and waking world, what concerns us here is not the specific interpretation of dreams, but the meaning of dreaming itself.

As indicated above, in the *Upaniṣads* and in the narratives associated with the sleeping Vishnu, an analysis of the dream state leads to important conclusions about the nature of the self and reality. In the monotheistic traditions, dreaming leads to different conclusions and is regarded with some ambivalence. These traditions, as already noted, suggest that whilst we sleep we are particularly vulnerable – both physically and spiritually – and the spiritual vulnerability is regarded as both a strength and a weakness. It is a strength because whilst we sleep we might be particularly open to communications from God, but it is a weakness because dreams can be deceptive. Dreams do not necessarily originate from God, but can also be the products of human desires or visitations from malevolent forces.

In Islam some dreams, sometimes referred to as 'true dreams' (*ru'ya*), are regarded as messages from God. There is a *hadith*[15] that indicates that Muhammad pronounced that, 'a good dream (that comes true) of a righteous man is one of forty-six parts of prophetism' (al-Bukhari 9:87:112, cited in Khan 2007). This figure is based on the idea that the revelations to Muhammad lasted 23 years, but that the revelations were preceded by six months in which Muhammad is reported as having true dreams. That is, Muhammad dreamt of things that subsequently came true. Furthermore, although Muslims believe that prophecy culminated and was completed with Muhammad, al-Bukhari records a *hadith* that states:

> I heard Allah's Apostle saying, 'Nothing is left of the prophetism except Al-Mubashshirat'. They asked, 'What are Al-Mubashshirat?' He replied, 'The true good dreams (that conveys glad tidings)'. (al-Bukhari 9:87:119, cited in Khan 2007)

In other words, in the times post-prophecy, Allah can communicate to the faithful through dreams.

Edgar argues that the concept of the true dream is 'a fundamental, inspirational, and even strategic, part of the contemporary jihadist movement' (Edgar 2007, p.59). Edgar (2006) suggests that it is commonly accepted that Mullah Omar, the former leader of the Taliban, was inspired to begin his armed struggle because of a dream in which the Prophet instructed him to save Afghanistan. In Islamic dream interpretation, dreaming of the Prophet automatically classifies the dream as true (Amanullah 2009, p.104). Many followers regard jihadists, like Mullah Omar, as holy because their dreams are true. There is, however, a kind of self-fulfilling cycle in which Omar is perceived as being holy because he has 'true dreams' and, because he is faithful, he has 'true dreams'.

True dreams are contrasted with false dreams (*hulm*), which can come either from Satan or simply from human desires. The dilemma is, of course, how to distinguish these different types of dream. Aydar suggests that only the pure can have 'true dreams' and understand their significance. On the other hand, the dreams of sinners are 'confused, meaningless and do not reflect reality' (Aydar 2009, p.86). Naturally, true dreams cannot contradict the Qur'an or the *hadith*.

There are also numerous references to dreams and dreaming in both the Hebrew and Christian Bibles. There are two distinct types of divine communication through dreams: unambiguous and ambiguous messages. In the Gospel of Matthew there are several *unambiguous* dreams associated with the birth of Jesus and his early childhood. For example, it states:

> An angel of the Lord appeared in a dream. 'Get up', he said, 'Take the child to Egypt. Stay there until I tell you, for Herod is going to search for the child to kill him.' (Matthew 2:13)

According to Matthew, Joseph had no doubt about the divine authenticity of this dream as the next verse indicates that Joseph fled with Mary and Jesus. However, only prophets can interpret *ambiguous* dreams. So, for example, Joseph (not the husband of Mary, but Joseph the son of Jacob, who wore the coat of many colours) is able to interpret the Pharaoh's dreams, which all his magicians had failed to do (Genesis 41:1–7). But caution is necessary and there are also warnings that God is against prophets 'who wag their own tongues' and 'who prophesy false dreams… They tell them and lead my people astray with their reckless lies' (Jeremiah 23:31–32). Therefore, whilst dreams can be a form of sacred communication that can inform the devout of important things in this world, they can just as easily lead people astray. Dream experts are required to identify whether a dream is a sacred communication, or merely a manifestation of human proclivities, or a deception by malevolent forces. The expert can also interpret the meaning of the dream. This suggests a further dilemma, how to differentiate between the true interpreter of dreams, who may be considered as a religious authority, and the charlatan, who may lead the faithful astray.

13.7. Sleep and Death

While dreams are regarded as a possible means of communication between the divine and humanity, many religious traditions note a correspondence between deep sleep and death. In the western world this can be traced back to classical Greece, where Hypnos (sleep) was believed to be the twin brother of Thanatos (death). In Arabic, sleep is referred to as the little brother of death. In the Qur'an the relationship between death and sleep is noted:

> It is Allah that takes
> The souls (of men) at death;
> And those that die not
> He takes during their sleep
> Those on whom He
> Has passed the decree
> Of death, he keeps back
> (from returning to life),
> But the rest He sends
> (To their bodies)
> *For a term appointed.*
>
> (*Sūrah* 39 – *Al Zumar.* 42)

The implication seems to be that Allah takes our souls at night as we sleep, and returns them on our waking, or retains our souls if it is the allotted time of death (see also *Sūrah* 6 – *Al An'ām*: 60). In other words, sleep is a temporary severance between the soul and the body, while death is a permanent separation of the spiritual and physical aspects of the individual. A further conclusion that can be drawn from this is that, whereas the body requires sleep, the soul does not sleep.

Certain branches of Christianity do, however, suggest that the soul sleeps after death, to be awakened on judgement day, although in Christian theology there is a debate about that. Martin Luther, for example, argued that the soul is immortal, but also disputed the Catholic concept of purgatory. This raised a theological dilemma: namely, what happens to souls between the death of the physical body and the resurrection and judgement at the end of time. Luther concluded that the soul sleeps and, in the way that the physical body feels nothing in the state of deep sleep, the soul feels nothing until awakened at the day of judgement.[16]

13.8. Conclusion

All religions make at least some passing comments on sleep. Whilst these comments and more extended discussions are mostly used to elucidate other theological or metaphysical concepts, they are also very informative about religious attitudes to sleep. I have argued that there are some broad areas of agreement about the place and nature of sleep between the monotheistic traditions that are different from the understanding of sleep in Indian traditions. I suggest that these different perspectives about sleep are a corollary of the different metaphysical understandings of creation and time. The monotheistic traditions view the cosmos as the creation of an omnipotent deity, and having a definite beginning and end time. Sleep is regarded as both a gift of God and indicative of the presence, mystery and power of God. At the same time sleep is also used as a metaphor for ignorance of the divine will, vulnerability and lack of vigilance. Both too much and too little sleep can be indicative of not being in accord with God's will.

In most Indian traditions creation is regarded in cyclical, rather than linear terms. This cycle of the manifestation and dissolution of the cosmos is regarded as being analogous to the cycle of waking and sleeping. These traditions suggest that a fundamental understanding of the nature of being can ensue from an analysis of the nature of sleep. In the discussions on the nature of sleep as a state of consciousness in the *Upaniṣads*, it is suggested that deep sleep is somehow closer to the nature of the liberating consciousness of the fourth state (*turīya*) than either the dream or the waking states.

In the monotheistic traditions sleep tends to be represented as natural and restorative. However, sleep is also often utilized to signify indolence and ignorance of the sacred, whilst being awake signifies vigilance and awareness of salvific teaching. In the cyclical view of the Indian traditions deep sleep is perceived as taking the sleeper closer to liberatory knowledge, whilst dreaming and being awake are regarded as further layers of consciousness, which occlude understanding. However, despite the fundamentally different metaphysical interpretations of sleep between monotheistic and Indian traditions, it is possible to conclude that all religions are ambivalent about sleep. This ambivalence manifests in the assertion that sleep is natural, and therefore an aspect of the sacred created order. On the other hand, religions suggest that it is sometimes necessary to transcend nature and the desire of the physical body for sleep in order to be in accord with the sacred.

Acknowledgements

Dr George Chryssides, Professor Ron Geaves and the Reverend Prebendary Dr Geoffrey Wynne have all very gracefully responded to my various questions. Their comments and suggestions have greatly assisted me in the writing of this chapter.

Notes

1. The term 'sacred' is used to indicate the belief in some non-empirical ground of being. The term 'God' is not used, as it is only appropriate for monotheistic traditions – particularly Christianity, Judaism and Islam.
2. Buddhism is included in the Indian traditions as, although there are comparatively few Buddhists in India, Buddhism originated in India.
3. In this chapter the convention CE (the Common Era) is used. This is the preferred term used by religious studies scholars for what in the past was identified as AD (Anno Domini: 'In the Year of the Lord') as this is a more inclusive term. BCE (Before the Common Era) is now used in preference to BC (Before Christ).
4. All translations of the Qur'an are taken from Ali (1999). The Qur'an is the collection of revelations to Muhammad, and is regarded by Muslims as the direct word of Allah, communicated through his messenger Muhammad. The Qur'an is not arranged chronologically or thematically. It is divided into 114 chapters known as *surāhs*, which are primarily arranged according to length, the second *surāh* being the longest. Each *surāh* has a title and is divided into verses.
5. All citations from the Bible are taken from the New International Version.
6. Swami is a honorific title that is generally given on initiation into a monastic or renunciate order.
7. *Atman* is a Sanskrit term, most commonly translated as 'Self' or 'true self'. It is a completely different concept to the Christian soul. It is suggested in certain Hindu philosophical traditions that we are neither truly our body or mind. *Atman* is the fundamental essence of our being, which is regarded as being equivalent to the essence of all creation known as *Brahman*. See Jacobs (2010, p.14).
8. Literally the 'power of the Self'.
9. In Punjabi this time is known as *Amrit Vela*, which can be more accurately translated as 'The Time of Nectar'. *Amrit* is an important concept in Sikhism. *Amrit* is the sugar water used in initiation – hence initiated Sikhs are referred

to as *Amrit Dhari* (see McLeod 1997, pp.144–145). *Amrit* is also a metaphysical concept that has connotations of those phenomena that lead away from worldly desires and towards liberation.

10. There are various conventions for referencing the Guru Granth Sahib (GGS) – the convention used here indicates the page and line number.

11. Muhammad was born in Mecca, probably around 570 CE when the dominant religious tradition was polytheistic. Muhammad preached a monotheistic message and denounced the worship of idols. This antagonized many of the Meccan leaders. In the face of increasing hostility Muhammad and his followers relocated to the town of Medina in 622 CE, where the community flourished. Eventually armed conflict ensued between the Meccans and the Muslim community in Medina. In 628 CE a peace treaty was signed between the Meccans and the Muslims ending the hostility.

12. It is suggested that *Brahman* (not to be confused with Brahma) underlies the phenomenal world of experience. The analogy used to explain the concept of *māyā* is that it is like misperceiving a piece of rope as a snake. Once it is realized that there is nothing other than Brahman, that everything that we experience is in fact as unreal as the misperceived snake, the aspirant will be liberated from the cycle of transmigration.

13. There are numerous Hindu texts, but none of them has the same canonical status as the Bible in Christianity or the Qur'an in Islam. Nonetheless, many Hindus identify the Vedas as the foundational texts of Hinduism. There are four Vedas, and each Veda is comprised of four genres of compositions. These genres are: the *Samhitās* which primarily consist of extravagant hymns of praise to the Vedic deities; the *Brāhmanas* which mainly are a consideration of ritual practice; the *āranyakas* which are rather obscure esoteric texts; and the *Upaniṣads* which include a great deal of philosophical speculation about the nature of reality. Whilst there is no absolute consensus it is often suggested that there are 108 important *Upaniṣads*.

14. If you repeat 'A', 'U' and 'M' rapidly the sound blurs into 'OM'.

15. The *hadith* are the secondary texts in Islam. Muhammad is regarded as the Muslim *par excellence* and consequently his life and sayings are important inspirations. Muhammad's personal pronouncements are not regarded as revelations, but are nonetheless important sources of authority, after the Qur'an. A saying or decision of Muhammad is referred to as a *hadith*, often translated as tradition. These individual traditions were collected into compilations, six of which are generally accepted as canonical (see Rippin and Knappert 1990, pp.7–8).

16. Many Christians do not agree with the concept of soul sleep. John Calvin, for example, published a tract entitled *Psychopannychia*, which has the marvelous sub-title: *A refutation of the error entertained by some unskillful persons, who ignorantly imagine that in the interval between death and the judgment the soul sleeps.*

References

Ali, A.Y. (1999) *The Meaning of the Holy Qur'an*. Beltsville, MD: Amana Publications.

Amanullah, M. (2009) 'Islamic Dreaming: An Analysis of Its Truthfulness and Influence.' In K. Bulkeley, K. Adams and P. Davis (eds) *Dreaming in Christianity and Islam: Culture, Conflict and Creativity*. New Brunswick, NJ: Rutgers University Press.

Ancoli-Israel, S. (2001) 'Sleep is not tangible, or What the Hebrew Tradition has to say about sleep.' *Psychosomatic Medicine 63*, 6, 778–787.

Aydar, H. (2009) 'Dreaming in the Life of the Prophet Muhammad.' In K. Bulkeley, K. Adams and P. Davis (eds) *Dreaming in Christianity and Islam: Culture, Conflict and Creativity*. New Brunswick, NJ: Rutgers University Press.

Bulkeley, K. (2008) *Dreaming in the World's Religions*. New York, NY: New York University Press.

Church of England (1771) *The Book of Common Prayer*. Available at http://books.google.co.uk/books?id=6Mo-AAAAcAAJ&pg=PR3-IA6&lpg=PR3-IA6&dq, accessed on 25 February 2011.

Danielou, A. (1991) *The Myths and Gods of India*. Rochester, VT: Inner Traditions.

Edgar, I. (2006) 'The "true dream" in contemporary Islamic/Jihadist dreamwork: a case study of the dreams of Taliban leader Mullah Omar.' *Contemporary South Asia 15*, 3, 263–272.

Edgar, I. (2007) 'The inspirational night dream in the motivation and justification of jihad.' *Nova Religio: The Journal of Alternative and Emergent Religions 11*, 2, 59–76.

Ekirch, A.R. (2006) *At Day's Close: A History of Nighttime*. London: Phoenix.

Eliade, M. (1969) *Yoga: Immortality and Freedom*, 2nd edn. New York, NY: Bollingen Foundation Inc.

Jacobs, S. (2010) *Hinduism Today*. London: Continuum.

Khan, M. (2007) *Translation of Sahih Bukhari*. University of Southern California: Centre for Muslim Jewish Engagement. Available at www.usc.edu/schools/college/crcc/engagement/resources/texts/muslim/hadith/bukhari, accessed on 31 January 2011.

McLeod, H. (1997) *Sikhism*. London: Penguin.

Nikhilananda, S. (1990) *The Upaniṣads: Volume Three – Aitreya & Bṛhadaranyaka*. New York, NY: Ramakhrishna Vedanta Centre.

O'Flaherty, D. (1984) *Dreams, Illusions and Other Realities*. Chicago, IL: University of Chicago Press.

Olivelle, P. (trans.) (1998) *The Upaniṣads*. Oxford: Oxford University Press.

Rinpoche, T. (1998) *The Tibetan Yogas of Dream and Sleep*. New York, NY: Snow Lion Publications.

Rippin, A. and Knappert, J. (eds) (1990) *Textual Sources for the Study of Islam*. Chicago, IL: University of Chicago Press.

Shiromani Gurdwara Parbandhak Committee (1994) *Sikh Rehat Maryada*. Available at www.sgpc.net/rehat_maryada/section_one.html, accessed on 25 May 2012.

Sikh Information (n.d.) *Amritwehla – Guru's Time*. Available at www.info-sikh.com/PageAmrit1.html, accessed on 25 February 2011.

Sivananda, S. (1998) *Mind: Its Mystery and Control*. Sivanandanagar: Divine Life Society. Available at www.dlshq.org/download/mind.htm, accessed on 7 February 2011.

Sivananda, S. (2000) *Easy Steps to Yoga*. Sivanadanagar: Divine Life Society. Available at www.dlshq.org/download/easysteps.html, accessed on 7 February 2011.

Smith, J. (1993) 'Sleep.' In M. Eliade (ed.) *The Encylopedia of Religion*. London: Macmillan.

Summers-Bremner, E. (2008) *Insomnia: A Cultural History*. London: Reaktion Books.

Weber, M. (2001) *The Protestant Ethic and the Spirit of Capitalism*. London: Routledge.

Zimmer, H. (1974) *Myths and Symbols in Indian Art and Civilization*. Princeton, NJ: Bollingen Paperbacks.

14

That Sweet Secession[1]

SLEEP AND SLEEPLESSNESS IN
WESTERN LITERATURE

Lee Scrivner

14.1. Introduction

What is this secession from conscious life we call sleep, this oblivious
third of our lives? We usually think little of it, but it is always hovering
around as a pending transaction or impending obligation. It visits us,
or we it, with fuzzy regularity largely beyond our control. Yet we must
submit to it somehow or perish. For if, as Prospero imagines, 'our little
life / Is rounded with a sleep' (*The Tempest*, IV. i. 157–158), life must
also be relentlessly intersected by little deaths, by the incessant, cyclic
return of slumber.

   We might first imagine sleeping to be one of those universal
human experiences such as breathing, which varies little from person
to person, from culture to culture, or from one historical period to
another. A quick glance at the historical, medical and literary record
of the past few millennia seems to bear this out. People, it appears,
have usually needed an average of six to eight hours of sleep per
night, and have often found getting to sleep difficult when under the
influence of strong emotions or irritating stimulations. Yet despite the
apparent universality of many aspects of slumber, a close analysis of

sleep in western literature reveals numerous practical and attitudinal transformations regarding this most elementary human condition.

A study of sleep's significance in literature would be incomplete, however, without also acknowledging that people have long been intrigued by literature's effect on sleep. Traditionally, good literature keeps one in wakeful anticipation, whereas 'uninteresting' or 'bad' literature or storytelling acts as a powerful soporific. In *One Thousand and One Nights* (Zipes 1997), for example, Scheherazade wards off her own execution by telling the Persian king tales so gripping they keep him wakefully eager to hear more. On the other hand, in Ovid's *Metamorphoses*, when Mercury must rescue the nymph Io from the ever-vigilant, hundred-eyed giant Argus Panoptes, it is only by reciting stories of inspired tediousness that the god is able to render the giant drowsy and thus slay him (see Martin 2004).[2]

The intersection of sleep and literature is made all the more complex by a consideration of the effects of literary representations of slumber. For most of its history, and especially before the invention of the electroencephalogram (EEG),* sleep has been thought of as a kind of nothingness, a lack. The sleeper has thus long been seen as devoid of appreciation, agency, sensation, or any sense of moral dilemma. So when characters in books sleep they are divested of many of the means by which an author typically simulates personality, lends emotional weight, establishes motive or otherwise renders their characters compelling. Accordingly, Shakespeare and a thousand other authors often only depict sleep as the longed-for yet unattainable goal of characters overburdened with cares:

> O sleep, O gentle sleep,
> Nature's soft nurse, how have I frighted thee,
> That thou no more wilt weigh my eyelids down
> And steep my senses in forgetfulness?
>
> (*Henry IV* Part II, III. i. 5–8)

This tradition of representing sleep as a kind of oblivion or nothingness is also underscored in Laurence Sterne's *Tristram Shandy* (1849). Here, the titular character expresses his desire to 'write a chapter upon sleep' in a chapter that largely confounds the consummation of this desire. Tristram's attempt offers little more than a catalogue of quotable clichés on the subject, where sleep is 'the refuge of the unfortunate' or 'the enfranchisement of the prisoner' – quotes that do not even seem to convince Tristram himself. Thus he is quick to refute the 'lie' that 'of all the soft and delicious functions of our nature, [sleep] is the chiefest' by claiming, 'I know pleasures worth ten of it' (pp.221–222). Finally, after largely sabotaging his so-called 'chapter upon sleep', he reveals that the condition might be best represented or appreciated by means of a kind of *via negativa*,[3] by rather considering sleep's absence. Paraphrasing the essay 'Of Experience' by the French Renaissance writer Montaigne, he ironically proposes that causing his sleep to be disturbed might allow him to 'better and more sensibly relish it' or better 'study and ruminate' upon it (p.222).

Such a methodology in investigating sleep further underscores the sense that many of its most salient features are to be found in those it lacks, its featurelessness. It is because sleep is so often depicted as a desired disengagement, a state devoid of sense perception, memory and emotion, that a literature of sleep, or a chapter on the literature of sleep, would be short indeed unless we, like Tristram or Montaigne, include in our study not merely sleep, but also its borderlands and shadowlands: historical and attitudinal mutations, circadian-rhythmic transformations, somnambulism and other pseudo-sleep states – even chronic insomnia. It is only through studying the effects of these near neighbours and antitheses of sleep that we can, like an astronomer studying the effects of a black hole, render palpable that thing which is otherwise phenomenologically void.

Proceeding roughly chronologically from the ancient to the modern period, this study considers a range of texts – medical and psychological treatises, ancient myths, Renaissance plays and modern novels – to show how authors have employed both sleep and sleeplessness to present us with questions about our paradoxical or troubled relation to nature's rhythms, our intentions, expectations and volition. It then chronicles the human sleep cycle's shift from an alignment with the periodic cycles in nature – waking in the day and sleeping at night – to its recalibration by the clocks and cogs of modernity during the second Industrial Revolution, the advent of 24-hour communications, night trains and shift work. Finally, it shows how, with the institution of the sleep laboratory, sleep was no longer seen as only an absence of identity, a disengagement or oblivion; it became a positive topography, an object with its own properties to be explored, causing both sleep and sleeplessness to be newly scrutinized, pathologized and commodified in our contemporary world.

14.2. Sleep and periodicity

Sleep's longstanding literary representation as a kind of negativity, lack or absence informs the tradition of the King in the Mountain in western folklore. This motif usually involves a national hero who never dies but only sleeps, often ensconced in a hill or mountain, in order that he might one day arise to deliver the given nation into a new epoch of peace and prosperity. Ireland's Fionn mac Cumhaill, for instance, sleeps in a cave under Dublin with his retainers and will one day return to defend the land. It is even supposed that the title of James Joyce's *Finnegans Wake* is an underhanded reference to this legend: *Finn again is awake* (MacKillop 1986, p.xi). Strikingly similar is the tale of the Swabian Holy Roman Emperor Frederick I Barbarossa, who sleeps in a cave under the Kyffhäuser range in Thuringia and who will one day awake to restore Germany (Detwiler 1976). According to another legend, the last emperor of Byzantium, Constantine XI, will likewise eventually rise from a deep slumber under his marble tomb to liberate Constantinople for the Greeks (Clucas 1988). The prevalence of these kinds of tales not only demonstrates the universality of nationalist sentiment, but also reminds us of an important aspect of sleep itself. Whilst death results in a permanent absence, a hero's death-like sleep retains a shred of hope, and is, in a sense, symbolic of nature's peek-a-boo periodicity, a reference to the fact that sleeping things are only absent temporarily and will eventually cyclically return again to wakefulness, to presence, like harvest moons or high tides.

Representations of sleep in some of the earliest literature in the West often thus underscore its periodic vacillation with wakefulness and the correspondence of this vacillation with other cycles in nature. The ancient Greeks made sleep the jurisdiction of anthropomorphic deities and weird demons whose actions determined both our shifting states of consciousness as well as the endless shift of day into night and back again. The Greek god of sleep, Hypnos, and Nyx, the goddess of the night, are chased away each morning by the 'bright consort of Tithonus', Eos, the dawn (Mozley 1928, p.63). Hesiod's *Theogony* describes a similar synchronization, where day and night 'draw near and greet one another as they pass the great threshold of bronze:...the one holds all-seeing light for them on earth, but the other holds in her arms Sleep the brother of Death' (Evelyn-White 1920, pp.133–134).

Amid these mythic wellsprings of western literature, the Greeks gradually developed a system of rational physics and medicine, assigning material rather than divine causes to cosmic, meteorological and bodily processes. The Greek system evolved into an enduring tradition of humoral and Hermetic lore that proposed that the sleep cycle in healthy humans corresponded, or should correspond, to the rhythmic fluctuations between opposed dualities in nature,[4] and physicians have continued to note such correspondences nearer to our own times:

> ...the succession of the seasons, and of day and night, the ebb and flow of the sea, the daily variations in the electricity of the air, in the rise and fall of the barometer, and the regular declination of the magnetic needle...illustrate the same law of periodical action, which is displayed in the unvarying alternation of sleep and waking. (Goodrich 1845, p.225)

Conversely, sleep patterns that happened to stray from or disregard these periodic, natural rhythms have long been considered an indicator of humoral imbalance and disease. Melancholia was commonly marked by intense 'watching', the pre-modern near-equivalent of insomnia, and Chaucer (2008, writing around 1370) thus depicts the melancholic's disregard for such 'natural' slumber in 'The Book of the Duchess' (p.330):

> Nature wolde nat suffyse
> To noon erthly creature
> Nat longe tyme to endure
> Withoute slep and be in sorwe.
> And I ne may, ne night ne morwe,
> Slepe; and thus melancolye
> And drede I have for to dye.

Though a correspondence between one's sleep and the night was seen as desirable, straying from such a strict synchronization was not in every case viewed as problematic. Roger Ekirch and other scholars have recently brought attention to evidence that, prior to the second Industrial Revolution in the mid-nineteenth century, people did not always pass the night in unbroken monophasic slumber. Rather, their nocturnal sleep was commonly bifurcated into a 'first sleep' and 'second sleep', and between these two periods of rest, people were typically wakeful for about an hour.[5] This so-called segmented sleep pattern allowed people to attend to basic bodily needs in the middle of the night, such as urination and hydration, and satisfy a range of desires from the contemplative to the criminal. Ekirch (2006), citing the opinion of the sixteenth-century French physician Laurent Joubert, claims that the wakeful period between the first and second sleep may have given the labouring classes an opportunity to more effectively copulate (being too exhausted on first going to bed). Similarly, the Swiss physician and alchemist Paracelsus recommended that one might use the segmented sleep pattern as an aid to digestion, and that one should sleep on the right side when first retiring to bed so that the liver was better positioned to heat the contents of the stomach, 'as a fire doth a kettle'; Paracelsus further proposed that 'after the first sleep 'tis not amiss to lie on the left side, that the meat may better descend' (Burton 1880, p.206).

However, some modern theorists and sleep researchers have posited a more spiritual role for this segmented sleep pattern. Thomas Wehr (1996) suggests that segmented sleep gave people a chance to reflect on their dreams and thus be more in touch with the 'wellspring of myths and fantasies' (p.341).[6] Yet imaginative literature that refers to this phenomenon of segmented sleep appears to both support and contradict Wehr's claim. Hawthorne's brief sketch 'A Bell's Biography' speaks of labourers, 'the sons of toil', who in the middle of the night, in a 'brief interval of wakefulness', hearken to the town bell that causes them to wonder: 'Is so much of our quiet slumber spent? – is the morning so near at hand?' (1837, p.223). A similar scene is more expansively rendered in another of Hawthorne's short sketches, 'A Haunted Mind', where 'you', the second-person subject of the sketch, emerge from a first sleep into an 'hour of wakefulness' at the pealing of a distant church clock's bell: 'You count the strokes – one – two, and there they cease.' Whereas in 'A Bell's Biography' the wakeful interval is depicted as fraught with anxiety over the lateness of the hour, in 'A

Haunted Mind' it becomes a meditative respite from all anxiety, even from time itself. It provides:

> ...one hour to be spent in thought, with the mind's eye half shut... Yesterday has already vanished among the shadows of the past; to-morrow has not yet emerged from the future. You have found an intermediate space, where the business of life does not intrude; where the passing moment lingers, and becomes truly the present; a spot where Father Time, when he thinks nobody is watching him, sits down by the wayside to take breath. (Hawthorne 1851, pp.80–81)

Later in 'A Haunted Mind' this nocturnal waking becomes a representation of the fleeting nature of life itself, which quickly passes into the permanent oblivion of death. Thus it provides both the occasion as well as the metaphoric vehicle through which one might better ponder one's mortality. In both this wakeful interval as well as in a human lifespan, 'you emerge from mystery, pass through a vicissitude that you can but imperfectly control, and are borne onward to another mystery' (Hawthorne 1851, p.86).

Yet sleep's metaphoric parity with death need not hinge on this segmented sleep pattern. Normal, diurnal wakefulness or even lucid dreams can be seen as a metaphor or a microcosm of an entire human lifespan, one that is, as in *The Tempest*, 'rounded with a sleep'. Emily Brontë (1818–1848), writing a decade after Hawthorne, employs the metaphor of sleep to emphasize the carefree oblivion of a longed-for death:

> Oh, for the time when I shall sleep
> Without identity,
> And never care how rain may steep,
> Or snow may cover me!
>   (Brontë, Brontë and Brontë 1905, pp.69–70)

14.3. Sleep as a paradox of will

As is evinced in both Brontë's poem and Hawthorne's 'A Haunted Mind', issues related to volition, the will and self-control, or the lack of all three, are central to the idea of what it is to be asleep, and often arise in its literature. Sleep has long been generally regarded as a state in which the powers of the will are held in abeyance. However, there were occasionally exceptions to this view of the utter helpless passivity of the sleeper. The nineteenth-century English psychologist James Sully, for instance, notes how during sleep, in a dream, one might remain 'conscious of voluntarily going through a series of actions' and maintain 'something resembling an exercise of voluntary attention' (1882, p.173). Furthermore, commentators in the popular press in the nineteenth century claimed that a kind of surrogate will is suggested in sleep by, amongst other things, the fact that some people are able to rouse themselves into consciousness at a predetermined hour (Chambers and Chambers 1879).

But for the most part, going to sleep involved forsaking the powers of volition and self-control. The German humourist Jean Paul Richter tells of the dangers of somnambulism, in which the unfortunate sleeper is taken over by an alien agency: people go to bed:

> …without reflecting that perhaps, in the first sleep, they may get up again as Somnambulists, and crawl over the tops of roofs and the like; awakening in some spot where they may fall in a moment and break their necks. (Richter 1874, p.80)[7]

Somnambulism thus displays a convoluted, vague relation to the will. One seems in control enough to amble about, yet unable to purposefully direct that movement. Such volitional ambivalence is similarly highlighted when a sleepwalking Lady Macbeth incriminates herself. A gentlewoman sees her unconsciously 'rise from her bed, throw her night-gown upon her, unlock her closet, take forth paper, fold it, write upon't, read it, afterwards seal it, and again return to bed; yet all this while in a most fast sleep' (*Macbeth*, V. i. 5–8), and it is the strange conflation in slumber of semi-purposeful acts with an auto-pilot obliviousness that makes her 'slumb'ry agitation' seem to the physician 'a great perturbation in nature' (*Macbeth*, V. i. 12–14).

Yet even outside of the context of somnambulism, sleep presents volitional ambiguities and paradoxes. Scottish philosopher Dugald Stewart recognizes that when we want to get to sleep we first must try to mimic a lack of will.[8] This seems to him fraught with much difficulty. Stewart wonders, how might one wilfully activate a lack of volition?

> If it were necessary that volition should be suspended before we fall asleep, it would be impossible for us, by our own efforts to

hasten the moment of rest. The very supposition of such efforts is absurd; for it implies a continued will to suspend the acts of the will. (Stewart 1802, p.333)

Another seeming paradox emerges in the realization that, though sleep was often considered to be a state devoid of will, it was also one in which one's psychosomatic energy – the so-called 'nervous agency' that in the nineteenth century was thought to fuel the will – was replenished. Furthermore, certain reserves of this nervous energy were required in order to voluntarily transit into sleep. It was once widely thought, for instance, that people of great nervous constitution and willpower could instantaneously fall asleep whenever they desired. Historical figures such as Napoleon and Wellington, it was said, could 'command sleep when it suited [them] to take rest' and go for great lengths without it 'when circumstances required such a privation' (Jones 1864, p.280).

The power of the will to induce sleep often enhanced the mystique of those who wielded it in the awed estimation of those who did not, especially since such a power had long been associated with magical or divine influence. The potions of Shakespeare's *Romeo and Juliet* and *Cymbaline* and the apple and spindle of *Snow White* and *Sleeping Beauty* demonstrate the prevalence and importance of magical soporifics in western literature, a tradition stretching back at least to ancient Greece. In Nonnus's *Dionysiaca*, for instance, Hypnos keeps Harmonia's wedding guests awake through the night by intentionally leaving behind his magic wand, 'because that was the rationer of sleep' (Rouse 1940, p.177). In the popular fiction of more recent times, the 'magic' driving the soporific wand's efficacy is replaced by technological knowhow. In Bulwer-Lytton's *The Coming Race* (1886), which is discussed further below, members of a technologically advanced, subterranean race use staffs to harness an atmospheric magnetism called Vril, which they use to wilfully force sleep upon the novel's narrator.

Often in western esoterica such magical wands and staffs – as appear in the myth of Hypnos, the tale of *Sleeping Beauty* and Bulwer-Lytton's novel – are stereotypically associated with an active, masculine principle. It may thus seem counterintuitive that in these cases the effects of such instruments facilitate the seeming passivity of sleep. Yet this apparent contradiction further underscores the aforementioned inherent contradictions in sleep itself – as a realization and rejuvenation of the will through seeming willlessness, as a death-like maintenance of life, and even in some cases, as an enhanced procreativity despite – or by means of – passivity. Each of these apparent contradictions is represented in the Greek myth of Endymion. Through Zeus' intercession, the mortal Endymion exchanges death for an eternal youth through divine sleep, yet in his slumber he is strangely active and vigilant.[9] In one of the most common versions of the myth, Endymion is loved by the goddess of the moon, Selene, who somehow mates with him whilst he sleeps and thus conceives 50 daughters, representing the lunar phases (Grimal 1996). The sexualized fertility of Endymion's suspended state makes his myth a masculinized and less violent precursor to the earliest known version of the tale of *Sleeping Beauty*, the fourteenth-century French romance of *Perceforest*. Here, the beautiful maiden Zellandine is not kissed awake by a handsome prince, but is rather raped by her lover Troylus and bears his child whilst sleeping (Haase 2008). Thus, though *Sleeping Beauty* and *Snow White* have come to represent ways in which a prolonged slumber sustains an innocent and inviolate femininity, such literature also underscores the fact that in sleep humans are at their most vulnerable, which makes ever urgent the question of how much one can trust one's bed mate.[10]

A modern novel, Jonathan Coe's *The House of Sleep*, explores these issues of vulnerability and trust, agency and lack thereof, when the main character and sufferer of narcolepsy, Sarah, discovers the voyeuristic tendencies of the novel's chief antagonist, Gregory:

> 'Well, when did you become so intimately acquainted with my eyelids?' and he answered, 'While you were asleep. I like watching you when you're asleep.' And this was the first intimation she had, the first hint, of his liking for standing over people in their beds, looking down on them as they slept, something she had regarded as interesting at first, the sign of an enquiring intelligence, until she began to wonder, in the end, whether there wasn't something sinister about it, fetishistic almost, this desire to look down on people as they lay helpless, unconscious, while he, the watching subject, retained full control over his waking mind. (Coe 1998, p.18)

Gregory's watchfulness ultimately takes the form of a strangely eroticized practice – called 'the game' – in which he rests his fingers over Sarah's eyelids to feel the movement of her eyes. He even parlays his fetish into a career: he goes on to run a centre for the study of sleep disorders, allowing him to feed his insatiable desire to observe his patients' inner lives in the involuntary twitching of their rapid eye movement (REM)* 'paradoxical sleep', and – further manifesting his controlling nature – even subjects some of them to dangerous sleep-deprivation experiments.

Coe's novel and the tale of Zellandine reveal ways in which sleepers and would-be sleepers are vulnerable to potential victimization by a malicious, wakeful presence. Yet the lack of wilful self-control in slumber has been conversely proposed as a means to protect the wakeful from would-be criminals. Shakespeare imagines that sleep would keep maliciously minded youth from acting on their inclinations: 'I would there were no age between ten and three and twenty, or that youth would sleep out the rest; for there is nothing in the between but getting wenches with child, wronging the anciency, stealing, fighting' (*The Winter's Tale*, III. iii. 59–60).

Finally, the loss of control in sleep is represented in literature by characters who fall asleep only to discover that, whilst they were sleeping serenely, a kind of temporal transformation has occurred. This seems to highlight one of sleep's central phenomena, that of the seeming disappearance of the normal sense of the passage of time. Thus Shakespeare's hypothetical sleeping juvenile delinquent in *The Winter's Tale* in effect uses sleep as a kind of time machine to propel him- or herself into a future in which he or she will be more civil. The literary implementation of sleep as just such a device for time travel had a particularly prominent heyday in the late nineteenth and early twentieth century. Novels such as Edward Bellamy's *Looking Backward: 2000–1887* (1951, first published in 1888), William Morris's *News From Nowhere* (2009, first published in 1890) and H.G. Wells's *When the Sleeper Wakes* (2004, first published in 1910) present main characters who sleep for generations and, upon awaking, discover a world that has been transformed into either a utopia or a dystopia. In the tradition of Washington Irving's *Rip Van Winkle* (1967, first published in 1819), then, the time-travelling slumber of these novels' protagonists allows the author of each to comment on the social and cultural conditions of their own day.

Indeed, literature has often proposed that so complete is one's surrender of self-control upon going to sleep that there is never any guarantee that one will find the world quite the same upon their return to consciousness. Not only may night-time be transformed, but so too can one's surroundings or one's self. One might wake to discover, such as in the case of Gregor Samsa in Franz Kafka's *The Metamorphosis* (Kafka 2007, first published in 1915), that one has transformed into a bug or even, as is playfully hypothesized by Sylvia Plath in *The Bed Book*, that one – or one's bed – has shrunken to the size of a pea (Plath and McCully 1976).

14.4. Sleep, industrial modernity and the rise of insomnia

The two main lenses through which we have thus far viewed sleep in this chapter – that of its periodicity and that of its relation to the will – must, in a sense, be superimposed when we consider sleep after the middle of the nineteenth century. In the Victorian period, people significantly enhanced their volitional powers through the railway and the telegraph, which made the world ever more instantaneously accessible, and thus transformed people's experience of time and space. For instance, after the institution of the transatlantic telegraph of 1866, many newspapers made arrangements for sending and receiving telecommunications after normal business hours, between 6 p.m. and 6 a.m. By 1877, the main telegraphic offices in New York and London had become like self-contained cities, devoted to 24-hour communication. Tom Standage describes them as having 'a press room, a doctor's surgery, a maintenance workshop, separate male and female dining rooms', as well as operators who 'work[ed] in shifts' and 'ensured that the whole system worked around the clock' (Standage 1998, p.99).

Considering the increasing precision with which people's time was thus managed in an age of trains and telegraphs, with ever more acute realization of, and attention paid to, the inconvenience or monetary cost of misspent time, there was an ever-increasing motivation for people's sleep schedules to be managed accordingly, with ever-greater precision. Meanwhile, Victorians' expectations also changed with regard to their own sleep habits. It seemed only natural that they, who were increasingly accustomed to thus expediting their will across continent-spanning wires or rails, should soon desire or expect to exact equivalent volitional control over something as near to them as their own bodies, over something as seemingly simple as falling asleep.

Bulwer-Lytton's novel, *The Coming Race*, first published in 1870, provides an example of a willed, technologically enhanced management of sleep in a setting where most other aspects of life are similarly managed. The aforementioned 'Vril staff' that is used to force sleep upon the narrator does not seem out of place amongst that society's other technological marvels – such as their urban lighting, lifts, telegraphs, automata and mechanical contrivances for flight – which similarly enhance what would seem to be an otherwise gloomy subterranean existence. After the narrator wonders how his 'cerebral organisation could possibly be duller than that of people who had lived all their lives by lamplight', he remarks: 'while I was thus thinking, [the Vril-ya] Zee quietly pointed her forefinger at my forehead and sent me to sleep' (Bulwer-Lytton 1886, p.47). This conflation of the narrator's wondering with Zee's actions seems to draw attention to the idea that any civilization that has become intellectually advanced enough to master its environment to the degree that the Vril-ya have, must also simultaneously exert an equivalent mastery over the body.

But such a mastery of the body was, sadly, only realized in fiction. Indeed, it was in the context of the new technologized cityscape of the 1860s that chronic insomnia first emerged as a pathological entity subject to increasing professional scrutiny and public concern. Ekirch (2006), Eluned Summers-Bremner (2008) and other commentators have recently focused on the effects on sleep of public lighting and increased time-consciousness in the nineteenth century. And indeed, many medical and cultural commentators of the Victorian period similarly attributed the increase of chronic sleeplessness to the nervous degeneration that occurred in the face of the overbearing stimulations of modern, urban life – its brighter lights, its faster paces, its more strident sounds, its shocking vibrations and electrifications.

Yet recent scholars have largely overlooked the fact that physicians and psychologists of the Victorian period also bemoaned the rise of insomnia from so-called 'brain-work' – the intellectual labour of accountants, bankers, journalists and lawyers – and the difficulty that this new breed of urban, professional 'thinkers' faced when attempting to cease to think. They remarked how an intense attention to a particular course of study or a difficult problem, or a heightened level of anxiety about technical minutiae, might cause the cerebral hyperaemia or neurasthenic enervation of insomniacs. The rise of insomnia, then, might be attributed not only to properties of technologic objects themselves – the brightness of electrical lighting, the loudness of a night train's whistle – but also, as is suggested in *The Coming Race*, to the intellectual involvement of the participants in and inventors of the ever more technically complex, 24-hour economy.

The literature of this period reveals a growing tension between this so-called brain work and sleep. In James Thomson's long poem 'The City of Dreadful Night', excessive human activity has transgressed the natural, periodic limits of daylight and prior business hours, whilst workers in the poem, such as the drudges driving an 'overburthened wain', struggle to accommodate this excess, heedless of normal, nocturnal sleep. Yet Thomson is especially explicit in his portrayal of the strain the over-active dystopian environment puts upon the mental powers:

> The City is of Night, but not of Sleep;
> There sweet sleep is not for the weary brain;
> The pitiless hours like years and ages creep,
> A night seems termless hell. This dreadful strain
> Of thought and consciousness which never ceases…
>
> (Thomson 1880, p.7)

Similarly, Charles Dickens's short story *The Signal-Man* shows how the onset of the railway and the telegraph taxed the brain and abolished sleep of one unfortunate railway employee. The unnamed signal-man listens and watches for telegraphic warning signals – an alarm bell and a red 'Danger-light' – that tell of trouble on the railway line. He 'passe[s] long winter nights there, alone and watching' (Dickens 1866, p.23). The narrator underscores the post's potential for exacerbating a worried insomnia, commenting on the poor man's deteriorating nervous condition in the face of the danger-light, and its persistent evocation of worry over an always-imminent disaster:

> That I more than once looked back at the red light as I ascended the pathway, that I did not like the red light, and that I should

have slept but poorly if my bed had been under it, I see no reason to conceal. (Dickens 1866, p.24)

Ironically, it is precisely the signal-man's monomaniacal exactitude – his uncompromising vigilance – that ultimately drives him mad and thus compromises his ability to perform his job. The theme of worried watchfulness is then taken yet further when the narrator becomes a kind of signal-man himself, faced with a similarly overwhelming responsibility for public safety. He debates with himself about whether he should warn others of the danger they face in the nervous signal-man's employment, a warning that would, paradoxically, spread new rail-related worries in an effort to counteract already existing ones. Significantly in Dickens's account, an insomniac vigilance is required of everyone in an industrialized, railway-riding society, in order to keep the whole system functioning properly.

Yet it is not just the perpetual vigilance necessitated by public safety in an age of mass transit that makes technological modernity so seemingly incompatible with sleep, nor even the oft-cited wakefulness of inventors of these selfsame modern technologies, such as the famously restless Edison and his co-workers – dubbed the 'insomnia squad' by his contemporaries. For a fuller understanding of the sudden emergence of 'brain-worker's' insomnia in the late nineteenth century, one must consider the psychological doctrines of the association of ideas that were popular in this period, and the potential difficulties that such doctrines were thought to pose for people who sought slumber in technologized environments.

The association of ideas, since its origins in the work of Aristotle, explains how thoughts quantitatively replicate in the mind based on some ideas' association – or topical contiguity – with other ideas. In the early part of the nineteenth century, the philosopher James Mill observed how thoughts quantitatively beget thoughts by virtue of a qualitative determination:

I see a horse; that is a sensation. Immediately I think of his master; that is an idea [conception]. The idea of his master makes me think of his office; he is a minister of state; that is another idea. (Mill 1829, p.52)

Thus, it is these ideas' topical interrelation that forms their zealous mutual attraction and causes each to pull its next-of-kin into the mind without much or any effort on the part of the thinking subject. The ease – or, indeed, inevitability – with which the mind makes associations in this way was thought to explain why urban brain-workers became increasingly restless as the nineteenth century wore on. Simply put, during and after the second Industrial Revolution people were surrounded by more and more things that were associated with or 'contiguous' with the idea of ceaseless activity. Prior to the middle of the nineteenth century, most objects of our attention suggested a periodic vacillation between activity and inactivity. After dusk in previous centuries, streets went generally dark, travel and communication all but ceased, towns fell relatively quiet. There were of course the occasional exceptions to this tendency, yet certainly after the second Industrial Revolution this quiet nocturnal life became increasingly intruded upon. As the late nineteenth century wore on in northern transatlantic urban centres, and the more live telegraphs and night trains actively snaked through cities under 24-hour lamplight, the more people's impressions and associations became suggestive of round-the-clock activity, or insomnia.

If this idea seems far-fetched, consider the story *Sounds in the Night* (Anonymous 1868), from a popular London magazine. It illustrates how a technologically active environment might facilitate a hyperactive association of ideas and intrude upon one's peaceful slumber. The story's narrator first attributes sleeplessness to too much 'brain work', then describes how, when he tries to sleep in his country-house, impressions of the distant city's technologies invade his bedroom's silence and initiate and perpetuate his obsessive mental associations. First comes the sound of a speeding night train. 'Listening attentively, I hear, clear and shrill, the scream of the railway engine as it plunges beneath our tunnel… "That is the 2:35 A.M. up express" I mentally say to myself' (pp.33–34).[11]

Yet it is not this engine's 'scream' itself that keeps the narrator awake thereafter, but the train of thoughts that it inspires. Immediately he begins to reflect on his own former railway journeys. He imagines the busy, round-the-clock coming and going of other railway travellers. 'How odd to think of the light, activity and bustle *there*, at this unearthly hour, and all still and motionless here at home.' His mind, however, is anything but 'still and motionless', for he continues to make associations. The narrator seems quite self-conscious of his reverie, explicitly remarking how his intellectually hyperactive condition exemplifies associationist psychology.

> I do not wonder that metaphysicians have dwelt so carefully on the subtle laws of association. How a casual sound awakens a mental association, and at the touch of this association the burial places of memory give up their dead. The sleepless hour is indeed the time for memory. (Anonymous 1868, p.37)

Similarly, Dickens introduces the idea of the wakefulness of those whose minds make associations involuntarily in his short sketch 'Lying Awake'. He reveals the musings of one who wants to sleep, but finds himself constantly drawn to and engrossed in memories and musings by the 'association of ideas' (Dickens 1853, p.145).

14.5. Sleep lab

For most of its history, sleep was considered as a unified whole. It was likened to a body of water or a curtain under or behind which one could submerge or hide one's self.[12] There has long seemed something comforting in this ability to so hide, to make identity disappear. In *Tristram Shandy*, the characterization of sleep as that which 'covers a man all over like a cloak' is more valued 'than all the dissertations squeezed out of the heads of the learned together upon the subject' (Sterne 1849, p.222).

Yet this view of sleep as singular, as a sensory negation or a mere oblivion, began to change in the late nineteenth century. The change was subtle at first, merely implied. Dickens, in 'Lying Awake' (1853), suggests a kind of fracturing of Cartesian unified subjectivity by means of an idiosyncratic description of his insomnia: 'Perhaps, with no scientific intention or invention, I was illustrating the theory of the Duality of the Brain; perhaps one part of my brain, being wakeful, sat up to watch the other part which was sleepy' (p.145). Yet such a brain, fractured thus between wakeful and sleepy binaries, soon became subdivided even further. In the 1880s, British physician Joseph Mortimer Granville characterized sleep rather as an aggregation of the self's various mental, sensory, muscular and visceral systems, each of which might maintain or involuntarily fall into its own independent sleep patterns: 'Sense organs must sleep, the viscera must sleep, and, above all, the nervous system composed as it is of a vast multitude of nerve-centres, each capable of a limited independence of action, must sleep' (Granville 1884, p.78). Granville then constructed out of this theoretical systemic heterogeneity a complex of potential 'false sleeps', wakeful states that mock true slumber. If just one of the body's constituent systems remained restless, despite all others being dormant, a false sleep would result. Only when these sovereign systems' various sleeps occurred unanimously and simultaneously could one win 'perfect' slumber. Singular, negative sleep was further eroded by around 1900. Kenton Kroker's (2007) fascinating history of sleep research, *The Sleep of Others*, explores how, shortly after the development of the EEG, it became a complex positive entity with functional characteristics; it was no longer 'little more than nothingness'; it adopted 'a kind of morphology that it had never had before' (pp.6–7).

Sleep as a complicated, multivalent terrain, worthy of careful, clinical study, becomes the focus of two recent novels that are partly set in sleep laboratories, Coe's *The House of Sleep* (1998) and William Boyd's *Armadillo* (1998). In *The House of Sleep*, the journalist Terry suffers from an impossibly severe case of insomnia and eventually becomes one of Gregory's patients. Gregory's account of the complex topologies of sleep, mapped by the EEG and a century of clinical research, reveal the fascinating world from which Terry in his sleeplessness has been effectively banished:

> Stage Two begins with the appearance of theta waves of three-and-a-half to seven-and-a-half cycles per second, along with spindles and K-complexes…and then we see slow delta wave activity beginning, which marks the start of unconsciousness proper. Stage Three is an interim stage, when the delta waves still account for less than half the recording on the EEG. Stage four is when the delta waves predominate… (Coe 1998, p.145)

Similarly, *Armadillo* portrays the strangely conflicted relationship between a sleep researcher, Alan, and his patient, the insurance adjuster, Lorimer. For both novels' sleep researchers, the world of sleep – manifested in its brainwave morphologies as well as in the vivid dreams that occasionally unfold there – becomes in some ways more attractive than the waking world. Thus both novels convey multivalent contradictions between the demands and fascinations of clinical research, the idea of productivity, the demands of one's career and the demands of sleep. Terry's prolificacy as a journalist, for example, is enhanced by his insomnia in that he is able to remain productive whilst his competitors, other would-be writers, are handicapped by their normal sleep patterns. Terry's career would thus suffer by any cure that Gregory might give.

Conversely, in Boyd's novel, Lorimer imagines that Alan's main priority is not to cure him of his disorder, but rather to simply exploit it for ever more intriguing research data, in order to satisfy his own curiosity and further his own careerist agenda: 'after six weeks of participation in the Institute's program, it was ever more clear to Lorimer that the dream segment of the research, rather than the curative outcome, most intrigued [Alan]' (p.90). Alan encourages Lorimer to mentally manipulate his lucid dreams whenever a particular love interest appears, explaining that it would help cure Lorimer's sleep disorder. Yet given that the conscious and wilful participation of the dreamer in a lucid dream makes sleep less deep, this therapeutic regimen would seem entirely counterproductive. Still, Alan's therapeutic approach underscores the longstanding desire to maintain the volitional powers despite sleep, to transform it into something more like wakeful life and to recoup, as Terry had done, the hours lost to involuntary and unproductive oblivion. Both novels thus show evidence of the modern desire to render sleep either productive or utilitarian, or else to abolish it completely in the face of an unflagging will.

Indeed, such a desire to maintain a round-the-clock wilfulness or productivity has marked much of the literature of sleep since the mid-nineteenth century, since the rise of technological modernity. In *The Coming Race*, oblivious or unproductive slumber becomes a kind of unfortunate vestige of a primitive age, a resource to be tapped. The narrator gets his language 'extracted' whilst he sleeps. He is then invited to compare such practices with those of his own civilization, asked if, in his world:

> …it was not known that all the faculties of the mind could be quickened to a degree unknown in the waking state, by trance or vision, in which the thoughts of one brain could be transmitted to another, and knowledge be thus rapidly interchanged. (Bulwer-Lytton 1886, p.26)

Such a colonization of sleep by utilitarian wilful consciousness has appeared more recently in James Cameron's film *Avatar* in which human characters manipulate their avatars while laying dormant in hi-tech pods. Thus oblivious or non-volitional sleep is entirely abolished. In both waking life as humans and whilst sleeping as Na'vi, Jake and Grace continue to enact their will, make decisions and remain involved in their surroundings, whether directly or vicariously. This scheme reveals one of the main misanthropic contradictions in the film: to live in seeming harmony with nature through the life of the Na'vi, Jake and Grace must disobey their own natural, circadian rhythms. Instead of finding harmoniously restful recuperation in themselves, they spend their sleep hours unnaturally enacting their wills through others' bodies. Christopher Nolan's film *Inception* (2010) also fantasizes about the colonization of sleep by the technologized will. In both films, sleep loses much of its intractable otherwordliness and becomes yet another environment in which one's waking volition might be enacted. In both films, one of sleep's principal defining characteristics is obliterated, and thus sleep essentially disappears.

14.6. Turning off

The contradiction in Cameron's film – the radically artificial co-opting of sleep in order to be more 'in touch with nature' – highlights the ever-increasing tension between the will and sleep in modernity. Since the invention of telecommunications a century and a half ago, and especially since the rise of the internet in the last two decades, our wills have been given a kind of transcontinental dominion. Our conscious lives thus more and more resemble that of Bulwer-Lytton's Vril-ya, in whose world 'the thoughts of one brain [are] transmitted to another' around the clock. Yet this new widening of the dominion of our wills has not occurred without some sacrifice, as gains in one terrain are usually not won without losses in another. Whilst using the internet to explore strange and faraway things, we often languish in ignorance of our own visceral life or the goings-on inside our heads or right outside our door; we lie supine whilst, like the humans of *Avatar* or *Inception*, we virtually control a supplementary distant 'space' and play within its prescribed logic.

If the internet represents this perpetual access of information and a virtual connectivity or control, and if literature represents an archiving of our fantasies, memories and histories, then sleep, as we have seen in this chapter, runs antithetical to them as the oblivion of this archive and a resistance to this round-the-clock inundation and facilitation. It will thus be interesting to see what forms the literature of sleep takes in the coming decades, in which our days and nights become ever more crowded with ideas and information and input, with spectacles and sounds vying for our limited capacities of attention. As much as it is in our nature to periodically relinquish our will, to allow ourselves to be taken over by our circadian rhythms and the phenomenology of nothingness, it will also always be in our nature to desire to account somehow for this longed-for blind spot in our lives.

This chapter was completed in October 2010.

Notes

1. From Laurence Sterne's *The Life and Opinions of Tristram Shandy, Gentleman* (1849).
2. See also: Simpson (2001, p.282).
3. Latin: 'way of negation' – a way of describing something by identifying what it is not. This method was famously used to describe God by philosophers and theologians such as Pseudo-Dionysius the Areopagite and Thomas Aquinas.
4. The humoral tradition was a Greek system of medicine in which health was largely determined by the balance of four bodily fluids or humors. Similarly, the Hermetic tradition underscored the importance of a harmonious balance of the four classical elements and a correspondence between rhythms in nature and the cosmos and those in the body. Sleep is acknowledged as part of this correspondence in such lore, which claims 'without the repose of the night our bodies would not resist the day's toil' (Kingsford and Maitland 1885, p.131).
5. Another kind of bifurcated sleep or polyphasic sleep, that of siesta cultures, is described in Brigitte Steger's chapter in this book (see Chapter 4).
6. See also Ackerman (2007, p.178).
7. To remedy this danger, the narrator fastens his right toe to his wife's left hand each night with tape – which he jokingly refers to as his 'marriage tie'.
8. Stewart, like Sully, also recognized that one might make decisions in one's dreams: 'That the power of volition is not suspended during sleep, appears from the efforts which we are conscious of making while in that situation. We dream, for example, that we are in danger; and we attempt to call out for assistance' (Stewart 1802, p.332).
9. Endymion is often depicted in literature and on sarcophagi as 'sleeping' with eyes wide open (see Yonge 1854, p.903–904).
10. Vulnerability is a topic considered elsewhere in this book (see Chapter 4).

11. Though the story is anonymously published in this journal, the author is likely the Reverend Frederick Arnold.

12. Examples of such a 'singular' sleep state are, of course, numerous, though the state might consist in varying degrees. See Frothingham (1866, p.202): 'Then comes sleep...pouring balm into hurt minds; immersing Nature in her bath of oblivion'. See also Stebbins (1859, p.380): 'Silence, darkness all around me, / Not a fire-beam on the wall – / Now, oh Night, thou voiceless soother, / Let sleep's curtain gently fall!'

References

Ackerman, J. (2007) *Sex Sleep Eat Drink Dream: a Day in the Life of your Body.* Boston, MA: Houghton Mifflin Co.

Anonymous (1868) 'Sounds in the Night.' *London Society 5,* 33–38.

Bellamy, E. (1951) *Looking Backward: 2000–1887.* New York: The Modern Library.

Boyd, W. (1998) *Armadillo: a Novel.* New York, NY: Alfred A. Knopf.

Brontë, E., Brontë, C. and Brontë, A. (1905) *Wuthering Heights, Agnes Grey and Poems.* London: Thomas Nelson and Sons.

Bulwer-Lytton, E. (1886) *The Coming Race.* London: George Routledge and Sons.

Burton, R. (1880) *The Anatomy of Melancholy: What it is with All the Kinds, Causes, Symptoms, Prognostics, and Several Cures of it. In Three Partitions.* Vol. 2. New York, NY: A.C. Armstrong & Son.

Chambers, W. and Chambers, R. (1879) 'Sleep-Sleeplessness.' *Chambers' Journal of Popular Literature, Science and Arts 790,* pp.98–99.

Chaucer, G. (2008) 'The Book of the Duchess.' *The Riverside Chaucer.* (Edited by L.D. Benson.) 3rd edn. Oxford: Oxford University Press.

Clucas, L. (1988) 'The Byzantine Legacy in Eastern Europe.' *East European Monographs.* New York, NY: Columbia University Press.

Coe, J. (1998) *The House of Sleep.* New York, NY: Alfred A. Knopf.

Detwiler, D.S. (1976) *Germany: a Short History.* Carbondale, IL: Southern Illinois University Press.

Dickens, C. (1853) 'Lying Awake.' *Household Words 6,* 136, 145–148.

Dickens, C. (1866) 'The Signal-Man.' *All the Year Round 16,* Extra Christmas Number, 20–25.

Ekirch, A.R. (2006) *At Day's Close: a History of Nighttime.* London: Phoenix.

Evelyn-White, H.G. (trans.) (1920) *Hesiod, the Homeric Hymns, and Homerica.* London: William Heinemann.

Frothingham, G.B. (1866) 'The Cry for Rest.' *Herald of Health and Journal of Physical Culture 8,* 5, 201–203.

Goodrich, S.G. (1845) *The World and Its Inhabitants.* Boston, MA: Bradbury, Soden & Co.

Granville, J.M. (1884) *Nerves and Nerve Troubles.* London: W.H. Allen.

Grimal, P. (1996) *The Dictionary of Classical Mythology.* Oxford: Blackwell.

Haase, D. (2008) *The Greenwood Encyclopedia of Folktales and Fairy Tales.* Vol. 3. Westport, CT: Greenwood Press.

Hawthorne, N. (1837) 'A Bell's Biography.' *Knickerbocker 9,* 3, 219–223.

Hawthorne, N. (1851) *Twice-Told Tales.* Vol. 2. Boston, MA: Ticknor, Reed and Fields.

Irving, W. (1967) *Rip Van Winkle.* London: Franklin Watts.

Jones, C.H. (1864) *Clinical Observations on Functional Nervous Disorders.* London: John Churchill & Sons.

Kafka, F. (2007) *Metamorphosis and Other Stories.* London: Penguin.

Kingsford, A.B. and Maitland, E. (1885) *The Hermetic Works: the Virgin of the World of Hermes Mercurius Trismegistus.* Madras: P. Kailasam Bros.

Kroker, K. (2007) *The Sleep of Others and the Transformations of Sleep Research.* Toronto: Toronto University Press.

MacKillop, J. (1986) *Fionn Mac Cumhaill: Celtic Myth in English Literature.* Syracuse, NY: Syracuse University Press.

Martin, C. (trans.) (2004) *Metamorphoses.* New York, NY: W.W. Norton.

Mill, J. (1829) *Analysis of the Phenomena of the Human Mind*. London: Baldwin and Cradock.

Morris, W. (2009) *News from Nowhere*. Oxford: Oxford University Press.

Mozley, J.H. (trans.) (1928) *Statius: Thebaid*. The Loeb Classical Library. Vol. 2. London: William Heinemann.

Plath, S. and McCully E.A. (1976) *The Bed Book*. New York, NY: Harper & Row.

Richter, J.P.F. (1874) 'Schmelzle's Journey to Flætz.' *Tales by Musæus, Tieck, Richter*. (Edited by Thomas Carlyle.) Vol. 2. London: Chapman and Hall.

Rouse, W.H.D., Rose, H.J. and Lind, L.R. (eds) (1940) *Dionysiaca*. Loeb Classical Library. Cambridge, MA: Harvard University Press.

Simpson, M. (ed.) (2001) *The Metamorphoses of Ovid*. Amherst, MA: University of Massachusetts Press.

Standage, T. (1998) *The Victorian Internet: The Remarkable Story of the Telegraph and the Nineteenth Century's On-Line Pioneers*. New York, NY: Walker and Co.

Stebbins, A. (1859) 'Firelight Fancies.' *Ladies' Repository 27*, 380.

Sterne, L. (1849) *The Life and Opinions of Tristram Shandy, Gentleman*. Leipzig: Bernhard Tauchnitz.

Stewart, D. (1802) *Elements of the Philosophy of the Human Mind*, 2nd edn. London: T. Cadell Junior and W. Davies, in the Strand.

Sully, J. (1882) *Illusions: a Psychological Study*. New York, NY: D. Appleton.

Summers-Bremner, E. (2008) *Insomnia: a Cultural History*. London: Reaktion Books Ltd.

Thomson, J. (B.V.) (1880) *The City of Dreadful Night and Other Poems*. London: Reeves and Turner. [The nineteenth-century poet James Thomson is widely known as B.V., which stands for his pseudonym *Bysshe Vanolis*. It also helps distinguish him from the eighteenth-century poet James Thomson.]

Wehr, T. (1996) 'A "clock for all seasons" in the human brain.' *Progress in Brain Research 111*, 321–342.

Wells, H.G. (2004) *When the Sleeper Wakes*. London: Phoenix.

Yonge, C.D. (trans.) (1854) *Deipnosophists*. Vol. 3. London: Henry G. Bohn.

Zipes, J. (ed.) (1997) *Arabian Nights: a Selection*. London: Penguin.

15
Sleeping on It

Andrew Green

15.1. Introduction

Snow (1959) suggested that the 'clashing point' of the two cultures, of science and the humanities, 'ought to produce creative chances'. He added (without giving any examples) that 'in the history of mental activity that has been where some of the break-throughs came' (Snow 1959, p.16). Break-throughs might be a tall order, but there are at least opportunities for new insights in browsing over, and reflecting on, the breadth of material presented in this book – 'sleeping on it', as it were.

This is no small task, however, and it is not possible to encompass all the material of the various chapters – that could amount to another book in itself – but this chapter draws upon what science and the humanities tell us about the options we have with regard to sleep. In doing so, there is no apology for the use of footnotes in the hope of maintaining a flow of ideas whilst still digressing on occasions to fill in some of the background, or to delve a little into subject areas that could not be covered directly in the book.

The division of this chapter into sections is somewhat arbitrary as overlap is inevitable: for example, sleeping at different times could involve either sleeping more or less than the norm. Broadly, however, this chapter considers: when we sleep, sleeping less, sleeping more, and how the boundaries between sleep and wakefulness can appear blurred.

15.2. When to sleep (and how much?)

We have no choice but to sleep, although someone lying awake in the small hours might disagree about the strength of that imperative. Whereas Randy Gardner set a record in 1965 by remaining awake for eleven days (264 hours), he was, according to Gillin (2002), 'basically cognitively dysfunctional' by the end of that time (see also Williams 2005, pp.20–21). Other chapters here suggest that there might be choice at least about when and how we sleep – or if not *choice* as such, that other options are possible. And it is here that the tension between the humanities and sciences in these chapters is most striking, that is, over what constitutes a 'natural' sleep pattern.

There is an assumption in western industrial society at least, that sleep should be in a single continuous period at night. For example, Carskadon and Dement (2011) describe 'normal human sleep' in those terms, without mention of other patterns, and although in Chapter 2 Paterson does not specify that monophasic sleep is the 'norm', she shows how circadian and homeostatic processes interact to produce a monophasic pattern – Borbély's two-process model. Steger notes (in Chapter 4) that Borbély subsequently implied that biphasic sleep – the siesta culture – is somehow 'immature', even though it is the same circadian process that predisposes us towards sleepiness in the afternoon.

There is some evidence, however, that an afternoon sleep was historically more widely acceptable in the UK and Northern Europe. Afternoon naps for the higher social classes (who could afford regular evening leisure activity) were not unusual according to Steger, and Green (2008) cites literary and historical evidence of siestas for hard working members of the lower classes in long summer days.[1] It is industrialization that 'typically involves eliminating the daytime siesta' (Walsh, Dement and Dinges 2011, p.716), but Steger shows that in some parts of the world, including some industrialized countries, napping – and napping in public – is much more acceptable than it is in the West. However, it is unclear how much of the napping she describes is planned and how much is opportunistic, and it has not been established whether such naps contribute to an individual's necessary total sleep time in 24 hours or whether it constitutes 'extra' sleep.

The distinction between 'replacement' and 'appetitive' nappers – the latter napping not for reasons of sleep need but for psychological benefits 'not directly related to the physiology of sleep', was made by Evans *et al.* (1977, p.687). They found different sleep architecture* during a 60-minute nap amongst appetitive nappers, replacement nappers and non-nappers (all college students). The non-nappers took significantly longer to get to sleep compared to either kind of napper, but the chief difference was that the appetitive nappers had more 'fragmented sleep' – moving between stages of sleep more often than the replacement nappers (though the total time in each stage was similar). Evans *et al.* (1977) concluded that napping could serve different functions. Similarly, Horne (1988) distinguished between core sleep and optional sleep, suggesting that we can take additional sleep beyond the biological necessity (see also Chapters 7 and 12). He argued that normal 7–8-hour sleepers could reduce their sleep by 1.5–2 hours, to 5.5–6 hours (Horne 1988, p.213), and proposed that it could be possible to take just 6 hours' sleep – though he stressed that it was an option only. Subsequently, Horne (2010) has observed that there is no evidence that habitually having less than 6.5 hours is harmful, 'unless it causes excessive daytime sleepiness' (Horne 2010, p.114).

The half-hour difference in Horne's estimates of duration in core sleep two decades apart is notable, since, in the interval, van Dongen *et al.* (2003) concluded from the findings of a sleep deprivation experiment (described in Chapter 7) that 6 hours is an insufficient core sleep duration. Cognitive deficits in participants, they argue, should not have developed in 6 hours of daily sleep, including appropriate slow-wave sleep (SWS),* if it were enough. However, Horne's (1988) original contention remains valid since, in effect, his conclusion was that there is *flexibility* in how much sleep one takes (see below).

Whilst the concept of the siesta is familiar to most people, including those who have never had one, it is modern night-time sleep that is the more different from traditional pre-industrial sleep patterns. Chapters 4, 5 and 14 all refer to the work of Ekirch (2001, 2006), and the compelling evidence that people in pre-industrial societies spent the night in two roughly equal spells of sleep either side of an hour or more of quiet wakefulness. It is tempting to speculate, in passing, that this provided the rationale for the saying that 'one hour's sleep before midnight is worth more than two after midnight'[2] (Cobbett 1829), a notion that is supported by the observation that our deepest and more restorative (slow-wave) non-rapid eye movement (NREM) sleep tends to occur earlier in the night's sleep (see Chapters 2 and 3). Ekirch (2001) notes that he found references to 'first sleep' (also known as 'first nap' or 'dead sleep') in 58 different sources dating from between 1300 and 1800, as well as similar references in French and Italian; the later period of sleep was known as 'second sleep' or 'morning sleep'. The literature of that period therefore provides clues to long-lost habits. One example cited by Ekirch is from mid-sixteenth-century writer William Harrison, who referred to 'the dull or dead of the night, which is midnight, when men be in their first or dead sleep' (Ekirch 2001); other sources more specifically refer to waking 'about midnight', but importantly, according to Ekirch, waking was spontaneous and routine. Furthermore, the segmented sleep pattern appears to have continued at least into the twentieth century in some cultures:[3]

> Anthropologists have found villages of the Tiv, Chagga, and G/ wi, for example, in Africa to be surprisingly alive after midnight with newly roused adults and children. Of the Tiv in central Nigeria, a study in 1969 recorded, 'At night, they wake when they will and talk with anyone else awake in the hut.' The Tiv even employ the terms 'first sleep' and 'second sleep' as traditional intervals of time.[4] (Ekirch 2001)

Thomas Wehr, whose work is cited in Chapters 5 and 14, supports Ekirch's contention. He noted how humans were thought to have different sleep from animals, and cites findings suggesting that during the sleep period other primates have between 17 and 20 per cent of wakefulness, compared to less than 1 per cent for young human adults. However, Wehr observed a further difference in that humans 'use artificial light to create an unending ~ 16-h photoperiod for themselves', and went on to suggest that 'consolidated sleep could be an artifact of modern lighting technology' (Wehr 1992, p.103).

Taking together the evidence from history, anthropology and science, an increasing weight of opinion suggests that we have evolved different ways of sleeping and that there is flexibility in the system. And of course there has to be some flexibility – at one level, so that sleep in different conditions and at different latitudes is possible (see Chapter 3), and at another level, so that we can respond to danger. Monophasic sleep now suits us: it is time-efficient and has proved convenient, but we still cannot all sleep at the same time. As Schwartz (1970) put it, 'no society could afford to permit sleep to overtake its entire membership' (p.494). It would be absurd to be able to sleep in the face of a threat, whether from a predator or an enemy or (less immediately) from hunger. The latter is more important to a small animal that feeds often, and experiments on mice, for example, by Fuller, Lu and Saper (2008), have shown that although the circadian rhythm entrained by the light/dark cycle is adequate when food is plentiful, the 'master' system can be overridden at times of great stress – including starvation. A 'feeding clock' was found in mice (in the dorsomedial hypothalamus) that could keep the animals awake until they had been able to eat. This illustrates the principle that it must be possible to override the master clock, and also offers potential for managing jet lag.[5]

It appears likely that segmented sleep and the existence of sleep cycles* with frequent brief wakenings would confer an evolutionary advantage. In a prehistoric community, or extended family, it would be probable that at any time in the night someone was likely to be awake, or close to being awake, and therefore more alert to danger. In modern times, it can be very reassuring for people experiencing poor sleep (e.g. new parents or people with chronic illness) to know that broken sleep, however unsatisfactory it might seem, is entirely natural.

15.3. Restricting sleep/sleeping less

Whatever the historic practices and the biological 'reality', in western industrial society most people would regard seven or eight hours' sleep some time between 10 p.m. and 8 a.m. as the norm. However, there are signs of change. People have increasingly *worked* around the clock to keep industry working and transport moving since the second Industrial Revolution,[6] as Chapter 14 shows, but in the later twentieth century, round-the-clock *leisure* also became possible. People have read long into the night for centuries – especially those bent on self-improvement (as, for example, two of Thomas Hardy's characters: Clym Yeobright and Jude Fawley[7]). 'Night-life' was always an option for those with leisure and resources (see Chapters 4 and 14), but frequent opportunities were not available for the majority until relatively recent times – in particular, the post-war period of the twentieth century.

The opportunities for night-time leisure are now many, and the modern sleeping environment is increasingly affected by new distractions or disincentives to sleep. Consider the possibilities for a child or young teenager in the UK in the 1950s who might have no option to delay sleep other than reading under the bedcovers with a torch after 'lights-out'. By the mid-1960s a much younger sibling probably had a battery-powered transistor radio and listened to pirate radio stations late at night. In contrast, their children, or grandchildren, might now have more technical equipment than would have been found in the cockpit of a light aircraft of the 1950s. Even if the modern child has no television in the bedroom (in the UK 70% do,[8] compared to 76% in the USA – see Chapter 5) they quite possibly have an array of other devices that might delay or curtail sleep, such as computers, games consoles, mp3 players and mobile phones.

Whether this is just normal behaviour or reflects medicalization* or the pathologizing of sleep habits (see Chapters 5, 6 and 14) is another question, but there does seem to be an increasing number of young people 'graduating' into the sleep clinic with problems of sleep disruption related to poor sleep habits. Some of the children who have grown up with mobile phones and the internet and are now reaching adulthood are finding it hard to maintain a sleep pattern that is conducive to work or independent living. This is not to suggest that the availability of technology and instant communication might *cause* sleep disorders, but it seems possible that they might exacerbate, or expose, an existing tendency to delayed or disordered sleep. For example, a person with delayed sleep phase syndrome (see Chapter 9) can now much more easily remain occupied late at night and further delay winding down for sleep, and thereby exaggerate the tendency to sleep late. If not actually sleepy at midnight, it is easy to become engrossed in something on the computer, or on the television, and delay settling for hours – soon perpetuating a habit.

However, there can be serious consequences of neglecting regular sleep schedules. The Selby rail crash in 2001 was caused by a sleepy driver whose vehicle left the road and ran onto the London to Edinburgh railway line and into the path of a train; he had stayed up talking through the night on the telephone to someone he had met through the internet instead of sleeping. The driver, Gary Hart, was gaoled for five years (Oliver 2002) for causing ten deaths by dangerous driving, although he claimed he could drive safely despite having little sleep. So, whilst it remains our choice to curtail sleep, we may face penalties if we cause harm as a result: society places some responsibility on us to have sufficient sleep and increasingly places restrictions on professional drivers. Walsh *et al.* (2011) describe some of the legislation in the USA relating to sleep and driving, including 'Maggie's Law' (named after Maggie McDonnell, a victim of a road accident where a driver had not slept for 30 hours), which states that a driver in the state of New Jersey can be charged with vehicular homicide if s/he causes a fatality after not sleeping for 24 hours or more. As Williams puts it, sleep 'becomes the duty or obligation of the good citizen in the service of both self and society' (Williams 2011, p.44). However, so far, whilst society might have an opinion of how much we should sleep, there has been no attempt to tell us *when* to sleep – unless we count daylight saving measures.

Curtailing sleep before driving is a common practice and many of us probably get up early in an attempt to beat the traffic with barely a thought about whether we have had sufficient sleep. In a review of literature on sleepiness and safety, Philip and Åkerstedt (2006) cite their work which showed that 'long distance driving was very frequently associated with sleep curtailment' (p.349). In their 1993 study 50 per cent of drivers at a rest area in France had reduced their sleep duration in the 24 hours before leaving for a long journey, and 10 per cent had not had any sleep in that period. To reduce the likelihood that drivers were self-selecting (tired drivers being more likely to stop in a rest area), they later sampled over 2000 drivers at an *autoroute* tollbooth. Again, 50 per cent had decreased their usual sleep time and 12.5 per cent had a sleep debt of more than three hours. In subsequent tests they found that, compared with controls, the sleep-deprived drivers 'showed a very altered level of vigilance with shorter sleep latencies measured during two consecutive naps' (Philip and Åkerstedt 2006, p.350).

However unwise it might be to curtail sleep in such a way, it is an example of how choices relating to time use are like other economic decisions that we make: we weigh up the costs and benefits of selecting one activity over another. Drivers either are unaware of the risks of curtailing sleep, misperceive them, or disregard them. According to economists Biddle and Hamermesh (1990), sleep can be considered as just another commodity, or another way of using our time – and there is a tradition of doing so since the mid-twentieth century at least.

In an exploration of time as an economic resource, Linder (1970) looked at ideas from the preceding decades that suggested that we might sleep less and make more of our time. Observing that 'we can cut down on the number of hours [of sleep] only for brief periods without nature taking her revenge' (p.48), he notes Lebhar's suggestion that we can increase our time budget by 'two hours a day snatched bodily from the waste-heap to be put to effective use' (Lebhar 1958, p.7). Lebhar argued that by sleeping for two hours less per day, more than two years[9] would be gained over the course of 26 years. Similarly, Ernst (1955) looked forward to a Utopia in 1976[10] when, apparently, we would need less sleep; he stated: 'Experiments indicate that under relaxed and satisfying habits [in 1976] six hours will be enough to replenish our bodily energies' (p.14). Lee (1964) reported the most extreme reduction in sleep in stating that 'the Russians are experimenting with a sleep machine called the "electrosone" which will pack a full night's sleep into just two hours or less' (p.163).[11] The world is still waiting.

None of the writers just mentioned were economists, who might be able to help explain, and draw conclusions from, the complex equations and statistical analysis of the time-use studies becoming increasingly available. It is also not possible to look here in detail at the part of the time-use literature that refers to sleep. However, two examples from recent accessible literature might be given in order to illustrate the richness of the available data, and to highlight the dramatic variation in sleep duration within and between societies. First, Robinson and Michelson (2010) show time-use data (gathered between 1998 and 2005) from 21 countries[12] around the world which suggest that the difference between the mean weekly sleep times of people in Bulgaria and people in Japan is as much as 8.7 hours: that is, on average, Japanese people appear to sleep for one-and-a-quarter hours less per night than Bulgarians. (The data do not indicate whether Japanese people compensate for this difference with *inemuri*, or daytime naps.) Second, Wittenberg (2005) cites a thesis by Gábor Szalontai that showed a difference in mean daily sleep time, of about 90 minutes, between poor African women and much more affluent white men in South Africa. It is suggested that 'all of this difference can be explained in terms of the relevant economic variables' (p.21).

The literature of economics might indeed be a source of explanations for behaviour that might curtail sleep. Szalontai suggests that 'adopting a view that sleep is solely a biological necessity and the amount of sleep is determined purely by physiological factors would be a very naïve view indeed' (Szalontai 2006, p.855). Yaniv's contention that jet lag is 'a rationally self-inflicted disorder which the individual finds too costly to avoid' (Yaniv 2004, p.7) seems uncontroversial (since maritime travel is seldom a practical option), but he also applies economics to the choice of bedtime, especially in relation to insomnia. Sleep restriction therapy – or bed restriction, as Yaniv terms it – is described in Chapter 9 (Box 9.2) and, as he observes, it *is* counterintuitive to ask a person who does not sleep enough to spend *less* time in bed. Yaniv argues that 'a more plausible approach would involve *increasing* time in bed in an attempt to acquire more sleep' (original emphasis), and suggests that the following equation provides 'rational support for such behavior' (Yaniv 2004, p.5).[13]

$$\frac{d\Theta^\star}{dR} = -\frac{1}{\Delta}\left[-U_{AS} + (1 + I_\theta)\,U_{SS} - I_\theta \Psi''\right] I_R$$

There appears to be a conflict here between economists and psychologists or sleep therapists. In the absence of an economist's contribution to this book it would be unfair to criticize such difficult equations, but the rationale for sleep restriction therapy is well established and there is much evidence for its effectiveness (Glovinsky *et al.* 2008; Spielman, Saskin and Thorpy 1987; Taylor *et al.* 2010). However, it would be a naïve sleep therapist that attempted to impose sleep restriction or stimulus control techniques (see Box 9.2) on a patient or client without taking account of their personal circumstances (social *and* economic). So, whilst the psychological principles behind such measures are sound, economic factors cannot be completely ruled out, since the values that people place on time, and what they can do with it, will affect their motivation and decisions.

Economic considerations – the premium put on time – might explain the use of modafinil* by students, amongst others. The potential effects on academic performance are noted in Chapter 6, but enhancing the ability to fit in college commitments and earn a living, as well as having a social life, are all clear incentives to use the drug. However, ethical questions are raised here as modafinil highlights a contradiction. In Chapter 13 Jacobs notes how, in the Calvinist tradition in particular, sleep could be seen to be equated with indolence, whereas modafinil could be considered a means of doing away with the need for such a waste of time. Accordingly, Williams *et al.* (2008) suggest therefore that, 'drugs such as modafinil *embody* the Protestant work ethic… or at the very least display an "elective affinity" to it' (p.29; original emphasis). However, they also draw attention to 'pharmacological Calvinism' – the belief, according to Conrad (2007), 'that it is better to achieve an objective such as pleasure, sexual satisfaction, mental stability and bodily fitness naturally than with drugs or medications' (p.92). This presents a dilemma. Whilst some of a Calvinist persuasion may welcome treatment for excessive sleepiness, it has been observed (from the standpoint of bioethics) that, 'pharmacological Calvinists fear that this could pathologize what is seen as normal sleeping time and daytime energy [and pose] difficult questions surrounding how much sleep and daytime energy is "normal"' (Cahill and Balice-Gordon 2005, p.3).

Such niceties do not apply in the case of military use of modafinil. As Kim puts it, 'the modern pressures of a complex, computer-driven and understaffed military machine requires [*sic*] soldiers be exploited for their maximum physical and mental facilities' (Kim 2007, p.65). Modafinil is therefore of particular interest to the military because it does not have potential for abuse (as do amphetamines, for example) and because it appears not to disrupt subsequent restorative sleep. Examining the range of pharmacological countermeasures against sleepiness, Caldwell and Caldwell (2005) note that modafinil appears best for maintaining wakefulness for up to 40 hours, especially when there may be an unexpected opportunity for sleep. However, they wisely conclude:

> …drugs are not a substitute for good work/rest scheduling… and…with regard to situations devoid of sleep opportunities, there has not been a drug of any description that has been found capable of indefinitely postponing the basic physiological need for 8 h of restful daily sleep. (Caldwell and Caldwell 2005, p.C48)

It seems therefore that even with pharmacological help, the best that we can do is postpone sleep – or perhaps increase the flexibility already permitted by the system.

15.4. Sleeping more – or sleeping differently?

Whilst there are many temptations and incentives to sleep less, there are fewer reasons why people would deliberately or voluntarily sleep more, unless making up for lost sleep. The story of the sleepers of Ephesus in Chapter 13 suggests that sleep could be thought of as a 'natural haven from adversity', as if a kind of hibernation. The antihero of *The Outsider* (Camus 1961, first published in 1942), in solitary confinement awaiting trial on a capital charge, trains himself to sleep away the hours. He reaches a point where there were 'only six hours to fill' (p.82). An early sleep researcher, Boris Sidis[14] (2010, first published in 1909), observed a tendency amongst prisoners in solitary confinement to sleep 'unless they find a source of mental activity by getting some external stimulation to awaken their mental life' (Sidis 2010, Chapter 3); he believed that monotony is 'the most important…condition common to sleep and subconscious states'. If there is a hint of a Protestant work ethic in this, the following observation of philosopher Dugald Stewart a century earlier is steeped in it:

> It is also a matter of common observation, that children and persons of little reflection, who are chiefly occupied about sensible objects, and whose mental activity is, in a great measure, suspended, as soon as their perceptive powers are unemployed, find it extremely difficult to continue awake, when they are deprived of their usual engagements. The same thing has been remarked of savages, whose time, like that of the lower animals, is almost completely divided between sleep and their bodily exertions. (Stewart 1802, p.330)

Similarly, in a footnote, Stewart also recalls Thomas Jefferson's observation of the disposition of slaves in the USA to 'sleep when abstracted from their diversions, and unemployed in their labour… *Notes on Virginia*, by Mr. Jefferson, p.225' (Stewart 1802, pp.330–331).

These examples of sleeping to pass the time are either fictional or from centuries ago, and suggest that in normal circumstances people would not choose to sleep to excess. It does not seem to have occurred to Stewart or Jefferson that a slave might sleep when not working because of having already worked long, hard hours (and lacking the resources to read philosophy). In modern times there is some evidence, as seen in Chapter 7, that prisoners, or at least detainees with mental health problems, might sleep to pass the time. However, much more research is necessary in order to establish, first, whether sleep duration does increase in conditions of extreme and persistent monotony and, second, to distinguish between the effects of mental illness or the side effects of treatment if those factors are present (cf. Chapter 10).

Nevertheless, many people with depression do speak of sleep as a refuge – sleeping away time, or certainly sleeping away the day (perhaps therefore sleeping at different times as opposed to necessarily sleeping more). A patient might describe a preference for the 'semi-oblivion of sleep' – or 'time out'. Another sufferer of depression, speaking at a conference on sleep and mental health,[15] described nocturnal wakefulness as 'prolonging the night-time refuge' from the pressures of work and family. Being up at night is a way of taking some 'me-time', and it is likely that some people choose a more nocturnal existence as an escape from dealing with society – now made easier in the UK with the increasing number of stores open for 24 hours, internet shopping and night-time activity already mentioned.

The idea that an extension of sleep could be an option was noted above in connection with sleeping less. Horne (2010) cites an observation by Kleitman and Kleitman in 1953 that adults in the far north of Norway slept for one hour less in the summer, and therefore slept more in the winter. It is understandable that people make the most of summer daylight and might sleep more on the cold dark nights of winter. Elsewhere in the world, however, people sleep to avoid the heat. The siesta has already been mentioned, but Worthman and Melby (2002) observe, from their survey of ethnographic studies, that 'customary siesta taking is well recognized and widespread, and usually is associated with increased nighttime activity so that sleep is rather more distributed around the clock' (p.85). High temperature is obviously a factor, but opportunity is another. It is possible for the traveller in East Africa, for example, to observe people dozing when work is slow, such as porters in a bus park in the long interval between morning departures and afternoon arrivals.[16] Trained professional staff might also sleep in quiet moments: in tropical rains or when there is an equipment failure, there might be nothing else to do but wait for the clouds to pass or the problem to be resolved. Consider, however, that they might have been up very early to work their allotments and might expect to work late at a second job – so perhaps it is, again, not so much a case of sleeping more, as one of sleeping differently.

In the end, it is difficult to see how people can voluntarily extend their sleep to any significant degree in ordinary circumstances. Someone with obstructive sleep apnoea (OSA) dozing off during the day might appear to sleep more, but the daytime sleep is not something they would choose, and might not represent *extra* sleep, because night-time sleep was insufficient. Someone having long sleep would seem to be either recovering from disrupted or lost sleep, or just sleeping differently (i.e. less at night and more in the day) – on the other hand, of course, they could just be a naturally long sleeper who might on occasion sleep less than necessary and then *seem* to sleep excessively.

15.5. Blurred boundaries

The extent to which excessive sleep, or sleep itself, is considered a waste of time may be debatable, but it has never been seriously suggested that we could do without it. Noting some of the likely purposes of sleep, Paterson (Chapter 2) suggests that sleep is an active physiological process,[17] and observes that the brain might continue to work in sleep as, for example, in 'sleeping on a problem'.[18] One person noted for this was Thomas Alva Edison: Scrivner (Chapter 14) alludes to his indefatigability but, whilst suggesting that Edison 'harboured a somewhat negative view of sleep, or…too much sleep' (Williams 2005, p.51), indicates that he was a 'famous napper'. It has been argued that Edison 'made extensive use of *hypnagogia* as a means of arriving at new ideas' (Mavromatis 2010, p.186, first published in 1987). Hypnagogia is a term coined by Mavromatis to include the hypnagogic and hypnopompic states,[19] between wakefulness and sleep, and the phenomena of them. He suggests there is evidence of a 'positive link between alpha-theta brainwaves, hypnagogic imagery and creativity' (p.187).[20] He cites a further example of creativity in hypnagogia – of the chemist August Kekulé who claimed to have seen images of the benzene molecule (whose structure he had been puzzling over) as he dozed by his fire.

Mavromatis (2010, first published in 1987) makes many claims for hypnagogia, and explores the relationship with dreaming and, in so doing, he inevitably strays into the territory of the 'paranormal' or 'supernatural'. However, whatever one believes about phenomena such as telepathy or out of body experiences, hypnagogia could provide the beginnings of an explanation for some of them since, as noted by Vaughn and D'Cruz (2011), hypnagogic hallucinations are difficult to distinguish from reality. One variety of hallucination is actually the origin of the word 'nightmare' (a wholly different experience from a terrifying dream in REM sleep), which occurs in NREM sleep: that is, the phenomenon of the Old Hag.[21] The nineteenth-century description of the nightmare by Robert Macnish goes on for several pages of colourful language, in which he conveys the horror of it, but the following extract, relating to the Old Hag, captures the tone:

> Or, he may have the idea of a monstrous hag squatted upon his breast – mute, motionless and malignant; an incarnation of the Evil Spirit – whose intolerable weight crushes the breath out of his body, and whose fixed, deadly, incessant stare petrifies him with horror and makes his very existence insufferable. (Macnish n.d., p.124, first published in 1834)

One can imagine the terror of someone believing such a vision to be real, particularly in times when beliefs in spirits were more widely held, but the fear is no less distressing today. It is possible to meet people who fear sleep and delay its onset as long as possible to avoid these experiences, and others such as night terrors.

The experience of the hypnagogic hallucination is all the more frightening if, as often it is, it is accompanied by sleep paralysis (see Chapter 9). It is where neuroscience meets folklore and has been extensively researched by Hufford in an almost forensic examination of frightening night-time experiences. He concludes that 'without sleep laboratories…folk tradition has apparently maintained an awareness of the distinction between REM intrusions into wakefulness and REM occurring in its proper place' (Hufford 1982, p.166). He notes the possibility that 'the victims are awake and that they do hear and see and feel odd-sounding things'. A more recent study by Parker and Blackmore (2002) also found that hypnagogic experiences are qualitatively different from dreaming. They say of the participants in their survey that 'although [they] often state that they are fully awake and able to look around the real environment, it is possible that they are experiencing a false awakening – that is dreaming they have woken up' (Parker and Blackmore 2002, p.57).

As noted, hypnagogic experiences (in NREM sleep) are clearly differentiated from dreams and, although people would not usually mistake dreaming for wakefulness there are also reports of problem-solving and the gaining of new insight in dreams. Wagner *et al.* (2004) cite examples of scientific advances said to be facilitated by dreams: Nobel Prize winner Otto Loewi 'woke up with the essential idea [to confirm experimentally his theory] of chemical neurotransmission' (p.352), and Dmitri Mendeleyev reported that his understanding of the rule for the periodic table emerged from a dream. According to Blackmore, René Descartes 'had a series of dreams which inspired him with the idea of a completely new philosophical and scientific system based on mechanical principles' (Blackmore 2010, p.12). As Scrivner (Chapter 14) observes, there is evidence that nineteenth-century writers maintained that some kind of consciousness could be retained in dreams. Dugald Stewart and psychologist James Sully held that decisions could be made in dreams and that it is possible to retain voluntary attention in dreams.

Chapter 7 shows how sleep is necessary for cognitive processes and there are suggestions, noted here, that these continue through dreaming. Very recently, van der Helm *et al.* (2011) have shown an association between REM sleep and overnight activity in the amygdala[22] (in response to emotional experience) and the reduction of 'next-day subjective emotionality' (p.2029). Consideration of disordered sleep also reminds us how the dividing line between sleep and wakefulness is not so clear – and the switch delicate. Arguably, all sleep disorders reflect the blurring of the boundaries between sleep and waking: for example, insomnia is remaining awake in sleep time, whilst in narcolepsy, cataplexy occurs when the muscle atonia of REM sleep intrudes into wakefulness or, in the case of sleep paralysis, atonia persists into wakefulness.

Jacobs (Chapter 13) shows how different religious traditions – especially the Hindu tradition – regard the relationships between sleep (and dreaming) and wakefulness, anticipating by centuries the scientific understanding of the three states of being – as in the case of prescient folk tradition noted above. Jacobs observes that we might misperceive wakefulness and dreaming. It may also be that O'Brien's humorous suggestion that we should 'invert our conception of rest and activity'[23] (O'Brien 1967, p.98, first published in 1939) is not so completely absurd, and that we should not think of sleep and wakefulness as *wholly* separate states. Recent research highlights how the predominant brain-wave activity of deep SWS can be present in wakefulness. Leemburg *et al.* (2010), investigating sleep restriction in rats, found that homeostatic regulation was preserved after five days of wakefulness (five days was chosen since it reflects the common practice of restricting sleep during the week and 'catching up' at weekends). As well as observing recovery slow-wave activity (SWA) after sleep restriction, they also observed SWA (usually associated with deep sleep) intruding into wakefulness and decreasing the build-up of sleep pressure. They note 'an intriguing possibility [...] that "wake slow waves" may decrease sleep need because they provide, at the cellular level, at least some of the benefits of sleep slow waves' (Leemburg *et al.* 2010, p.15943). However, they go on to note that increased wake SWA (caused by prolonged wakefulness or by drugs) still results in cognitive deficits – so there is still no escaping the need for sleep.

Commenting on such research on the (distant) possibility of 'learning' to sleep less, Van Someren (2010) asks whether it will bring us closer to understanding the function of sleep. At the same time he questions the validity of that question in asking 'what would be the function of wakefulness?' (Van Someren 2010, p.16004). That might best be addressed in a chapter on philosophy, but it raises an important point: we question the purpose of sleep although that is partly to presuppose that there is a degree of separation. However, 'perhaps the states of sleep and wakefulness reflect mainly an organizational principle, evolved to separate processes, ranging from the molecular to the behavioral, that would, if taking place simultaneously or close in time, be detrimental to the organism?' (Van Someren 2010, p.16004). That is, however blurred the boundaries between sleep, dreaming and wakefulness may seem, all three are necessary and have evolved with a purpose.

15.6. Conclusion

This chapter has attempted to draw some conclusions from an extensive range of contributions and, if that were not difficult enough, it is now necessary to draw a conclusion from those conclusions. Sleep is something on which most disciplines have something to say, but with the recent increasing interest in sleep by all disciplines represented here (and others that are not), the overall message becomes less clear. It seems that the more that we discover, the less able we are to make pronouncements with such certainty as those of Dugald Stewart two centuries ago (see above). However, we can safely conclude that sleep is not, to borrow Scrivner's words (Chapter 14), 'a kind of oblivion or nothingness'.

The sciences provide increasing evidence that sleep is essential for the maintenance of physical and psychological health and the enhancement of daytime performance – in effect, confirming the experience of everyone. They also provide ever more detailed descriptions of the mechanisms that regulate sleep and wakefulness, and explanations of how they might be disrupted. The humanities challenge the concept of 'normal sleep' and show us that sleep practices vary through time, between cultures and within societies, and that sleep is not always fully in accordance with what is assumed to be the pattern that has evolved throughout human history. Furthermore, they contend that sleep has to some extent become medicalized – implying that the definition of sleep disorder is shaped by societal norms, and perhaps influenced by economic and commercial pressures.

The two cultures might therefore appear to be at odds with each other: science telling us that there are norms, and that deviation amounts to disorder, whilst the humanities point to the possibility of difference. However, it is the chapter here that is perhaps the most complex for the non-scientist (Chapter 3) that offers a middle way by explaining how we (and other animals) can adapt our sleep to environmental differences. The process of evolution seems to have allowed us a significant degree of adaptability or flexibility over how and when we sleep. It remains to be seen whether evolution has equipped us with sufficient adaptability to meet the challenges posed by 24-hour society.

Acknowledgement

The author thanks Claire Durant of the Psychopharmacology Unit of the University of Bristol for her helpful comments on this chapter.

Notes

1. In *The Return of the Native* (Hardy 1974a, first published in 1878) – set in the 1840s when Hardy was a child – Yeobright had to take up manual labour:

   > His custom was to work from four o'clock in the morning till noon; then, when the heat of the day was its highest, to go home and sleep for an hour or two; afterwards coming out again and working till dusk at nine. (p.273)

   According to Cannon (2007), medieval stonemasons would work on cathedral construction from dawn until dusk during the summer but stop to sleep at midday.

2. Cobbett (1829) attributes this saying to 'country-people', and also argues that young people should sleep more in the winter since 'an hour in bed is better than an hour spent over fire and candle in an idle gossip'. (There are no page numbers in the edition referred to here: this advice is in section 38.)

3. See also Worthman and Melby (2002) who describe fluid boundaries between wake and sleep in some traditional societies and note that the !Kung of Botswana and the Efe of the Democratic Republic of the Congo (formerly known as Zaire) go to sleep when they feel like it but may get up later if they hear something going on.

4. Linder (1970) refers to an observation by anthropologist Paul Bohannen that the Tiv do not measure time, although they do 'count recurrent natural units such as days, markets, moons and dry seasons' (p.19).

5. It is suggested that this principle could aid recovery from jet lag since fasting for 16 hours is sufficient to engage the feeding clock: the international traveller should therefore resist the temptations of airline food and eat at the locally appropriate time on arrival at the destination (http://news.bbc.co.uk/1/hi/health/7414437.stm, accessed on 22 October 2011: 'Avoiding food "may beat jet lag"').

6. The second Industrial Revolution is usually considered to have been from the mid-nineteenth century until the start of the First World War and is defined by a renewed speed of ground-breaking inventions. According to Mokyr (1998) it can be dated 1870–1914.

7. In *The Return of the Native* (1974a, first published in 1878) and *Jude the Obscure* (1974b, first published in 1896) respectively. Hardy himself did his self-improvement at the other end of the day: as an apprentice architect he would typically read for two hours from 6 a.m. before walking to work at 8 a.m. He would also take his fiddle in the evening and accompany his father and uncle to play at village festivals – thereby having a life he later described as 'twisted of three strands – the professional life, the scholar's life and the rustic life, combined in the twenty-four hours of one day' (Gittings 1978, p.70). It is not known how much sleep Hardy had in those days, in the late 1850s, but this seems like further evidence of a creative individual restricting sleep.

8. Available at http://news.bbc.co.uk/1/hi/education/4669378.stm, accessed on 25 September 2011.

9. Lebhar (1958) points out that since in this additional time one would not need to sleep for the full eight hours either, a further saving of several months could be made.

10. Ernst was a lawyer and he admitted that the choice of 1976 for his Utopia was somewhat arbitrary – being the bicentennial year of the USA. Older readers in the UK will probably recall 1976 for extremes of weather rather than for social or technological advances. Ernst's prognostications appear to be more an exercise in optimism than a measured examination of scientific and sociological trends.

11. Lee (1964) was a theologian and optimistically asked the reader to 'imagine the revolutionary implications for leisure time once this device, now being tested in American medical centers, is perfected!' (p.19). It seems that the electrosone never was perfected; studies by Feighner, Brown and Olivier (1973) and Flemenbaum (1974) did not produce encouraging results. The electrosone therefore appears to have gone the way of the jet pack, monorails, meals in tablet form that would save us having to eat broccoli, and other things promised, along with the 'white heat of scientific revolution'. For contemporary press reports on the electrosone, see:

    http://news.google.com/newspapers?nid=2199&dat=19630117&id=b1
    IyAAAAIBAJ&sjid=kuUFAAAAIBAJ&pg=4993,1094398

    http://news.google.com/newspapers?nid=1876&dat=19720922&id=6o
    EsAAAAIBAJ&sjid=V80EAAAAIBAJ&pg=7267,4527866

    http://news.google.com/newspapers?nid=1915&dat=19700722&id=S
    _8gAAAAIBAJ&sjid=ZXQFAAAAIBAJ&pg=1131,3699001 (accessed on 30 April 2012).

12. Mainly in Europe, but also Australia, Brazil, Canada, Japan, Korea and the USA.

13. The reader is referred to Yaniv for explanation, but some of the factors in this equation are:

    A – wakeful activity
    S – time in bed asleep
    θ – bedtime
    I – time in bed before sleep
    R – Psychological stress
    U – utility
    Ψ – discomfort stemming from insomnia

14. Sidis was described in a magazine article as a 'neurologist, psychologist, and various other kinds of scientific "ologist"' (Sumner 1923). Sumner's article is worth looking up: although Sidis had some ideas that have not stood the test of time, some of his observations about insomnia are still sound – for example:

    Nine tenths of your difficulty in going to sleep is due to your fear that you won't go to sleep. And nine tenths of the bad effects of a sleepless night are not the result of your loss of sleep, but of your worry over it. (Sumner 1923, p.15)

15. At the Royal Society of Medicine in London, November 2011.

16. Author's observations.

17. Not a new idea – and one that was expressed almost 100 years ago by Addington Bruce (n.d., first published in 1915):

    It is now known that sleep, contrary to the belief formerly so widely entertained, is no mere passive, negative state, the product of toxic or other harmful elements, but it is an active, positive function, a protective instinct of gradual evolution and dependent for its operation partly on the will and partly on the environment. (p.8)

18. An alternative view of this, put forward by C.P. Snow in his role as novelist, is that we actually need time to appear to have considered a choice, or to think how to justify a decision that was quickly made – or perhaps make up excuses for making what might seem like an unwise choice: 'When one asked for time to "sleep on it"…one was, nine times out of ten,…searching for rationalisations and glosses to prettify a decision which was already made' (Snow 1979, p.704, first published in 1970).

19. *Hypnagogic* relates to the transition from wakefulness to sleep, and *hypnopompic* relates to the transition from sleep to wakefulness. Mavromatis coined the term *hypnagogia* to encompass experiences on going to sleep *and* waking.

20. As evidence of Edison's alleged use of hypnagogia, Mavromatis quotes an unreferenced passage (see below) in a slim volume on relaxation by Ed Bernd Junior, which indicates that the mind is more creative under alpha brainwave activity. The description of dozing off is not consistent with what is found in Nigel Hudson's Chapter 8 in this book:

    Edison used to work very hard in his research – at beta, the faster brain wave frequencies. Then when he would reach a 'sticking point' he would take one of his famous 'cat naps'. He would doze off in his favourite chair, holding steel balls in the palms of his hands. As he would fall asleep – drifting into alpha – his arms would relax and lower, letting the balls fall into pans on the floor. The noise would wake Edison and very often he would awaken with an idea to continue the project. (Bernd 1977, pp.28–9)

    Since Edison was not having his EEG monitored it is probably unwise to attribute any particular brainwave pattern to him, but Nigel Hudson, in a personal communication, suggests an alternative explanation: 'It may be that Edison was entering a state of enhanced concentration similar to a trance during these so-called cat-naps. If he started to drift into sleep, the dropping of the steel balls would wake him and so prevent him from actually falling asleep.'

21. The Old Hag is the origin of the term nightmare. According to Jones (1931, p.243), it originally meant 'night-fiend' or, more specifically, 'night-hag' or 'nighte-wytche'. *Mara* is the Anglo-Saxon for incubus or succubus (a male or female demon, respectively, believed to have sexual intercourse with a sleeping woman or man) – or more literally translated as 'crusher', representing the crushing weight on the breast. For a detailed examination of the change of meaning of nightmare – to a largely REM sleep phenomenon – see Hufford (1982). What Hufford could not foresee, however, is the subsequent debasement of the term in everyday language, as in 'the traffic on the M25 was a nightmare'

– a far cry from (mostly) Macnish's graphic description. (See also Henry Fuseli's 1781 painting 'The nightmare': available at http://mydailyartdisplay.wordpress. com/2011/08/08/the-nightmare-by-henry-fuseli, accessed on 11 November 2011.)

22. A mass of nuclei in the temporal lobe of the brain involved in processing emotions and in memory consolidation. (The name amygdala relates to the almond shape of the structure – the Latin name of the almond tree being *Prunus amygdalus*.)

23. O'Brien argues that the sleeping state should be predominant:

> What is wrong with Cryan and most people, said Byrne, is that they do not spend sufficient time in bed. When a man sleeps, he is steeped and lost in a limp toneless happiness: awake he is restless, tortured by his body and the illusion of existence. Why have men spent the centuries seeking to overcome the awakened body? Put it to sleep, that is a better way. Let it serve only to turn the sleeping soul over, to change the blood-stream and thus make possible a deeper and more refined sleep… We must invert our conception of repose and activity… We should not sleep to recover the energy expended when awake but rather wake occasionally to defecate the unwanted energy that sleep engenders. This might be done quickly – a five-mile race at full tilt around the town and then back to bed and the kingdom of the shadows. (O'Brien 1967, p.98, first published in 1939)

References

Bernd, E. Jr (1977) *Relax, it's Good For You.* Palestine, TX: Alvis Productions Inc.

Biddle, J.E. and Hamermesh, D.S. (1990) 'Sleep and the allocation of time.' *Journal of Political Economy 98*, 5, pt 1, 922–943.

Blackmore, S. (2010) *Consciousness: an Introduction,* 2nd edn. London: Hodder Education.

Bruce, H.A. (n.d.) *Sleep and Sleeplessness.* Kila, MT: Kessinger Publishing, LLC. (Original work published in 1915.)

Cahill, M. and Balice-Gordon, R. (2005) 'The ethical consequences of modafinil use.' *Penn Bioethics Journal 1*, 1. Available at www.bioethicsjournal.com/past/pbj1.1_cahill.pdf, accessed on 23 October 2011.

Caldwell, J.A. and Caldwell, J.L. (2005) 'Fatigue in military aviation: an overview of U.S. military-approved pharmacological countermeasures.' *Aviation, Space, and Environmental Medicine 76*, 7 Suppl., C39–C51.

Camus, A. (1961) *The Outsider.* (Translated by S. Gilbert.) Harmondsworth: Penguin. (Original work published in 1942.)

Cannon, J. (2007) *Cathedral.* Constable: London.

Carskadon, M.A. and Dement, W.C. (2011) 'Normal Human Sleep: An Overview.' In M.H. Kryger, T. Roth and W.C. Dement (eds) *Principles and Practice of Sleep Medicine,* 5th edn. St Louis, MO: Elsevier Saunders.

Cobbett, W. (1829) *Advice to Young Men, and (Incidentally) to Young Women in the Middle and Higher Ranks of Life: In a Series of Letters, Addressed to a Youth, a Bachelor, a Lover, a Husband, a Citizen or a Subject.* London: William Cobbett. Available at http://books.google.com/ books?id=fU4JAAAAQAAJ&pg=RA1-PT283&dq=cobbett+advice&hl=en#v=onepage&q& f=false, accessed on 4 October 2011.

Conrad, P. (2007) *The Medicalization of Society: on the Transformation of Human Conditions into Treatable Disorders.* Baltimore, MD: Johns Hopkins University Press.

Ekirch, A.R. (2001) 'Sleep we have lost: pre-industrial slumber in the British Isles.' *American Historical Review 106*, 2. Available at www.historycooperative.org/journals/ahr/106.2/ah000343.html, accessed on 22 October 2011.

Ekirch, A.R. (2006) *At Day's Close: A History of Nighttime*. London: Phoenix.

Ernst, M.L. (1955) *Utopia 1976*. New York, NY: Rinehart & Company.

Evans, F.J., Cook, M.R., Cohen, H.D., Orne, E.C. and Orne, M.T. (1977) 'Appetitive and replacement naps: EEG and behaviour.' *Science 197*, 4304, 687–689.

Feighner, J.P., Brown, S.L. and Olivier, J.E. (1973) 'Electrosleep therapy: a controlled double blind study.' *Journal of Nervous and Mental Disease 157*, 2, 121–128.

Flemenbaum, A. (1974) 'Cerebral electrotherapy (Electrosleep): an open-clinical study with a six month follow-up.' *Psychosomatics 15*, 1, 20–24.

Fuller, P.M., Lu, J. and Saper, C.B. (2008) 'Differential rescue of light- and food-entrainable circadian rhythms.' *Science 320*, 5879, 1074–1077.

Gillin, J.C. (2002) 'How long can humans stay awake?' *Scientific American*, 25 March. Available at www.scientificamerican.com/article.cfm?id=how-long-can-humans-stay, accessed on 4 October 2011.

Gittings, R. (1978) *Young Thomas Hardy*. Harmondsworth: Penguin Books.

Glovinsky, P.B., Yang, C.-M., Dubrovsky, B. and Spielman, A.J. (2008) 'Nonpharmacologic strategies in the management of insomnia: rationale and implementation.' *Sleep Medicine Clinics 3*, 2, 189–204.

Green, A. (2008) 'Sleep, occupation and the passage of time.' *British Journal of Occupational Therapy 71*, 8, 339–347.

Hardy, T. (1974a) *The Return of the Native*. London: Macmillan. (Original work published in 1878.)

Hardy, T. (1974b) *Jude the Obscure*. London: Macmillan. (Original work published in 1895.)

Horne, J.A. (1988) *Why We Sleep*. Oxford: Oxford University Press.

Horne, J.A. (2010) 'Sleepiness as a need for sleep: when is enough, enough?' *Neuroscience and Biobehavioral Reviews 34*, 1, 108–118.

Hufford, D.J. (1982) *The Terror That Comes in the Night: an Experience-Centred Study of Supernatural Assault Traditions*. Philadelphia, PA: University of Pennsylvania Press.

Jones, E. (1931) *On the Nightmare*. London: Leonard & Virginia Woolf at the Hogarth Press. Available at http://ia700506.us.archive.org/20/items/onthenightmare032020mbp/onthenightmare032020mbp.pdf, accessed on 9 November 2011.

Kim, D.Y. (2007) 'Modafinil: the journey to promoting vigilance and its consideration by the military in sustaining alertness.' Available at www.docstoc.com/docs/76136036/Modafinil-the-military%E2%80%80A6.rtf, accessed on 12 June 2012.

Lebhar, G.M. (1958) *The Use of Time*, 3rd edn. New York, NY: Chain Store Publishing Corp.

Lee, R. (1964) *Religion and Leisure in America*. New York, NY: Abingdon Press.

Leemburg, S., Vyazovskiya, V.V., Olcesea, U., Bassetti, C.L., Tononia, G. and Cirella, C. (2010) 'Sleep homeostasis in the rat is preserved during chronic sleep restriction.' *Proceedings of the National Academy of Sciences of the USA 107*, 36, 15939–15944.

Linder, S.B. (1970) *The Harried Leisure Class*. New York, NY: Columbia University Press.

Macnish, R. (n.d.) *The Philosophy of Sleep*. BiblioLife. (Original work published in 1834.)

Mavromatis, A. (2010) *Hypnagogia: the Unique State of Consciousness Between Wakefulness and Sleep*. London: Thyros Press. (Original work published in 1987.)

Mokyr, J. (1998) 'The Second Industrial Revolution, 1870–1914.' Available at http://faculty.wcas.northwestern.edu/%7Ejmokyr/castronovo.pdf, accessed on 29 October 2011.

O'Brien, F. (1967) *At Swim-Two-Birds*. Harmondsworth: Penguin Books. (Original work published in 1939.)

Oliver, M. (2002) 'Selby crash motorist receives five year sentence.' *Guardian*, 11 January. Available at www.guardian.co.uk/uk/2002/jan/11/selby.railtravel, accessed on 3 October 2011.

Parker, J.D. and Blackmore, S.J. (2002) 'Comparing the content of sleep paralysis and dream reports.' *Dreaming 12*, 1, 45–59.

Philip, P. and Åkerstedt, T. (2006) 'Transport and industry safety: how are they affected by sleepiness and sleep restriction?' *Sleep Medicine Reviews 10*, 5, 347–356.

Robinson, J.P. and Michelson, W. (2010) 'Sleep as a victim of the "time crunch" – a multinational analysis.' *electronic International Journal of Time Use Research 7*, 1, 61–72. Available at http://ffb.uni-lueneburg.de/eijtur/pdf/volumes/eIJTUR-7-1.pdf#page=62, accessed on 14 October 2011.

Schwartz, B. (1970) 'Notes on the sociology of sleep.' *The Sociological Quarterly 11*, 4, 485–499.

Sidis, B. (2010) *An Experimental Study of Sleep* (Kindle edition). Evergreen Review Inc. (Original work published in 1909.)

Snow, C.P. (1959) *The Two Cultures and the Scientific Revolution: The Rede Lecture.* Cambridge: Cambridge University Press.

Snow, C.P. (1979) *Strangers and Brothers,* Vol 3. London: Charles Scribner's Sons.

Spielman, A.J., Saskin, P. and Thorpy, M.J. (1987) 'Treatment of chronic insomnia by restriction of time in bed.' *Sleep: Journal of Sleep Research & Sleep Medicine 10*, 1, 45–56.

Stewart, D. (1802) *Elements of the Philosophy of the Human Mind,* 2nd edn. London: T. Cadell Junior and W. Davies, in the Strand.

Sumner, K. (1923) 'The secret of sound sleep.' *American Magazine 95*, 14–15; 98–104. Available at www.sidis.net/soundsleep.htm, accessed on 8 November 2011.

Szalontai, G. (2006) 'The demand for sleep: a South African Study.' *Economic Modelling 23*, 5, 854–874.

Taylor, D.J., Schmidt-Nowara, W., Jessop, C.A. and Ahearn, J. (2010) 'Sleep restriction therapy and hypnotic withdrawal versus sleep hygiene education in hypnotic using patients with insomnia.' *Journal of Clinical Sleep Medicine 6*, 2, 169–175.

van der Helm, E., Yao, J., Dutt, S., Rao, V., Saletin, J.M. and Walker, M.P. (2011) 'REM sleep depotentiates amygdala activity to previous emotional experiences.' *Current Biology 21*, 23, 2029–2032.

van Dongen, H.P.A., Maislin, G., Mullington, J.M. and Dinges, D.F. (2003) 'The cumulative cost of additional wakefulness: dose-response effects on neurobehavioural functions and sleep physiology from chronic sleep restriction and total sleep deprivation.' *Sleep 26*, 2, 117–126.

Van Someren, E.J.W. (2010) 'Doing with less sleep remains a dream.' *Proceedings of the National Academy of Science 107*, 37, 16003–16004.

Vaughn, B.V. and D'Cruz, O.F. (2011) 'Cardinal Manifestations of Sleep Disorders.' In M.H. Kryger, T. Roth and W.C. Dement (eds) *Principles and Practice of Sleep Medicine,* 5th edn. St Louis, MO: Elsevier Saunders.

Wagner, U., Gais, S., Haider, H., Verlager, R. and Born, J. (2004) 'Sleep inspires insight.' *Nature 427*, 6972, 352–355.

Walsh, J.K., Dement, W.C. and Dinges, D.F. (2011) 'Sleep Medicine, Public Policy and Public Health.' In M.H. Kryger, T. Roth and W.C. Dement (eds) *Principles and Practice of Sleep Medicine,* 5th edn. St Louis, MO: Elsevier Saunders.

Wehr, T. (1992) 'In short photoperiods, human sleep is biphasic.' *Journal of Sleep Research 1*, 2, 103–107.

Williams, S.J. (2005) *Sleep and Society: Sociological Ventures into the (Un)Known.* London: Routledge.

Williams, S.J. (2011) *The Politics of Sleep: Governing (Un)consciousness in the Late Modern Age.* Basingstoke: Palgrave Macmillan.

Williams, S.J., Seale, C., Boden, S., Lowe, P. and Steinberg, D.L. (2008) 'Waking up to sleepiness: Modafinil, the media and the pharmaceuticalisation of everyday/night life.' *Sociology of Health and Illness 30*, 6. Available at http://wrap.warwick.ac.uk/489/1/WRAP_Williams_OVERDOSING_ON_WAKEFULNESSR3ANON.pdf, accessed on 15 October 2011.

Wittenberg, M. (2005) *Industrialisation and Surplus Labour: a General Equilibrium Model of Sleep, Work and Leisure.* Cape Town: School of Economics, University of Cape Town. Available at www.commerce.uct.ac.za/Economics/staff/mwittenberg/2005/lewismodel.pdf, accessed on 14 October 2011.

Worthman, C.M. and Melby, M.K. (2002) 'Toward a Comparative Developmental Ecology of Human Sleep.' In M.A. Carskadon (ed.) *Adolescent Sleep Patterns: Biological, Social, and Psychological Influences.* Cambridge: Cambridge University Press.

Yaniv, G. (2004) 'Insomnia, biological clock, and the bedtime decision: an economic perspective.' *Health Economics 13*, 1, 1–8.

Glossary

Actigraphy: measurement of rest and activity using an accelerometer, or actigraph, usually worn on the wrist or ankle to detect movement. Although people are not totally still in sleep, or continually moving in wakefulness, the pattern of sleep/wake cycles can be discerned over the course of a few weeks (see Chapter 8).

Electroencephalogram (EEG): a recording of the tiny electrical potentials generated by neurons in the brain (see Chapter 8).

Medicalization: a term from sociology describing a process in which non-medical problems come to be seen as medical problems and treated as an illness or disorder.

Modafinil: a drug used in the treatment of narcolepsy that promotes wakefulness (see Chapter 11).

Multiple sleep latency test (MSLT): an assessment which times how long a person takes to go to sleep and to enter rapid eye movement (REM) sleep, used particularly in the diagnosis of narcolepsy (see Chapter 8).

Pittsburgh Sleep Quality Index (PSQI): a self-rated questionnaire widely used to measure sleep quality in research and in clinical practice (see www.sleep.pitt.edu/includes/showFile.asp?fltype=doc&flID=1296).

Polysomnography (PSG): recording of multiple physiological variables during overnight sleep, especially the EEG, used to measure the stages of sleep for the purpose or diagnosis of sleep disorder or research (see Chapter 8).

Rapid eye movement (REM) sleep: the stage of sleep in which dreaming takes place. The body is effectively paralysed, apart from the muscles involved in respiration and moving the eyes. As far as electrical activity in the brain is concerned, it resembles wakefulness (see Chapters 2 and 8).

Sleep architecture: the pattern of sleep stages throughout the night. When the succession of different stages of sleep is shown graphically, the picture resembles a city skyline.

Sleep cycle: the succession of stages of sleep from stage 1 (S1) (or N1) to REM that is repeated throughout the night, often separated by a brief awakening (see Chapter 2).

Sleep efficiency: a figure, expressed as a percentage, reached by dividing the amount of sleep achieved by the amount of time spent in bed (total sleep time/time in bed x 100). A good sleeper's efficiency is usually over 90 per cent whereas that of someone with insomnia may be as low as 50 per cent.

Sleep hygiene: a term attributed to Peter Hauri to include the kind of lifestyle and environmental factors that could interfere with sleep, which individuals could 'tidy up' for themselves.

Sleep onset latency: the time it takes to fall asleep.

Sleep-onset REM periods (SOREMPs): periods of REM sleep occurring on first going to sleep (as opposed to the usual progression through non-REM sleep) and characteristic of narcolepsy.

Slow-wave sleep (SWS): stage 3 and 4 (S3, S4) sleep (or stage N3) – deep sleep (see Chapters 2 and 8).

Zeitgeber: literally 'time-giver', a cue that resets the body clock to keep it entrained with the 24-hour cycle of light and dark, the chief one of which is daylight (see Chapter 3).

The Contributors

Helen L. Ball

Helen Ball is Professor of Anthropology and Fellow of the Wolfson Research Institute at Durham University where she founded and directs the Anthropology Sleep Laboratory. Although she has studied parent–infant sleep for the past 15 years, her interest in child sleep was ignited by Caroline Jones's PhD research, and she is now involved in several projects on sleep in children, and in adults. She continues to study issues of infant feeding and sleeping from an evolutionary perspective. She serves on the National Childbirth Trust Research Advisory Board and on the La Leche League Panel of Professional Advisors.

Andrew Green

After gaining a degree in geography, Andrew Green trained in occupational therapy in York and began working in psychiatry in 1986. He has worked since 1992 in Neuropsychiatry at the Burden Neurological Hospital – subsequently, the Burden Centre for Neuropsychiatry at Frenchay Hospital – in Bristol, and during this time gained an MSc from the University of Exeter and an MPhil from the University of Southampton. He first took an interest in sleep disorders on being asked to contribute to a therapy group for patients with insomnia in 1999 and now spends most of his time working with patients with a wide range of sleep disorders.

Dietmar Hank

Dietmar Hank is a consultant in learning disability psychiatry and is Honorary Consultant in Neuropsychiatry at the Burden Centre, Frenchay Hospital, Bristol. He trained in psychiatry in South Wales and Bristol and gained an MSc in Psychological Medicine at Cardiff University and Postgraduate Diploma in Neuropsychiatry at the University of Birmingham. His special interests are neurodevelopmental and sleep disorders.

Jane Hicks

Jane Hicks originally trained in general practice but is now a liaison psychiatrist with an interest in sleep disorders. She has been involved in the writing of national guidelines for narcolepsy but more recently completed her MD thesis on the pharmacological and behavioural management of insomnia. She worked at the Burden Centre for Neuropsychiatry in Bristol for over ten years and was instrumental in developing a successful CBT-I group. This has become a clinical service for patients with chronic insomnia and has been effectively trialled in primary care.

Nigel Hudson

Nigel Hudson is a neurophysiological scientist and service manager at the Neurophysiology Department at Plymouth Hospitals NHS Trust. He has 40 years' experience in neurophysiology and has been recording sleep EEGs for the whole of this time. For the past 20 years he has been involved with a multidisciplinary sleep service and has been recording and reporting polysomnograms and multiple sleep latency tests. He is a member of the British Sleep Society and current President of the Association of Neurophysiological Scientists.

Stephen Jacobs

Stephen Jacobs is Senior Lecturer at the University of Wolverhampton teaching both religious studies and cultural studies. He gained a PhD in 2000 at the University of Wales, Lampeter. His thesis was a study of Hindu reform groups in the late nineteenth and early twentieth centuries. He has published a textbook on contemporary Hinduism (*Hinduism Today*: 2010) and articles on media and religion. He is currently undertaking ethnographic research on the Art of Living Foundation, an important Hindu-derived meditation movement. Since studying Hindu philosophy in India, he has been interested in the metaphysical speculation about the nature of sleep found in the *Upaniṣads*.

Caroline H.D. Jones

Caroline H.D. Jones is a medical anthropologist. Her PhD, at Durham University's sleep laboratory, examined the link between short sleep duration and obesity in young children, using a mixed methods approach. In 2010 she spent some time researching parents' knowledge of, and attitudes to, children's sleep at Brown University's Pediatric Sleep Clinic, Rhode Island, USA. She is interested in the interplay between biology and culture in shaping children's sleep habits, and associated health. She is currently a senior researcher at the Department of Primary Care Health Sciences, Oxford University.

Robert Meadows

Rob Meadows is a lecturer in sociology at the University of Surrey, which he joined in 1999 to work in the Human Psychopharmacology Research Unit of the Medical Research Centre, having previously gained degrees in law, sociology and social anthropology, and socio-legal studies. In 2003 he joined the Sociology Department as Research Fellow and co-investigator on an Economic and Social Research Council (ESRC)-funded project looking at couples' sleep. He became a senior researcher and part of the core management team on a large-scale project on ageing and sleep. During this period (2002–2008) he also worked part time on his PhD, which looked at the ways in which couples negotiate their sleep.

Hazel O'Dowd

After qualifying in 1994, Hazel O'Dowd worked for 11 years as a clinical psychologist in both mental health and general medicine. She then established the Frenchay CFS/ME adult service in Bristol, which is one of the largest of its kind in the UK. Treatments follow the National Institute for Health and Clinical Excellence guidelines, of which sleep management is an integral part. She sits on the executive board of the British Association for CFS/ME and is part of their national training team. Dr O'Dowd has also been involved in several studies researching interventions for CFS/ME that have included components on modifying sleep disruption and sleep-related patient distress.

Louise M. Paterson

Louise M. Paterson trained in pharmacology at the University of Bristol, where she obtained her BSc (2000). She continued her studies at Bristol and was awarded a PhD in Pharmacology in 2004. Her interest in sleep research began with an investigation of the effects of caffeine and sleep-promoting medications on sleep in animal models and healthy volunteers. This was followed by a series of post-doctoral positions in translational sleep research in healthy volunteers and patients. In 2009 she moved to Imperial College, London, where she is pursuing her interest in combining sleep research with human brain imaging.

Lee Scrivner

Lee Scrivner is Lecturer in Humanities at Bosphorus University in Istanbul. He received his PhD in 2011 from the University of London. His thesis traced the rise of insomnia as a pathological entity and a cultural phenomenon in the late nineteenth and early twentieth centuries. He is interested in both sleep and insomnia from multidisciplinary angles and, more generally, the interplay of mind and body, especially as it relates to technology. He also holds degrees in English (BA) and British and American Literature (MA) from the University of Utah, and has taught English at the University of Nevada, Las Vegas and the University of London, Birkbeck.

Brigitte Steger

Brigitte Steger, PhD, is University Lecturer in Modern Japanese Studies at the University of Cambridge. She has published widely on social and cultural issues of sleep, including daytime sleep. Her regional focus is Japan, both past and present. She has recently conducted research on everyday life and sleep in tsunami evacuation shelters in north-east Japan (see www.ames.cam.ac.uk/general_info/biographies/japanese/Steger.htm).

Alex Westcombe

After completing a degree in psychology and physical education, Alex Westcombe worked as a researcher in psychosocial aspects of cancer and then retrained as a clinical psychologist in Bristol, graduating in 2005. Since then he has worked exclusively in clinical health psychology, particularly in long-term pain and fatigue. The role of sleep within physical health conditions has been an interest throughout his career.

Sue Wilson

Sue Wilson has been studying sleep for about 20 years. She has used the measurement of sleep patterns in the EEG to characterize the effects of drugs in the brain, and has published on drug effects on sleep in depression, anxiety, addiction and sleep disorders such as insomnia and parasomnias. She participates in the sleep and neuropsychiatry clinic at The Burden Centre, Frenchay Hospital, Bristol, assessing sleep in patients with insomnia, parasomnias and other sleep disorders. She recently co-ordinated a national consensus group on treatment of sleep disorders.

Katharina Wulff

Katharina Wulff, PhD, is a Senior Research Scientist in Clinical Neurosciences at the University of Oxford. Trained in both animal and human biological rhythms, the focused interest of her research is the investigation of mechanisms underlying abnormal biological rhythms and sleep in ocular pathologies, neuropsychiatry and neurodegenerative disorders of the brain and their consequences for mental and emotional well-being. She uses simultaneous, long-term measurements of rest/activity, light exposure, endocrine patterns and sleep EEG to detail relationships with time of day and season, and has published on sleep and circadian rhythm disruption in mental disorders.

Subject Index

mechanism and control 29,
45–7
and temporal regulation of sleep
57–8
see also timing of sleep
circadian rhythm sleep disorders
29, 163, 174, 176, 184
and traumatic brain injury
202–3
clock gene 56, 61
cocaine 222
Coe, Jonathan 108, 277–8, 285–6
cognitive behaviour therapy 193,
240
for insomnia 174, 175–6, 216
continuous positive airway pressure
see CPAP
core body temperature 42, 57
core sleep *see* optional sleep and
core sleep
cortisol 43
co-sleeping with babies and
children 71–2, 73, 92–3
CPAP 178
users' experience 114–15
creativity in sleep 303, 305

daytime sleepiness/excessive
daytime sleepiness (EDS)
52, 168, 176, 177, 178,
180, 197, 201, 202, 222,
231–2, 233
daytime sleep and napping 74,
77–81
of children 97–8
in east Asia 73, 78–80, 81, 82
in history 75–6, 292
for passing time 302–3
power nap/strategic nap 80–1,
82, 83
replacement and appetitive naps
292–3
death
fear of, in sleep 70
relationship with sleep in
religion and mythology
248, 257, 263–4
sleep as a metaphor for 274
see also mortality
delayed sleep phase syndrome
(DSPS) 184, 296
and traumatic brain injury 202
delta activity/waves 22, 153, *159*
in schizophrenia 196, 271,
272, 277
delta sleep *see* slow-wave sleep/
SWS
dementia 113, 168
Alzheimer's disease 49, 197–8
depression 49, 172, 174, 193–5,
238–9, 240–1, 302
desynchronization 57
Dickens, Charles 169, 177, 281–2,
284
Dinges, David, 80
Dopamine 59, 210, 213, 221, 222
dream sleep *see* REM sleep

dreaming 24, 31–2,
and opiates 220
control of in Tibetan dream
yoga 255
and Hindu tradition 257,
258–9
lucid dreaming in literature 286
and creativity 305
and REM sleep behaviour
disorder 181
dreams
ambiguous and unambiguous
in Hebrew and Christian
Bibles 262
as sacred communication 260–2
as a source of myths 273
true and false in Islam 261–2
see also nightmares
driver safety and performance 108,
133, 134, 135, 215, 233,
296–7
drugs 209–24
addiction/dependence 215–16
modes of action 212
see also antidepressant drugs;
antihistamine drugs;
antipsychotic drugs;
hypnotic drugs; wake-
promoting drugs
duration of sleep
in animals 34–5, *130*
in children 93–5, 143
core sleep and optional sleep
293
estimation of 124–5, 231
international differences 298
and monotony/lack of
occupation 302–3
in persons with mental health
problems 129–31
in residents in forensic
psychiatry units 129–30
in time use studies 125–32
inverse relationship with work
129

economics 129, 296–8
ecstasy 223
Edison, Thomas Alva 169, 282,
303, 310
EEG 22, 24, 36, *37*, 149–64
awake (stage W) *157*
development of 150–2
and diagnosis of sleep disorders
160
frequency bands 152–3
REM sleep *159*
and sleep 154–9
sleep-related phenomena 153–4
stage N1 sleep *158*
stage N2 sleep *158*
stage N3 sleep *159*
see also PSG
Ekirch, Roger 83, 88, 272–3,
293–4
electrocardiogram 162

electroencephalography/
encephalogram *see* EEG
electromyography (EMG) 22, 156,
157, 159, 162
electrooculography (EOG) 22, 156,
157, 159
electrosone 298
encephale isole 154–5
entrainment, range of 50
entrainment of circadian clocks
50–1
environment *see* sleeping conditions
Ephesus, sleepers of 250
epilepsy/epileptic seizures 152,
160, 178
Epworth Sleepiness Scale (ESS)
227–8
and Fatigue Severity Scale 232
excessive daytime sleepiness (EDS)
see daytime sleepiness
exercise, effects on sleep 138–40
exploding head syndrome 181

fatigue, definitions and meanings
229
fatigue and sleep 233–4, 236
Fatigue Severity Scale (FSS) 229
and Epworth Sleepiness Scale
232
feedback loops 43
fibromyalgia 238–9, 240
'first night effect' in PSG 164, 235
flexibility in sleep times *see* timing
of sleep
fragmented sleep
in animals 35
and ecstasy 223
in persons with intellectual
disability 199
in older people 21, 25, 112
in schizophrenia 49, 195
free running of sleep/wake cycle
50, 52, 56, 57
Freud, Sigmund 31

GABA 59–60, 210, 212
and alcohol 219
and hypnotic drugs 213–14
receptors 214
GAD 190–1
and insomnia 191–2, 204
galvanometer 151
gamma-aminobutyric acid *see*
GABA
gamma-hydroxybutyrate 180
Gardner, Randy 39, 292
gender differences 25, 109–11
generalized anxiety disorder *see*
GAD
glutamate 210, 211, 219
God
associated with light
never sleeps 253, 256
sleep as gift of 248
sleep as sign of faith in 253–4
gods' sleep in Hinduism 256
Greek (ancient) medicine 272

Author Index

CPI Antony Rowe
Eastbourne, UK
June 20, 2023